The Lost Self

The Lost Self

Pathologies of the Brain and Identity

Edited by

TODD E. FEINBERG
JULIAN PAUL KEENAN

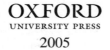

OXFORD
UNIVERSITY PRESS
2005

OXFORD
UNIVERSITY PRESS

Oxford University Press, Inc., publishes works that further
Oxford University's objective of excellence
in research, scholarship, and education.

Oxford   New York
Auckland   Cape Town   Dar es Salaam   Hong Kong   Karachi
Kuala Lumpur   Madrid   Melbourne   Mexico City   Nairobi
New Delhi   Shanghai   Taipei   Toronto

With offices in
Argentina   Austria   Brazil   Chile   Czech Republic   France   Greece
Guatemala   Hungary   Italy   Japan   Poland   Portugal   Singapore
South Korea   Switzerland   Thailand   Turkey   Ukraine   Vietnam

Published by Oxford University Press, Inc.
198 Madison Avenue, New York, New York 10016
www.oup.com

Oxford is a registered trademark of Oxford University Press

Library of Congress Cataloging-in-Publication Data

The lost self : pathologies of the brain and identity / edited by
Todd E. Feinberg, Julian Paul Keenan.
p.   ;   cm.
Includes bibliographical references and index.
ISBN-13 978-0-19-517341-3
ISBN 0-19-517341-4
1. Depersonalization.   2. Self.   3. Identity (Psychology)   4. Cognitive
neuroscience. [DNLM: 1. Brain—physiopathology.   2. Ego.
3. Mental Disorders—physiopathology.   WL 103.5 L881 2005]
I. Feinberg, Todd E.   II. Keenan, Julian Paul.
RC553.D4L67 2005
616.8 — dc22   2004024803

2   4   6   8   9   7   5   3   1

Printed in the United States of America
on acid-free paper

Preface

I originally came to the study of the self as a clinician. In the course of my training and practice I had the opportunity to examine an array of interesting patients who had disordered selves as a result of brain pathology. For instance, I could not help but be struck by the oddness of a female patient of mine who suffered a stroke and then sang pop tunes to her paralyzed arm in the hope of bringing it back to life, or the woman who tried to throw her similarly motionless limb in the garbage in her hospital room. Some patients I witnessed screaming at their reflections in a mirror; others told tales of imaginary alter egos, or grappled with one of their arms as it tried to strangle them. Over the last 20 years the core of my work has involved the study of these cases and their disorders.

Three years ago I met Julian Keenan, co-editor of this volume, who is one of a growing breed of neuroscientists engaged in the experimental study of the self. Dr. Keenan has employed diverse imaging and nonimaging experimental methods in examining the brain correlates of the self in normal subjects. Together, in this volume we bring to the reader contributions from an eclectic group of original thinkers who explore the current state of our knowledge of the philosophical, neuropsychological, and neurobiological basis of the self and in particular how the self is transformed by brain pathology.

As I read these chapters, I was struck by how far the scientific study of the self has come. As is often—if not always—the case in science, it is also clear how far we have to go, but I hope the reader will agree that the journey has begun.

Many people in many roles have helped with this project. We especially thank Fiona Stevens, our editor at Oxford, for helping with the development of this project from its inception. Her expert guidance, advice, and support were invaluable. Thanks are due as well to Edith Barry. We also thank Jill Gregory for her beautiful cover art and her help with the figures in several chapters.

Contents

Contributors

Simon Baron-Cohen, Ph.D.
Autism Research Centre
Cambridge University
Department of Psychology and Psychiatry
Cambridge, United Kingdom

Sarah-Jayne Blakemore, Ph.D.
Royal Society Dorothy Hodgkin Research
  Fellow
Institute of Cognitive Neuroscience
University College London
London, United Kingdom

William Christiana, B.A.
Cognitive Neuroimaging Laboratory
Department of Psychology
Montclair State University
Upper Montclair, NJ

John DeLuca, Ph.D., ABPP
Director of Neuroscience Research
Kessler Medical Rehabilitation Research
  and Education Corporation
West Orange, NJ and
Professor of Physical Medicine and
  Rehabilitation, and of Neurosciences
UMDNJ-New Jersey Medical School
Newark, NJ

Martha J. Farah, Ph.D.
Bob and Arlene Kogod Term Professor of
  Psychology
Department of Psychology

University of Pennsylvania
Director Center for Cognitive
  Neuroscience
Philadelphia, PA

Todd E. Feinberg, M.D.
Professor of Clinical Psychiatry and
  Behavioral Sciences and Clinical
  Neurology
Albert Einstein College of Medicine
Chief, Yarmon Neurobehavior and
  Alzheimer's Disease Center
Beth Israel Medical Center
New York, NY

Esther Fujiwara, Ph.D.
The Rotman Research Institute
Baycrest Centre for Geriatric Care
Toronto, Ontario, Canada

Joseph T. Giacino, Ph.D
Associate Director of Psychology
JFK Medical Center
Center for Head Injuries
Edison, NJ and
Department of Neuroscience
Seton Hall University
South Orange, NJ

Seth Gillihan, M.A.
Department of Psychology
University of Pennsylvania
Philadelphia, PA

GEORG GOLDENBERG, M.D.
Neuropsychologische Abteilung
Krankenhaus München Bogenhause
München, Germany

KEVIN GUISE
Cognitive Neuroimaging Laboratory
Department of Psychology
Montclair State University
Upper Montclair, NJ

J. ALLAN HOBSON, M.D.
Professor of Psychiatry
Harvard Medical School
Laboratory of Neurophysiology
Massachusetts Mental Health Center
Brookline, MA

JULIAN PAUL KEENAN, PH.D.
Director, Cognitive Neuroimaging
   Laboratory
Assistant Professor
Department of Psychology
Montclair State University
Upper Montclair, NJ

TROELS W. KJAER, M.D.
Clinical Neurophysiology Clinic
Copenhagen University Hospital
Copenhagen, Denmark

HEDY KOBER, B.A.
Department of Psychology
Columbia University
New York, NY

HANS C. LOU, M.D.
Department of Functionally Integrative
   Neuroscience
Aarhus University Hospital
Aarhus, Denmark

SARAH MALCOLM, B.A.
Cognitive Neuroimaging Laboratory
Department of Psychology

Montclair State University
Upper Montclair, NJ

HANS J. MARKOWITSCH, PH.D.
University of Bielefeld
Department of Physiological Psychology
Bielefeld, Germany

ROY J. MATHEW, M.D.
Professor of Medicine-Psychiatry
Department of Internal Medicine
Texas Tech Health Sciences Center
Odessa, TX

BRUCE L. MILLER, M.D.
A. W. & Mary Margaret Clausen
   Distinguished Professor of Neurology
Director, UCSF Memory & Aging Center
   and Alzheimer Disease
Research Center
San Francisco, CA

SUKHVINDER OBHI, PH.D.
Department of Psychology
University of Western Ontario
London, Ontario
Canada

KAREN SPANGENBERG POSTAL, PH.D.,
ABPP-CN
Neuropsychology Consultants
Andover, MA

ALYSA RAY, B.A.
Department of Psychology
George Washington University
Wasghington D.C.

ANTTI REVONSUO, PH.D.
Professor, Department of Psychology
Center for Cognitive Neuroscience
University of Turku
Turku, Finland

DAVID M. ROANE, M.D.
Associate Professor of Clinical Psychiatry
Albert Einstein College of Medicine
Chief, Division of Geriatric Psychiatry
Beth Israel Medical Center
New York, NY

R. SHAYNA ROSENBAUM, PH.D.
Postdoctoral Fellow
Rotman Research Institute
Baycrest Centre for Geriatric Care
Toronto, Ontairo, Canada

JOHN R. SEARLE, PH.D.
Mills Professor of Philosophy
Department of Philosophy
University of California, Berkeley
Berkeley, CA

WILLIAM W. SEELEY, M.D.
Clinical Fellow in Behavioral Neurology
UCSF School of Medicine
San Francisco, CA

MARK SOLMS, PH.D
Chair of Neuropsychology
University of Cape Town and
Groote Schuur Hospital
Cape Town, South Africa

DONALD T. STUSS PH.D.
Director, Rotman Research Institute
Professor of Psychology and Medicine
University of Toronto
Toronto, Ontario, Canada

1

Introduction

TODD E. FEINBERG AND JULIAN PAUL KEENAN

Over the last decade there has been an explosion of interest in the science of consciousness. Less attention had been paid, however, to the neurobiology and neuroscience of the self. But what is "consciousness" if it is not a product of a self? It is an often ignored fact that without a self that is the subject of consciousness, consciousness does not exist; and the degree to which explicit consciousness exists depends to a large extent upon the degree that there is a subject, a self, that is the source of that consciousness.

It is not surprising, therefore, that the term *self* is as difficult to define as the term *consciousness*. According to Levin:

> The self is the ego, the subject, the I, or the me, as opposed to the object, or totality of objects—the *not me*. *Self* means "same" in Anglo-Saxon (Old English). So *self* carries with it the notion of identity, of meaning the selfsame.It is also the *I*, the personal pronoun, in Old Gothic, the ancestor of Anglo-Saxon. Thus, etymologically *self* comes from both the personal pronoun, *I*—I exist, I do this and that—and from the etymologically root meaning "the same"—it is the same I who does this, who did that. (Levin, 1992, p. 2)

The philosopher Galen Strawson, who has written about as much as any philosopher on the nature of the self, points out there is a grand multiplicity of meanings of the term *self*.

> It is difficult to know where to begin, because there are many different notions of the self. Among those I have recently come across are the cognitive self, the conceptual self, the contextualized self, the core self, the dialogic self, the ecological self, the embodied self, the emergent self, the empirical self, the existential self, the extended self, the fictional self, the full-grown self, the interpersonal self, the material self, the narrative self, the philosophical self, the physical self, the private self, the representational self, the rock bottom essential self, the semiotic self, the social self, the tranparent self, and the verbal self. (Strawson, 2000, p. 39)

That's a lot of selves! However, Strawson goes on to consider that essentially the self is, first and foremost, a *subject* of experience. To this James adds that the self should be conceived as possessing a dual aspect as both the subject *and* an object of experience. The self as subject and object were two sides of the same coin:

> Whatever I may be thinking of, I am always at the same time more or less aware of *myself*, of my *personal existence*. At the same time it is *I* who am aware; so that the total self of me, being as it were duplex, partly known and partly knower, partly object and partly subject, must have two aspects discriminated in it, of which for shortness we may call one the *Me* and the other the *I*. (James, 1892; p. 43)

The forgoing suggest that the self is both a subject and an object of itself. In this book we consider both of these aspects of the self, but we focus on special and particular aspects of the self, namely: What happens to the self in certain neuropathological conditions? And what can these conditions teach us about the neurobiology of the self?

The next four chapters introduce the reader to some general questions regarding the philosophy and neuroscience of the self. In Chapter 2 John Searle, one of the pioneers of the philosophy of consciousness, considers first what philosophers mean by the "self." He points out that that traditionally, the problem of the self in philosophy is generally viewed as the problem of personal identity. He goes on to identify four different criteria for deciding the question of personal identity: the identity of the body, the identity of consciousness recorded in memory, the stability and continuity of personality, and "the relative coherence of the spatio-temporal continuity of the physical body through change." Searle notes that of these criteria, the problem of human consciousness poses a particular problem for our understanding of the self. He argues that considering the self as a feature of a "unified conscious field" is the best approach to understanding its ontology.

Martha Farah and Seth Gillihan then provide a selective review of the cognitive neuroscience of the self, with particular reference to imaging studies in normal subjects. The authors first discuss the difficulties encountered in performing this type of research. For example, they cast a critical eye on the definitions of the self, the interpretation of the data, the controls that are employed as comparisons for the self, as well as the methods used in analyzing neuroimaging data. The authors then divide studies of the self under four main headings: self-awareness and first-person perspective, autobiographical memory, agency, and self-concept. These distinctions allow for a succinct and cohesive review of the literature. While the authors have a number of concerns regarding current studies of the cognitive neuroscience of the self, they predict that neuroscientists will soon overcome the methodological difficulties they now encounter.

Next, Feinberg presents his model of the neurological underpinnings of the self in Chapter 4. The author has previously argued that in order to explain the unity of the self and consciousness, it should be viewed as the result of multiple, nested, hierarchically arranged neurological levels. In Chapter 4 he draws upon the prior neurological models of Maclean, Mesulum, and others and organizes the neural hierarchy of the self into roughly seven nested hierarchical levels. While the highest and most abstract aspects of the self are made possible by the hierarchically highest and most phylogenitically recent neural structures, all levels of the neural hierarchy may make a contribution to the self. Finally, he suggests that *meaning* provides the constraint necessary for the unity of the mind's "inner eye," and *purpose* provides the constraint necessary for the highest and most intentional actions.

The next three chapters examine the self and self-related functions with reference to particular neuropsychological functions and neuroanatomical regions. In Chapter 5 Stuss and his colleagues address the frontal lobes and the self. These writers suggest, as does Feinberg in Chapter 4, that the self is hierarchically organized and propose that there are four hierarchical levels related to the self. The highest level of the self, involved in self-awareness, is subserved by the frontal lobes. These authors argue that executive processes typically associated with the frontal lobes may actually be dissociable from both self-awareness and theory of mind. They consider which candidate frontal regions might be critically involved in certain overlapping self-related functions such as autonoetic consciousness, theory of mind, and autobiographical memory, processes that they argue are more closely linked to the self than are executive functions per se.

As pointed out by Stuss and coworkers in Chapter 5, autobiographical memory is surely essential to the self as an enduring entity. In Chapter 6 Fujiwara and Markowitsch provide a further in-depth examination of autobiographical memory as it relates to the self. The authors begin by detailing the cognitive neuropsychology and neuroanatomical basis of autobiographical memory. They find that autobiographical memory is subserved by a large and interconnected network of neural structures including core memory regions such as the hippocampal formation, areas involved in self-related processing, especially the medial prefrontal cortex, and regions involved in the integration of sensory and emotional processing including the posterior association cortex and posterior cingulate gyrus. They find, in line with other authors in this volume (see, for example, Chapters 8 and 9), that nondominant hemispheric functioning plays a special role in self-related functions. They describe disorders of autobiographical memory in patients with neurological lesions as well as in patients with psychiatric disorders and consider how these clinical conditions inform us about the nature and neurobiology of autobiographical memory. In particular, they describe how autobiographical memory dysfunction in neurological and psychiatric patients converge in psychogenic amnesia and consider what this observation tells us about the relationship between autobiographical memory, emotion, and the self.

Goldenberg in Chapter 7 next considers the neuropsychological and neuroanatomical basis of the body image. He describes what he argues are the two central aspects of the body image with reference to the self: the awareness of the current configuration and permanent structure of one's own body, and the knowledge of the structure of human bodies in general. He explores the cognitive and neural bases of these two properties of the body image and along the way discusses in depth some pathologies of the body image including phantom limb phenomena, personal neglect, autoscopy, and autotopagnosia. He ultimately argues that the body image is not innate but rather acquired through experience of one's own and others' bodies.

The next six chapters focus on clinical disorders of the self. Feinberg and coworkers, in Chapter 8 describe a group of neurological disorders that bear particular relevance to the understanding of the self: *delusional misidentification* and *delusional reduplication* syndromes. The authors first describe several subtypes of these conditions. Then, in an extensive review of previously published cases of these conditions, they examine their clinical, neuropsychological, and neuroanatomical features. The authors describe a particularly high incidence of right frontal pathology in these cases and consider what specific role the nondominant hemisphere might play in the creation and maintenance of the self.

In a related chapter Karen Spangenberg Postal in Chapter 9 examines cases of delusional misidentification of the self in a mirror. She describes a typical case of this disorder, examining it from the clinical, neuropsychological, and neuroanatomical points of view. She then examines the disorder in the context of psychiatry and self research as a whole. She concludes, similar to Feinberg and colleagues in Chapter 8, that the mirror sign, like other varieties of delusional misidentification, is more common in patients with right hemisphere disease and results from a complex interplay of neurocognitive and emotional factors.

In Chapter 10 Seeley and Miller consider how the self and self-related functions break down in dementia. They first present a brief overview of the phylogeny and ontogeny of the self and suggest which particular brain structures might be critical to the creation of the self. Using this model, they describe the manner in which the self may become disorganized and even dissolve in the presence of a dementing illness.

Simon Baron-Cohen next discusses the self in autism and Asperger Syndrome. Baron-Cohen, one of the leaders in this area, begins Chapter 11 with a brief introduction to autism followed by a discussion of the components of empathy. He stresses that empathy involves both cognitive and emotional aspects and describes these features of empathy within the context of Leslie's scheme of understanding minds. Baron-Cohen then considers empathy in relationship to autism and Asperger syndrome by tracing the developmental course of these disorders throughout the lifespan. The chapter concludes with a discussion of the "extreme male brain theory" previously proposed by Baron-Cohen.

Chapter 12 is an examination of schizophrenia and agency by Sarah-Jayne Blakemore. In schizophrenic patients there is a tendency to misattribute behaviors initiated by the self to an external agent. Blakemore describes experimental examinations of this tendency, focusing especially on PET imaging during voluntary action. Blakemore suggests that two regions appear important for the sense of agency, specifically the cerebellum and the parietal cortex. She suggests that excessive activity of a cerebellar–parietal network results in misattribution of agency such that self-generated actions are thought to have an external origin.

In Chapter 13 Hedy Kober and colleagues examine depersonalization as it relates to the self. The chapter addresses intriguing question regarding the brain areas that are related to disturbed self-processing in this disorder. Kober and her colleagues attempt to find common ground among studies that differ widely in method and study populations. They first examines Keenan's right-hemisphere model of the self. This is followed by an examination of the early studies of depersonalization and the brain. Modern neuroimaging studies are then considered, including experiments using PET and fMRI imaging. After a discussion of Mathew's work (see Chapter 15) and the treatment of depersonalization disorders, the authors conclude with a description of a patient treated for depersonalization disorder using TMS.

The last series of chapters address how the self is transformed in dreams, under the influence of psychoactive agents, and during meditation. First, Antti Revonsuo examines how the sleeping brain represents the self in dreams in Chapter 14. He initially enumerates the various ways that the dream self resembles or differs from the waking self. For example, while the dream self possesses a body image like the waking self and sees the world from a similar point of view as the waking self, the dream self suffers from transient amnesia and confabulates. Revonsuo also examines the interesting feature of bizarreness in dreams and suggests that the data indicate that the dream self is in certain respects *less* bizarre than other non–self-related dream content, and he relates this observation to the patterns of REM sleep activation. In the concluding sections of the chapter, Revonsuo argues for a novel "threat simulation theory" of dreaming, in which the biological function of dreaming is a sort of "dress rehearsal" for potentially real, life-threatening events. This somewhat controversial opinion differs from the Freudian point of view that dreams often and largely serve a wish-fulfilling function.

In Chapter 15 Roy Mathew examines alterations of the self that are due to an array of psychoactive drugs. Mathew, with a decidedly non-Western emphasis, places the use of psychoactive agents into historical context and describes his own work with PET and cannabis as a model for depersonalization (also discussed in Chapter 13). After a discussion of the effects of mescaline, cocaine, and ecstasy on the self, the author makes a grand effort to relate the scientific concepts of dissociation, depersonalization, and the core self to Eastern spiritual, religious, and philosophical traditions, and all of this to the neurobiology of the self.

Hans Lou and Troels Kjaer introduce the study of meditation as a vehicle for discovering the neural correlates of the self in Chapter 16. The chapter begins with a thorough introduction to experiments designed to isolate the neural components of meditation. The authors introduce their own work on meditation in which they found precuneal, medial frontal, and striatal activation during meditation. The authors conclude that a network involving medial parietal, medial prefrontal, and right lateral parietal regions are critically involved in self-representation.

Finally, in a fascinating final chapter, world-renowned sleep and dreaming researcher J. Allan Hobson provides a harrowing yet moving personal perspective on his own "journey of the self." In February of 2001, Dr. Hobson suffered a brain stem stroke. Approximately 5 months after partial recovery from this first neurological insult, due to the combined effects of pneumonia, cardiac failure, and adverse drug reactions, Hobson went into a hallucinatory delerium. His description of this period is simultaneously fascinating and frightening and provides a marvelous window into the manner in which the mind and self can be transformed by the brain's metabolic milieu. Upon reflection Hobson concludes that in spite of his mental transformation during the time of his illness, the nature of his experiences and his ability to describe and understand them speaks to the resilience and durability of the self in the face of the ravages of neurological illness.

We hope readers enjoy the work of this eclectic group of writers and the varied approaches they take to the immensely complicated but endlessly fascinating topic of the self.

References

James, W. (1892). *Psychology: The Briefer Course.* Reprinted in: G. Allport (Ed.), *Psychology: The Briefer Course.* Notre Dame, IN: University of Notre Dame Press, 1985.

Levin, J.D. (1992). *Theories of the Self.* Washington, DC: Taylor & Francis.

Strawson, G. (2000). The phenomenology and ontology of the self. In: D. Zahavi (Ed.), *Exploring the Self. Philosophical and Psychopathological Perspectives on Self-Experience* (pp. 39–54). Amsterdam: John Benjamin.

2

The Self as a Problem in Philosophy and Neurobiology

JOHN R. SEARLE

There are a large number of different problems concerning the self in psychology, neurobiology, philosophy, and other disciplines. I have the impression that many of the problems of the self studied in neurobiology concern various forms of pathology—defects in the integrity, coherence, or functioning of the self. I will have nothing to say about these pathologies because I know next to nothing about them, and they are discussed elsewhere in this volume. I will only mention some pathologies, such as those of split brain patients, that are directly relevant to the philosophical problems of the self.

The Philosophical Problem of the Self

In philosophy, the traditional problem of the self is the problem of personal identity. Indeed, in the standard *Encyclopedia of Philosophy* (Edwards, 1967), the entry "self" just says "see personal identity." The problem of personal identity is the problem of stating the criteria by which we identify someone as the same person through changes. Thus, for example, the problem of personal identity arises in such a question as: What fact about me, here and now, makes me the same person as the person who bore my name and lived in my house 20 years ago? There are a number of criteria of personal identity, and they do not always yield the same result. I will get to these shortly.

I think that in fact there are at least two philosophical problems concerning the self. Besides the problem of personal identity, there is the problem of whether it is necessary to postulate the existence of a self that goes beyond the recognition of the body and of the sequence of experiences that occur in the body. In our philosophical tradition, and especially in our religious tradition, it is common to suppose that in addition to our bodies we also possess souls, that souls are the essence of ourselves, and that, therefore, for each of us, his or her self consists of a soul.

On this view what we think of as our mental life, both conscious and unconscious, is something that goes on not in our bodies but in our souls, which can also be called our selves or our minds. According to Descartes, an influential exponent of this tradition, each of us is identical, not with a body, but with an entity we can call mind, soul, or self, and we only happen to be contingently attached to a body during the course of a lifetime. Once we die, the soul will depart from the body and have a separate existence. I think the temptation to confuse the problem of personal identity with this second problem of the self derives from the fact that we suppose that if we had an affirmative solution to the second problem it would automatically provide a solution to the first. If we knew that in addition to our bodies we each had a soul, or self, or mind, and this entity was the very essence of our being, then the continuation of the self, so described, would immediately provide a solution of the problem of personal identity. You are identical with the person who lived here 20 years ago because you are the same soul or self.

So much for the tradition. Where are we today? Well, I do not know anybody who believes in the existence of an immortal soul except those who do so for some religious reason. A famous neurobiologist who believed in the soul was Sir John Eccles; there are a number of philosophers who also believe in the existence of an immortal soul, but like Eccles their belief is part of their general religious conviction. From my experience most philosophers do not believe in the existence of the soul. Furthermore, what is more important for the purposes of our present discussion, most philosophers do not believe in the existence of the self as something in addition to the sequence of our experiences, conscious and unconscious, and the body in which these experiences occur. I think most philosophers accept Hume's skepticism about the existence of the self (Hume, 1951, p. 251 ff). Hume asked himself the following question: When I turn my attention inward and focus on what is going on in my mind, what do I find? Hume says that I do not find any self or soul or person in addition to the sequence of my experiences. If, for example, I clutch my forehead and concentrate very seriously on what is happening in a way that will try to locate my self, what I locate will be the pressure of my hand on my forehead and a lot of other such experiences, "impressions" and "ideas" as Hume calls them. Hume's view, which has been very influential and is probably the most common view in philosophy about the self, is that each of us consists of a physical body, and each of us has a sequence of experiences within that body.[1] But that is it, as far as human life is concerned. There is no self or soul left over, nor is there any need to postulate any such entity.

Well, what about personal identity? There are a variety of criteria that we do, in fact, employ in deciding questions of the identity of a person across time and change. It seems to me that, in fact, we employ at least four different criteria for deciding questions of identity. The first and most important is the identity of the body. I am the same person as the person who bore my name decades ago because my present body is spatiotemporally continuous with the body that existed under my name at that time. Of course, there are philosophical puzzles: None of the molecules in my body today is the same as those in my body of decades ago, so how can the body be the same if all the microparts are different? Furthermore, philosophers are good at inventing puzzling science fiction thought experiments. Suppose that bodily fusion and fission were common. What would we say if humans routinely split into two or three or five bodies, as amoebae now split into two? But in spite of these puzzles, we have a pretty clear notion of bodily identity that works across time and change. Well, why isn't that enough? Unlike the identity of material objects such as cars and houses, we are convinced that the identity of the body is not enough to constitute a personal identity. We all understand Kafka's story of Gregor Samsa who wakes to find *himself* in the body of a giant insect, and it is easy to imagine science fiction scenarios of brain transplants in which I might find myself having a different body. Furthermore, possession of the same brain might not by itself be enough for personal identity. Suppose that I had the same brain but that all the information in my brain were transferred to another person's brain, and the information in his brain were transferred to mine. We might feel that I now inhabit his body, and he inhabits mine. I am not saying that these science fiction fantasies are sufficiently clear, or even coherent. I only point to them because they indicate that where our own personal identity is concerned, we think there is more to it than just the body.

Well, what more? Locke said that the essential thing to personal identity is what he called "consciousness" (Locke, 1947, pp. 182–201). Most interpreters think that by *consciousness* he meant our present memory experiences of a continuity between our present self and the earlier self that had the experiences on which our present memories are based. In short, Locke's consciousness criterion is usually, and I think correctly, interpreted as a memory criterion. The idea is that in addition to the continuity of the body, we need a continuity of consciousness as recorded in memory. In addition to the third-person criterion of bodily continuity, we need the first-person criterion of the experience of the personal identity of the self. And this is how all human personal identity differs from the identities of cars, houses, etc.

A third criterion, commonly used in ordinary life, is relative stability and continuity of personality. In cases in which we feel that a person's personality has altered dramatically and drastically, we are inclined to feel "she is not the same person any more." To take a famous case, when an iron bar went through the skull of the nineteenth century railway worker Phineas Gage, he miraculously survived, but his personality was totally different. Before he had been friendly, gregarious, and reliable; afterwards he became hostile, surly, and capricious. From a purely practical point of view, we would continue to regard him as the same person. For example, he would still owe the taxes of Phineas Gage and still own the property of Phineas Gage, but from a neurobiological point of view and a philosophical point of view, we would want to know very much what had changed in Phineas Gage so as to render him a totally different personality from what he had been before.

A fourth criterion is the relative coherence of the spatiotemporal continuity of the physical body through change. There is a standard pattern by which one and the same body grows and ages until eventual death, but suppose that the entity, though spatiotemporally continuous, varies wildly and unpredictably in its physical form. Suppose my body might change into that of a car or a house or a mountain. We think we understand Gregor Samsa's body changing into that of a large insect, but how far are we prepared to go? I do not think we need to answer that question in advance. The point I am making now is that we in fact employ four different sets of criteria in our concept of personal identity—spatiotemporal continuity of body, continuous memory, continuity of personality, and coherence of physical change—and that the everyday concept works well enough because these hang together to give consistent answers in real life.

So far so good, or so it might seem. It seems there is no such thing as the self in addition to all the stuff I have been talking about—continuity and coherence of the living body together with continuous memory sequences and coherent personalities, but I do not think this conclusion is correct. I have reluctantly come to the conclusion that the nature of human consciousness requires the postulation of a non-Humean self, and this postulation poses problems for neurobiology that go beyond the standard neurobiological problems of consciousness but will enable us to re-pose the question of consciousness in important ways.

The Neurobiological Problem of Consciousness

Sometimes, but unfortunately not very often, we can get a scientific solution to a long-standing philosophical problem. A famous case is the problem of life. The problem was: how can mere inert, inanimate matter be alive? Traditionally, there were two possible answers, the mechanist answer, according to which life could be reduced to mechanical processes, and the vitalist answer, according to which something more was needed, an *élan vital,* a vital force, that infused life into inert matter. We cannot take this problem seriously anymore, and it is hard for us to recover the passion with which it was debated a mere century ago. The point is not that the mechanists won and the vitalists lost, but rather that we got a much richer conception of biochemical mechanisms—a conception that did not exist when the debate raged in the nineteenth and early twentieth centuries.

I hope something like this is also happening to the problem of consciousness. The problem here is: how can mere unconscious bits of matter in the brain cause consciousness? On this problem we have a head start over the problem of life because we know before we ever get started on the investigation that processes in the brain do, in fact, cause consciousness. All the same, much, though not all, current neurobiological research suffers from a mistaken conception of the problem, and that in turn derives from a mistaken conception of the self. In order to work up to the self, I have to say a bit about consciousness.

I sometimes still hear it said that "consciousness" is hard to define. But if we are just talking about a definition that gives us not a scientific analysis, but rather locates the target of our investigation, then it seems to me that consciousness is not hard to define. Here is a definition: consciousness consists of those states of feeling, sentience, or awareness that typically begin when we wake from a dreamless sleep and continue throughout the day until those feelings stop, that is, until we go to sleep again, go into a coma, die, or otherwise become "unconscious." On this account dreams are a form of consciousness that occur to us during sleep. What, then, are the features of consciousness that we would like to be able to explain on this definition? Conscious states, so defined, are *qualitative* in the sense that there is always a certain qualitative feel to what it is like to be in one conscious state rather than another. We all know the difference between listening to Beethoven's Ninth Symphony and drinking cold beer. The difference is precisely the kind of qualitative difference that I am talking about. We know furthermore that all such conscious states are *subjective* in the sense that they exist only as experienced by a human or animal subject. Conscious states require a subject for their very existence. They do not exist in a neutral or third-person fashion; they have an existence that depends on their first-person subjective qualities, and that is just another way of saying that a conscious state must always be someone's conscious state. In philosophy this point is sometimes put by saying consciousness has a "first-person ontology." *First-person* here means there must be an *I,* some subject that experiences the consciousness, and *ontology* just refers to the mode of existence that something has. A third feature of consciousness is less frequently remarked on, but I think it is absolutely essential to understanding the other two. Conscious states always come to us as part of a unified conscious field, so when I am listening to Beethoven's Ninth Symphony while drinking beer, I do not just have the experience of listening and the experience of drinking; rather, I have the experience of drinking and listening as part of one total conscious experience, and this is characteristic of consciousness generally, that consciousness always and only occurs as part of a unified conscious field. This is why, by the way, the split brain experiments are so important to the study of consciousness. As far as we can tell from the experiments of Sperry and Gazzaniga (Gazzaniga, 1985), a patient whose corpus collosum has been cut gives all the external symptoms of having two separate conscious fields, one in each hemisphere, and these are only imperfectly united into a single conscious field; sometimes they exist as separate conscious fields.

Among philosophers, Immanuel Kant attached a great deal of importance to the unity of the conscious field. He called it "the transcendental unity of apperception" (Kant, 1997). I think the unity of our conscious field is important to our analysis of the concept of the self, and I will say more about it later. For the moment, I just want to call attention to the fact that these three features, qualitativeness, subjectivity, and unity, are not independent of each other. Each implies the next. You cannot have a qualitative experience such as tasting beer without that experience occurring as part of some subjective state of awareness, and you cannot have a subjective state of awareness except as part of a total field of awareness, even if the only thing in this particular impoverished field is the state of awareness itself. So we might say, initially at least, that the problem of consciousness is precisely the problem of qualitative, unified subjectivity. The three features are simply different aspects of the one common essential trait of consciousness. Now there are lots of other traits of consciousness that should be investigated, and I have investigated the philosophical aspects of them at some length in a number of books (Searle, 1984, 1992, 1997, 2004). However, for the purposes of this chapter, I will focus on only these three, and particularly on the last, because they are most relevant for our examination of the problem of the self.

Notice an interesting feature of the unified conscious field. Within the field we can change our attention at will. Without moving my head or even my eyes, I can focus my attention on this or that feature of my visual field. And even with my eyes closed I can think now about this problem, now that problem, moving the focus of my attention, again, entirely at will. This ought to seem puzzling to us. The brain creates a conscious field just as the stomach and digestive tract create digestion. So what has conscious *will* got to do with it? To put the question crudely, when I say I can shift my attention at will, who does the shifting? Why should there be anything more to my conscious life than the existence of a conscious field? Where is there anything more? I will come back to these questions because I think they are essential to understanding the problem of a self.

How can we solve the problem of consciousness as a problem in neurobiology? First of all we have to state exactly what the problem we wish to be able to solve is, and here I think the answer can be stated quite simply. The neurobiological problem of consciousness is: How exactly do brain processes cause our conscious states in all their enormous richness and variety, and how exactly are these conscious states realized in the brain? Why do conscious states exist at all, and where and how do they exist in the brain? It took a long time for many neurobiologists to see that this was a crucial question in neurobiology; indeed, I would say it is the number one question in the biological sciences today. Right now there is a great deal of research on precisely this topic.

Most researchers are seeking the neuronal correlate of consciousness (NCC). The idea is this: in order to solve the problem of consciousness, we should find out first what is going on in the brain at the neurobiological level at a time when a subject is conscious. What neurobiological features are correlated with the conscious features? We now think, perhaps with too much optimism, that recent improvements in our investigative techniques, especially single-cell recording and fMRI, will give us a richer research apparatus for discovering the NCC. The idea, though often not explicitly stated, is that the investigation will proceed according to a pattern that has been fairly common in the history of science. The first step is to find a neuronal correlate of conscious states. This would be the NCC. The second stage is to investigate whether the NCC is actually a *causal* correlation, and we do this by the usual tests. In an otherwise unconscious subject, can you produce consciousness by producing the NCC? In an otherwise conscious subject, can you shut off consciousness by shutting off the NCC? If you have affirmative answers to these questions, then it is a reasonable supposition that the correlation is more than accidental; it is, in all likelihood, a causal correlation.

The third stage, and we are a long way from reaching it, is to formulate a general theory, a general statement of the laws or principles by which the correlation functions causally in the life of the organism. This research, as I said, is off and running. I am quite optimistic about its long-term prospects, though I have to admit progress has been very slow. In general, there are two lines of research that go on in this field, one of which seems to me much more promising than the other, although the more promising, unfortunately, is harder to conduct as an actual research project. The most common line of research is what I call the "building-block approach" (Searle, 2000). The idea of this approach is to think of the unified conscious field as made up of all of its different components. Right now, for example, I am experiencing the color red as I look at a red box on my table, I am hearing the sound of my voice, I am feeling a slight aftertaste of coffee in my mouth, and so on. The idea of the building-block approach is to think of the entire conscious field as made up of such building blocks (the experiences of color, of sound, of taste, etc.). On this view, if we could find the NCC for even one building block and understand the mechanisms by which that NCC caused consciousness, that presumably would give us an entering wedge that would enable us to crack the whole problem of consciousness. The mechanisms by which the NCC for a particular conscious state produce that conscious state will presumably be generalizeable to other conscious states. The analogy with genetics is obvious: You do not have to know how every phenotypical trait is the expression of some gene or set of genes in order to appreciate the power of the DNA conception of genetics. You have to understand the general mechanisms involved, and then you can apply them to particular cases. Most research on consciousness that I am aware of follows the building-block approach.

Another approach, pursued by a minority of investigators, is what I call the "unified-field approach." We want to know not so much what causes the experience of red, though that is part of our overall investigation, but rather how the brain becomes conscious in the first place. What exactly is the difference between the unconscious brain and the conscious brain, and how exactly do those differences cause the brain to be in a state of consciousness? The state of consciousness, as I have argued earlier, is a matter of a unified conscious field, so the question for this approach is: how does the brain produce the unified conscious field?

I said that I think the unified field approach is superior. Why? Science typically has proceeded by the practice of breaking larger problems down into smaller problems by using an atomistic approach to large problems. Why would this not work for consciousness? Perhaps it will, but there is an immediate objection: the building-block approach identifies building blocks that can exist only in a subject who is already conscious, but if that is right then it looks as if the NCC for the experience of the color red does not give us the NCC for the experience of consciousness; rather, it gives us the NCC for a particular mode *within a preexisting conscious field*. On the unified field approach we should think of perception *not as creating* consciousness, but as *modifying* the preexisting conscious field (Llinas, 2001). On the building-block approach perception creates consciousness just like that, out of nothing except neuronal processes. On the unified field approach perception does not create consciousness but modifies the consciousness of the preexisting conscious field.

Why am I so convinced that the building-block approach is the wrong approach? The answer is that if we take the building-block approach as giving us the NCC for consciousness and not for particular modifications of the conscious field, then it would make predictions that seem implausible. The approach would predict that in an otherwise unconscious subject, if you could introduce the NCC for the experience of the color red the subject would suddenly have a conscious flash of red and then lapse back into total unconsciousness. That seems to me extremely unlikely. From what we know about the experience of red, it occurs only in subjects who have a preexisting consciousness, that is, who are conscious already when they experience red, and so on with perception in general. Alarm clocks, for example, do not create just a single percept but rather create a field in which that percept is the central entity.

Whether the building-block or the unified-field approach is better is an empirical question not to be settled by philosophical analysis, and I am prepared to be proven wrong. Perhaps the building-block approach will succeed in the end, but right now I think it is a source of difficultly. In fact, it turns out it is not at all hard to find various kind of NCCs for particular sorts of experiences, and many researchers have done that (Kinwasher, 2001). But we still have not solved the problem of consciousness by these findings because we still do not have an answer to the question: what makes the brain conscious? The reason I have belabored this point is because I think there are lessons to be learned about the neurobiological problem of the self from reflecting on the neurobiological problem of consciousness.

The Requirement of the Self as a Formal Feature of the Unified Conscious Field and Its Implications for Neurobiology

There are famous objections to Locke's idea of memory as the essential criterion for personal identity. One objection is this: It would be circular to make memory a criterion for the identity of the self, because in order to establish that the memories in question are correct memories, one first has to establish that the person who has these memories is really identical with the person whose experiences he claims to remember. Thus, if I now sincerely claim that I remember writing the *Critique of Pure Reason,* that by itself goes no way at all toward showing that I am, in fact, identical with the actual author of the *Critique of Pure Reason,* because one would first have to establish that I did write the *Critique* before one could know that the memories are accurate. For exactly the same reason, the fact that I now claim to remember writing *Speech Acts* by itself goes no way at all toward showing that I am identical with the actual author of *Speech Acts.* Hence, it looks as if memory is no good as a criterion of the self because, to establish that the memory is an accurate memory as opposed to an illusory one, one first has to establish the very identity that the memory was supposed to establish. I think this is a fair objection if we treat memory as a criterion of personal identity, but that need not be our only interest in memory. It seems to me, for this discussion, that what we are interested in is not how to establish conclusively that I am identical with such and such a person who lived so many years ago, but rather what facts about my conscious states give me a sense of myself as a single continuing entity through time? It is this sense of the self that is more relevant to problems in neurobiology.

I now think that with the introduction of memory I am prepared to state the philosophical problem of the self, and how it bears on neurobiology, a little more precisely. It is a remarkable feature of the conscious field, which I identified earlier, that the elements of the conscious field are not, so to speak, neutral. They are not just given to me as independent phenomena, but rather they exhibit certain special traits that I now will to specify further. First, it is an absolutely astounding thing about the conscious field that, given the same conscious field, I can shift my attention at will. Even without changing the direction of my eyes, I can focus my attention now on the coffee cup on the table, now at the computer screen in front of me, now at the bookcase on my right. The shift of attention within a constant conscious field is something I can do at will. A second feature, which derives from the first, is that I can change the entire conscious field at will, simply by doing something different, such as moving my head, or closing my eyes, or standing up and leaving the room. The fact that I have the ability to do things seems to be an essential part of the normal human conscious field, and we can easily imagine a different mode of existence in which I was utterly passive and I simply experienced events occurring to me but had no sense whatsoever of having any control over them. When I engage in conscious voluntary action, I have a sense of my own freedom. I have the sense that I am doing this, but I could, right here and now, be doing something different. In such cases I have the impression that the causes of my action, in the form of the reasons on which I am acting, are not causally sufficient to determine the action. In normal nonpathological cases the action is *motivated but not determined,* because there is a *gap* between the perceived causes and the action. This gap has a name in philosophy, it is called the freedom of the will. It does not matter for our present purposes whether the sense of freedom is a mark of real freedom or only an illusion. I cannot think the gap away, for even if I become a convinced determinist and refuse to make any choices on the grounds that everything is determined anyway, my refusal to make any choices is intelligible to me as my action only under the presupposition of freedom. I have freely chosen not to make any free choices. The third feature of the conscious field is that I do, in fact, have a sense of myself as a particular person situated at a particular time and place in history with a certain set of particular experiences and memories. We need to put these various features together into a unified account of the self before we can state questions that could be addressed by neurobiology.

The sequence of conscious experiences (as identified by Hume) together with the fact that these experiences come to us as part of a unified conscious field (as identified by Kant) is still not enough to give us the characteristic experiences that constitute our idea of the self. Even if we add to the Hume-Kant story the idea that some of these experiences are memories of earlier experiences (as identified by Locke), we still do not have our conception of the self. What is missing? Let us go back to the point I made earlier, that we can shift our attention at will and indeed initiate actions at will. Who does the shifting, and who does the initiating? One thing I have noticed in teaching these matters to undergraduates and discussing them with professionals is that *everybody* feels the attraction of the homunculus fallacy. It is very tempting to think that there is a little guy in my head who does my thinking, perceiving, and acting. Of course, the homunculus fallacy is a fallacy, because it leads to an infinite regress. If my vision can only occur because the little man in my head watches the TV screen in my head, then who watches the TV screen in the little man's head? But, and this is the crucial point, though the homunculus is a fallacy, the urge to postulate the homunculus is powerful and well founded. The problem is that we cannot make sense of our conscious experiences if we think of them as just a sequence of events (impressions and ideas à la Hume) related by present memory experiences of earlier experiences (à la Locke) and part of a unified conscious field (à la Kant). We need to postulate, initially at least, a locus of the initiation of action. My decisions and actions are not just events that occur, but rather *I decide* and *I act*. But now we have to proceed very carefully, or else we will start sounding like the worst kind of German philosophers (Was ist das Ich?). So far we have postulated only a purely formal entity. It is simply an x, something capable of initiating and carrying out actions. Notice, however, that the entity that initiates actions must be the very same entity as the entity that reflects on reasons for action, and indeed the same entity that has perceptions and memories that form the basis of the reasons on which it reflects and decides on actions. Just as we had to postulate a purely formally specified entity that decides and acts, so the connection between perception, memory, and reasons for action requires us to postulate that the *same* entity that performs the action has all of these other features. Why? Well, if the entity that decides and acts is different from the one that perceives, remembers, and reflects, then we would not get the connection necessary to make sense of our actions. If I act on a reason R, then R must be *my* reason for acting. For example, if I jump out of the way because I see a truck bearing down on me, then the entity that initiates the jumping has to be the same one that does the seeing, otherwise the seeing gives no reason for the jumping. Furthermore, once the action has been performed, the same entity that did the performing is the one who has responsibility for the performance and thus gets the credit or the blame. We can pull all these threads together as follows.

The universal urge to postulate a homunculus is based on very profound features of our ordinary conscious experiences. In order to make sense of those experiences we have to suppose,

There is some x such that

x is conscious

x persists through time

x has perceptions and memories

x operates with reasons in the gap

x, in the gap, is capable of deciding and acting

x is responsible for at least some of its behavior.

The x in question is the self in at least one sense of the word. Notice that the postulation of the self is not the postulation of a separate entity distinct from the conscious field but rather it is a formal feature of the conscious field. The point I am making is that if we reflect on the features of the conscious field, we see that we cannot accurately describe it if we think of it as a field constituted only by its contents and their arrangement. Rather, the contents require a principle of unity, but the principle is not a separate entity. To suppose we had both a conscious field *and* a self would be a category mistake, like supposing that the country most of which is between Mexico and Canada consists of 50 states *plus* the United States of America. Rather, the postulation of a self is like the postulation of the point of view in visual perception. We cannot make sense of our perceptions unless we suppose that they occur from a point of view, even though the point of view is not itself perceived. Similarly, we cannot make sense of our conscious experiences unless we suppose that they occur to a self, even though the self is not consciously experienced. The self is not a separate thing or entity any more than the point of view is.

Let us now pull these various threads about the self together. Let us remind ourselves first that we are talking about a problem in animal biology. There is no dualism or spiritualism hiding in our account. The irreducibly mental unified conscious field is a biological, and therefore "physical," or "natural," feature of the brain. There is nothing spooky or unnatural about it. We have discovered under analysis that our bodies with their brains are capable of causing and sustaining a unified conscious field, and this unified field is qualitative and subjective, unlike other aspects of our biological life. I have claimed that the sense of permanence and coherence that we each get in our conscious field also requires memory.

But, interestingly, the unified conscious field, even given a sense of continuing identity via memory, is not enough to account for the facts of our ordinary nonpathological experience. To account for those facts we need to postulate a (purely formal) self, x. What are these facts, and why do they force us to postulate a self? The first fact is that because of the gap, decisions and actions do not just happen. There has to be something that makes the decision and performs the action. In my case decisions and actions are not things that just happen to me, rather *I* make the decisions and carry out the actions. And the second fact is that the existence of an agent, something that can decide and act, is not by itself enough. The very same entity that decides and acts has to be the entity that perceives, remembers, imagines, reflects etc. I not only act but the same I that acts also reflects, perceives, remembers, and so on. So, at least for nonpathological cases, we are forced to postulate a single entity x that constitutes the self and has all the psychological properties that constitute the unified conscious field. The self in question, the x, is conscious and is capable of deciding and acting in the gap, but the same x that decides and acts must be capable of thought, because the decisions and actions are based on reasons. And those reasons themselves are based on perception, memory, and other cognitive capacities. Hence, the x that does the deciding, acting, and thinking must be the x that exercises all these other cognitive capacities.

Several philosophers, famously Kant, have said that all consciousness is self-consciousness. If that means that every first-order conscious state requires a second-order state about the first state, it is wrong. I can, for example, just enjoy a beer. I do not have to also enjoy my enjoying of the beer. But there is a sense in which it is right. All (nonpathological) consciousness, first- or second-order, has to be possessed by a self. The self is not the object of consciousness. If I drink the beer, the object of my consciousness is the beer I am drinking, not the self that does the drinking, nor is the self the content of the consciousness. If I drink the beer, the content of my consciousness is the experience of beer drinking, not the experience of the self. There is no experience of the self, but in order that there be a conscious experience of beer drinking that has object and content, there has to be a self that experiences the content and is aware of the object.

We will understand this point better if we pursue the analogy with vision. In order to make sense of my visual perceptions, I have to postulate a visual apparatus that is necessary for visual perception but is not itself part of the object nor the content of visual perception. This apparatus will include a point of view as well as a spatially located mechanism that does the seeing. But neither the point of view nor the mechanism are seen, nor are they part of the experience of seeing. Exactly analogously, in order to make sense of the conscious field, we have to postulate a self that is not part of the conscious field, nor is it one of the objects of the conscious field.

Finally, what has all this got to do with neurobiology? How does the brain, indeed, how could the brain, produce all the features I have been describing? A neurobiological account of consciousness cannot stop with the NCC, even with an NCC that is known to function causally in producing consciousness. In order to have a scientific account of consciousness, we will need more than an account of how the brain produces subjective states of sentience and awareness. We will need to know how the brain produces the peculiar organization of experiences that expresses the existence of the self.

How would one go about conducting such research? I am too ignorant of brain functioning to have an intelligent opinion, but here is one suggestion. In other areas of brain science we have learned a lot from studying the pathological cases. Just as with vision we have learned much from blind sight, and with memory we have learned much from bilateral removal of the hippocampus, so in the study of the self we might start with some of the pathologies discussed elsewhere in this book.

Note

1. Strictly speaking, Hume did not believe that we were justified in supposing that bodies had a "separate and distinct" existence, but that is another issue that is independent of his skepticism about the self.

References

Edwards, P. (Ed.) (1967). *The Encyclopedia of Philosophy* (vol 7, p. 345). New York: Free Press.

Gazzaniga, M. (1985). *The Social Brain: Discovering the Networks of the Mind.* Perseus Group Books.

Hume, D. (1951). *A Treatise of Human Nature,* book I, part III, section VI "Of Personal Identity." Oxford: Oxford University Press.

Kant, I. (1997). *Critique of Pure Reason,* trans. Paul Guyer and Allen W. Wood. Cambridge: Cambridge University Press.

Kinwasher, N. (2001). Neural events and perceptual awareness. *Cognition, 79,* 89–113.

Llinás, R. (2001). *I of the vortex, From Neurons to Self,* Cambridge, MA: MIT Press.

Locke, J. (1947). *An Essay Concerning Human Understanding,* A.S. Pringle-Pattison (Ed.), Oxford: Oxford University Press.

Searle, J.R. (1984). *Minds, Brains and Science,* Cambridge, MA: Harvard University Press.

Searle, J.R. (1992). *Rediscovery of the Mind,* Cambridge, MA: MIT Press.

Searle, J.R. (1997). *The Mystery of Consciousness,* New York: New York Review of Books.

Searle, J.R. (2000). Consciousness, *Annual Review of Neuroscience, 23,* 557–578.

Searle, J.R. (2004). *Mind: A Brief Introduction,* New York: Oxford University Press.

3

The Cognitive Neuroscience of the Self: Insights from Functional Neuroimaging of the Normal Brain

SETH J. GILLIHAN AND MARTHA J. FARAH

The study of the brain, like the study of any other complex system, is aided by the use of multiple different methods. After centuries of studying higher brain function by relying primarily on a single type of evidence, namely, the effects of brain lesions on human cognition, it has recently been possible to study brain function in healthy, normal humans. Functional neuroimaging provides a second powerful method for understanding the neural bases of human cognition alongside the venerable lesion method.

One of the most ambitious applications of imaging to date has been the study of our sense of self. Case studies of patients with neurological and psychiatric disease have suggested that the sense of self is a discrete, separately lesionable component of the mind and brain. This has motivated cognitive neuroscientists to attempt to identify self-related processing in functional brain scans. Can self-awareness be visualized as a distinctive pattern of brain activity? What have we learned in this way about the neural systems underlying the psychological self? What problems have we encountered in imaging self-related cognition, and which of these continue to limit our understanding of the brain bases of self? The goal of this chapter is to address these questions by reviewing and critiquing the current functional neuroimaging literature on the self.

We begin by defining the subject of study. The concept of *self* is difficult to define in a noncircular way. We take it as a given that self-related cognition must be distinct from cognition about people other than the self. The operational definition of the self, that is, the experimental methods that have been used to capture self-related processing in the lab, provides another indication of what is meant by the *self* in cognitive neuroscience literature. By this measure our sense of self includes awareness of our own current mental state, first-person perspective, autobiographical memory, sense of agency, and self-concept. Note that this definition of self is focused on the psychological rather than the corporeal self. The imaging literature on each of these aspects of the psychological self will be reviewed here.

Self-Awareness and First-Person Perspective

One of the earliest imaging studies to address the self was reported by Lane and colleagues (1997). They had subjects view emotionally evocative pictures and focus attention on either their own emotional responses to the pictures or the objective spatial properties of the pictures. When attention was focused on the subjects' own responses compared to the pictures' spatial properties, there was significantly more activation evoked in a number of areas, including the anterior cingulate cortex, which the authors inferred must play a role in the sense of self.

Gusnard and colleagues (2001) operationalized self-awareness in a similar way, comparing an "internally cued condition" in which subjects judged whether each image in a series gave them a pleasant, neutral, or unpleasant feeling and an "externally cued condition" in which they judged whether the image depicted a scene that was indoors or outdoors. These authors found increased medial prefrontal activity (dorsal to midsections) associated with the internally cued condition, in addition to greater activity in the frontal operculum/left insula.

A difficulty in interpreting the results of these two studies comes from the many dissimilarities between the self and nonself comparison conditions. In both the Lane et al. and the Gusnard et al. studies, the self-processing task had an affective component, while the comparison task did not, and this alone might be expected to recruit medial prefrontal brain regions (Bush, Luu, & Posner, 2000; Drevets & Raichle, 1998). In fact, affective evaluation has been found to activate these areas outside tasks that call for self-reflection (Zysset et al., 2002).

The first-person perspective was studied by Vogeley et al. (2001) by reading subjects scenarios in two different conditions. In the "theory of mind" condition (TOM), the story concerned someone else, and afterward the subject answered questions about the person's actions, beliefs, and perceptions. In the "self" condition subjects read similar stories and were then asked questions about their own actions, beliefs, and perceptions within the story. For example, the subject read a story about leaving his or her umbrella at home, and later in the day it starts to rain; the subject then answered the question, "What do you think?" A baseline condition, with no person's psychological perspective (self or other), was included in the design, and baseline activations were subtracted from the self and TOM condition activations. Not surprisingly, the self and TOM tasks involved some common areas of activation, in the right prefrontal cortex (PFC). In addition, the self condition activated certain distinct areas, namely the right temporoparietal junction and bilateral anterior cingulate cortex. The authors concluded that "this study provides experimental evidence for an at least in part independent cerebral implementation of self perspective in the context of theory of mind" (p. 180).

The design of this study is, in principle, well suited for isolating the self perspective, as it contrasts thinking about one's own thoughts and experiences with thinking about those of another person in the context of an otherwise similar task. However, the findings must be interpreted with extreme caution because of the authors' use of a fixed effects model for their statistical analyses, particularly given the small number of subjects (eight) and of stories per condition (eight). Fixed effects models tend to overestimate the reliability of findings obtained from groups of subjects and do not address the question of whether the experiment, if done again with different stimulus items and different subjects, would replicate (Aguirre, 2003; see also Hildebrand, 1986). Therefore, we cannot know whether specific subjects' responses to the task or incidental features of a few of the stories in the TOM and self conditions are responsible for the reported differences.

Autobiographical Memory

Autobiographical memory is central to our sense of self and has been studied in three imaging studies of the self (for further discussion on the self and autobiographical memory, see Chapter 6, this volume). Fink and coworkers (1996) scanned subjects while they listened to a narrative describing a memory of their own (autobiographical) and a narrative describing another person's memory (nonautobiographical). The autobiographical condition evoked greater activation in the right temporal lobe, anterior insula, and other right hemisphere areas. As the authors point out, their two conditions differ in several ways, aside from the presence versus absence of autobiographical memory per se. Some of these differences nevertheless pertain to self-specific processing, for example, the difference in personal relevance between the two types of memory and the difference in perspective between imagining oneself or another person in the narrative. Unfortunately, the conditions also differ in ways that are not at all related to the self: The autobiographical narratives were generated by the subjects, whereas the nonautobiographical narratives were not (see Slamecka & Graf, 1978, for generation effects in memory), and the autobiographical narratives had last been encountered weeks before the scan, whereas the nonautobiographical narratives had been presented to them just one hour before the scan. Additionally, the hemispheric encoding/retrieval asymmetry (HERA) model (Tulving et al., 1994) suggests that the right hemisphere is preferentially involved in episodic memory retrieval, and many studies have supported this claim (see Nyberg, Cabeza, & Tulving, 1996, for a review). Therefore, the greater activation in right hemisphere regions could be a function of the episodic retrieval in the autobiographical condition, rather than a result of self-related processing per se.

Conway and colleagues (1999) compared the PET activations associated with retrieving autobiographical memories and a simple paired-associate memory control task. Prior to the scan, subjects chose autobiographical memories to recall in response to specific cue words. When the cue word was presented during the scan, they were to recall the memory and respond with a word that would later help them report the details of the memory to the experimenters. As a control task subjects were taught word pairs such as "flower-clock" before the scan and when cued with one word during the scan were to respond with the associated word. The comparison between the two tasks revealed greater activation of large areas of the left hemisphere during autobiographical recall, including inferior, middle, and superior frontal gyri, posterior to middle temporal gyrus, anterior occipital lobe, and posterior

parietal lobe. As before, however, the memory control task differed from the autobiographical recall task in a number of ways, including the absence of any meaningful narrative linking the associated words, and therefore the activation differences
do not necessarily result from the difference in autobiographical content per se.

Maguire and Mummery (1999) avoided many of the difficulties of the previous studies by designing "true or false" memory questions tailored to each individual subject and systematically varying the personal relevance and temporal specificity of these questions. Examples included, "You were Mike's best man at his
wedding" (personally relevant, specific time), "Ray is the youngest of your broth-
ers" (personally relevant, no specific time), "Zola Budd tripped Mary Decker" (not
personally relevant, specific time), and "Presenter Chris Evans has red hair" (not
personally relevant, no specific time). We do not know how the memories used in
the different conditions varied from one another in terms of familiarity, affective
content, and so forth. However, at the very least the questions allowed the researchers to compare self-related and non-self-related memories in the context of
generally similar tasks and materials. The relevant contrast showed activation of
medial prefrontal, temporal, and parietal cortex bilaterally as well as left hippocampus and temporal pole.

In sum, imaging studies of autobiographical memory have been limited by confounding between the autobiographical content of memory and other aspects of
memory, and the brain regions implicated have varied. Even the best-matched experimental design (that of Maguire & Mummery, 1999) did not control or measure
potential confounding. Nevertheless, that study did operationalize self- and non–
self-related processing in similar ways using real-world memory, and its findings
therefore offer a useful and interesting starting point for future investigations.

Agency

The sense of agency is the recognition of being the cause of an action (see Blakemore & Frith, 2003, for a review of agency and the self; see also Chapter 12, this
volume). Alterations in sense of agency associated with an action potentially can
reveal self-specific representations, either through experimental manipulations of
the sense of agency or in pathological states that affect the sense of agency.

Schizophrenia appears to involve alterations in the sense of self (Kircher &
David, 2003), including the overextension of agency to the actions of others (delusions of influence) and the attenuation of agency (thought insertion and delusions
of alien control). Of direct relevance to the localization of agency, a PET study that
compared schizophrenic patients while experiencing delusions of alien control and
after resolution of this symptom found that the delusion of alien control was associated specifically with right parietal cortex hyperactivation (Spence et al., 1997).

A PET study of imagined movement provides another perspective on the neural substrates of agency. Ruby and Decety (2001) instructed subjects to imagine
either themselves or the experimenter engaged in such actions as "stapling a sheet
of paper" or "peeling a banana." Imagined self-action, compared to experimenter

action, activated the left inferior parietal lobule, posterior insula, and post-central gyrus as well as bilateral inferior occipital gyrus; imagined experimenter action activated left posterior cingulate cortex and right precuneus, inferior parietal cortex, and frontopolar gyrus.

A more direct approach to mapping the anatomy of agency, taken by a number of recent studies, is to vary the congruence between subjects' intended and perceived actions (Farrer & Frith, 2002; Jeannerod et al., 2003). For example, Farrer and Frith scanned subjects while they used a joystick to control the motion of a visually presented cursor, conferring a sense of agency, or used a disconnected joystick while watching the cursor move under the experimenter's control, a condition violating agency despite its similarity to the first in sensori-motor processing. Results were consistent with those of Ruby and Decety (2001), implicating bilateral insula activity in the experience of agency and bilateral parietal activity, including right inferior parietal cortex and left lateral premotor cortex, in the experience of external control. Leube and colleagues (2003), using a similar experimental paradigm, reported right superior parietal cortex activity when subjects experienced a mismatch between their own action and the observed action of a hand, along with right inferior frontal activation; they also reported visual system activity, which they interpreted as being a result of visual differences in stimuli across conditions. Similar activations in the visual system (occipital cortex) were reported when subjects watched themselves perform an action with their hand versus watching a foreign hand perform the same action.

McGuire, Silbersweig, and Frith (1996) carried out the verbal analog of this design, comparing reading aloud while hearing one's own natural voice and reading aloud while hearing either a transformed voice or the experimenter's voice. There was increased activity in lateral temporal cortex bilaterally, greater on the right, during the incongruent voice conditions.

Taken together, these studies suggest a specific neural substrate involved in the experience of an action as caused or not caused by the self. For limb movements, the trend is for insular and right parietal cortices to be implicated in the sense of agency and violation of agency, respectively (see also Chapter 12, this volume, for further discussion of the neural substrate of self-generated action). For speech lateral temporal cortex rather than parietal cortex is implicated, with greater response on the right side.

Self-Concept

A straightforward way of assessing self-concept is for subjects to classify trait adjectives, such as "tall," "sincere," and "wealthy," as self-descriptive or not. Variations on this general approach were used in a large number of studies in cognitive psychology and account for the largest number of imaging studies of the self to date.

The early research in cognitive psychology demonstrated that people have better memory for self-descriptive words and that the mere act of considering whether a trait word applies to oneself results in better memory. Initially, this "self-reference effect" was interpreted as evidence for a distinct cognitive representation of the self, separate from representations of other people (Rogers, Kuiper, & Kirker, 1977). According to this interpretation, words encoded self-referentially were associated with the self-concept or self "schema" (as well as with the other semantic structures that would normally be associated with or without any mention of the self), and this additional association provided more robust memory representation and retrieval.

However, this interpretation was called into question once it was noticed that the self-referential encoding conditions of these early experiments differed in a number of ways from the control conditions. When the self-referential encoding was compared to other-referential encoding in studies that more closely equated the familiarity, affectivity, concreteness, elaboration, and organization of the self and other schemata, the self-reference effect vanished (see Symons & Johnson, 1997, for a review). We recount the history of the self-reference effect in cognitive psychology here because the methodological problems that undermined that research also affect the functional neuroimaging studies that used the same approach.

In the often-cited PET study by Craik and coworkers (1999) normal subjects made self-referent judgments about trait adjectives (*self* condition) and three other comparison judgments: whether the adjective described a famous person (*other*), was positive or negative (*general*), and how many syllables it had (*syllable*). This last task was used as a baseline that was subtracted from the other conditions. Results from comparisons among these three semantic judgments yielded only one significant difference in relative regional cerebral blood flow (rCBF): the *self* condition produced more activation of the right anterior cingulate area than did the *general* condition. The contrast of potentially greatest interest, namely that between *self* and *other* judgments, was not significant. Indeed, the authors point out "every significant activation in the *self-syllable* contrast was also found in either the *other-syllable* contrast or the *general-syllable* contrast, or both" (p. 30). In further analyses aimed at isolating self-related processing, they found activation of medial and right frontal areas when the *self* condition was compared to the combination of the other three conditions. However, the latter combination includes the *syllable* condition, and it is not clear what meaningful hypothesis is tested by a contrast with the three different nonself conditions together. Perhaps the most salient aspect of the results was, in the authors' words, the "striking . . . similarity among the *self, other,* and *general* conditions when compared with the *syllable* condition" (p. 31).

In a later study from the same group (Fossati et al., 2003), a *self* condition much like that of the previous study was contrasted with a condition labeled *other* but in fact equivalent to the *general* condition in Craik and coworkers (1999), in that it required subjects to judge whether the trait words were positive or negative. The researchers systematically varied the emotional valence of the trait words and contrasted activation in what they termed the *self* and *other* conditions for positive and negative traits. They found self-related activity in dorsomedial prefrontal cortex bilaterally as well as left posterior cingulate, regardless of the emotional valence of the traits being judged.

Kircher and colleagues (2000) also imaged subjects making judgments about trait adjectives. However, rather than isolating self-processing by contrasting self-reference judgment with other types of judgment, Kircher and colleagues contrasted two types of self-reference judgment: judgments of words that were self-descriptive and judgments of words that were not. They explain that this change was made in order to avoid "diluting" the self-judgment condition with the processing of non-self-descriptive adjectives. However, it is not clear whether this design would increase or decrease experimental power. On the assumption that the self-concept must be consulted in order to decide whether an adjective is or is not self-descriptive, Kircher and colleagues' design involves contrasting two conditions that both evoke self-processing. Indeed, by analogy with models of the lexical decision task, in which the lexicon is searched exhaustively for nonwords to be correctly rejected (Forster, 1992), one might even hypothesize more self-related processing in the non-self-descriptive condition.

Nevertheless, Kircher and coworkers (2000) found activation differences between conditions. Several activations, mostly in the left hemisphere, were specific to the affirmative judgments. The authors point out the similarity between this pattern of activation and one from a different task within the same study that involved making self-other face recognition judgments. As reviewed earlier, this study found more activation in the right limbic system and left PFC, among other areas, when subjects discriminated morphed versions of their own face from an unfamiliar face, relative to discriminating morphed versions of their partner's face and an unfamiliar face. Kircher and coworkers interpreted these results as evidence for a specific area that is involved in representing an internal self concept that can be accessed both visually and verbally.

If judgments of self-descriptive and non-self-descriptive trait adjectives both engage the self-concept, as we have suggested they might, then what could account for the differences found in this study? There are two non-self-specific possibilities. First, the words in the two conditions were rated differently by subjects on both likeability and "meaningfulness" (see Jones, Sensenig, & Haley, 1974, for a similar association between self-relevance and positive words). Second, subjects were making different responses to the different blocks of words, affirmative to self-descriptive words and negative to non-self-descriptive words, and this might also account for activation differences.

In a later study by Macrae and colleagues (2004), subjects also were instructed to judge whether stimulus items were self-descriptive; greater activation was reported in left medial prefrontal cortex for self-descriptive words. Likeability and meaningfulness of trait terms were not reported, but assuming they followed the usual trend, self-related traits would be higher on both measures. These differences could account for the reported activations.

In a second study by Kircher and colleagues (2002), the researchers introduced an *incidental* self-processing task. For this task subjects were presented, as before, with words that were either self-descriptive or not, but the task was to judge whether the word was a physical or psychological trait. As before, the activation associated with the non-self-descriptive words was subtracted from the activation

associated with self-descriptive words. This comparison was taken to isolate incidental self-processing, in that self-concept was not being accessed intentionally, and
the resulting pattern of activation differed from the intentional self-processing of the
previous experiment. Specifically, the incidental processing of self-descriptive traits
(versus non–self-descriptive traits) showed activations in both the left and right
hemispheres, including significantly more activation in the right middle temporal
gyrus and inferior parietal lobe, and left inferior frontal gyrus and superior temporal
gyrus. The only areas of overlap between intentional and incidental self-processing
were two small regions of the left hemisphere, one in the fusiform gyrus and one
in the superior parietal lobule. While this experiment potentially could illuminate
brain areas involved in incidental self-processing, the confound between self-
descriptiveness, likeability, and meaningfulness remains, along with the potential
for the many other confounds noted in relation to the SRE. Therefore, we cannot
conclude based on these results that the activations for self-descriptive traits are
due to self-specific processing.

Johnson and colleagues (2002) used fMRI with a task similar to the classic
self-reference method, with short descriptive statements substituted for single
words. Subjects verified statements such as "I catch on quickly" and "I get angry
easily." This task was contrasted with the control task of verifying factual statements such as "You need water to live." Self task activity was significantly higher
in medial PFC and posterior cingulate. These results are difficult to interpret due
to the nature of the control conditions; the control condition used by Johnson and
colleagues differed in its social content, and the areas activated are associated with
social/emotional cognition in tasks lacking self-related processing (Adolphs, 2001;
Adolphs, Tranel, & Damasio, 2003), with the medial PFC in particular associated
with knowledge about people (Mitchell, Heatherton, & Macrae, 2002). In order to
conclude that self-reflection per se is responsible for the activation, it must be contrasted with a condition involving a specific other person.

Three recent studies have employed an "other person" control condition. Kelley and coworkers (2002) used a trait adjective judgment task in which they included
three conditions: deciding whether the adjectives described the subject (*self* condition) or President George W. Bush (*other* condition), or deciding whether the adjective was printed in capital or lowercase letters (*case* condition). If self-related
processing evokes additional activation in the same regions as other-related processing, the authors would interpret this as evidence favoring the view that the
self-reference effect merely reflects the greater semantic organization and elaboration of the self schema relative to other schemata. In contrast, if distinct brain
regions are activated during self-processing, this would indicate that, in the authors' words, "the self-reference effect results from properties of a unique cognitive self" (p. 786). The *self* and *other* conditions activated similar regions in the
left frontal lobe (dorsal and inferior frontal cortex), compared to the case condition. However, regions of the medial PFC were activated in the *self* condition, but
not in the *other* condition. The authors concluded that "self-referential processing
is functionally dissociable from other forms of semantic processing within the
human brain" (p. 785).

Kjaer, Novack, and Lou (2002) took a similar approach, asking subjects to reflect on their own personalities and physical traits for short periods, as well as on the personality and physical traits of the Danish queen. They found increased neural activation in medial parietal cortex and in left orbitofrontal cortex when subjects reflected on their own personality traits, and in anterior cingulate cortex during reflection on their own physical traits, relative to the corresponding traits of the queen. Lou and colleagues (2004) carried out two more experiments with a similar task using only mental traits. In the first they had subjects again recall their own traits, the Danish queen's traits or their best friend's traits, while undergoing fMRI. This time they found medial prefrontal activation common to both self and other conditions, with lateral regions in parietal and temporal cortex distinguishing self from other. A second experiment, using TMS to disrupt processing, found selective effects of parietal TMS for the self condition relative to the best friend condition.

In some of the foregoing studies, medial PFC was activated in association with the self concept. However, processing of the traits of others also activated this area and even did so to the same extent in one study (Craik et al., 1999). It is therefore possible that medial PFC plays a role in person processing in general and is sometimes more strongly engaged by the self conditions of experiments for reasons similar to the causes of the self-reference effect described earlier. Recall that the self-reference effect in memory was originally obtained in experiments contrasting self- and other-related processing, but when differences between self and other in familiarity, differentiation, elaboration, and so forth were controlled for, the effect vanished. Given the known association between the medial and orbital regions of the PFC and both person knowledge (Mitchell et al., 2002) and affective processing (Davidson & Irwin, 1999), it is possible that the activation of these areas is a function of amount and type of knowledge rather than self versus other knowledge per se. Although the experiments of Kelley and coworkers (2002) and Kjaer and coworkers (2001) include control conditions involving people, in both cases the control person is a public figure about whom the subjects would have less knowledge as well as less affective response. Of course, it may not be possible to equate the self and other conditions of any task for all of the potentially confounding factors. Nevertheless, it should be possible to more closely equate them, for example by the use of a close other such as a spouse. The approach of parametrically varying familiarity and other attributes would also yield information concerning the role of these factors in self-related brain activity. The literature on the self-reference effect in cognitive psychology demonstrates the feasibility and the importance of attaining experimental control over these factors.

Conclusions: Conceptual and Empirical Challenges

In the past few years a number of functional neuroimaging studies have been published on the neural bases of the self. A strength of this literature is the variety of ways in which the self has been operationalized. Researchers have not confined themselves to a single experimental technique for eliciting self-related processing, but instead have imaged different kinds of tasks that seem related to one another mainly by their relevance to the self. These include awareness of own current mental state, first-person perspective, autobiographical memory, sense of agency, and self-concept.

Unfortunately, the results of this research to date have been inconclusive. One respect in which this is true is that different studies identify different brain regions with self-related processing, and some identify none at all. Of course, such an outcome does not necessarily indicate scientific failure; the neural systems underlying the self could be complex, and it is not at all implausible that the role of the self in, say, agency might be quite distinct from the role of the self in autobiographical memory.

A more fundamental problem with the results reported to date is the generally poor matching of baseline to experimental conditions. Cognitive neuroimaging usually tells us about the difference in brain activation between two conditions or states. To image self-related processing, one would compare activation during self-related processing with activation during baseline processing that involves all of the same perceptual, cognitive, and motor demands as the self condition except for self-processing per se. In reality, it can be difficult even to decide what such a baseline would be, much less implement it. Nevertheless, the disparities between the experimental and baseline conditions in many of the studies reviewed here are large enough to be problematic. In some studies self-related processing was compared to semantic processing of information that did not pertain to people at all. The activation patterns isolated by these comparisons therefore could as likely be related to person-specific processing as self-specific. Of those studies that did compare cognition about the self to cognition about others, few equated the self and other (baseline) conditions in familiarity, affective associations, and other respects.

The challenge of matching experimental and baseline conditions is not unique to imaging experiments. As we have argued elsewhere (Gillihan & Farah, in press), much of the patient research on the psychological self displays the same problem. For example, a patient with selective impairment of semantic knowledge about the self must be shown to have preserved, or at least significantly better, semantic knowledge about other subjects, taking into account the intrinsic difficulty of the two kinds of semantic knowledge test. In general, most neuropsychological case studies of the self have not provided well-controlled comparisons between self- and nonself-related processing.

The imaging results reviewed here suggest that, with the exception of sense of agency, we lack decisive evidence for or against the existence of a neural system dedicated to the self. The trend for medial prefrontal activation in other forms of self-related processing may reflect the role of this area in affective and person-related processing in general, with the self simply being the person we know best and care most about. If this interpretation is correct, how can we explain the compelling intuition that the self is a distinct and unitary entity?

One possibility is that our sense of self, like our conscious awareness in general, is a subjective mental state whose relation to the objective information processing of the brain is obscure. Pinker (1997) has proposed that the human mind represents the world syntactically, by parts and their relations, whereas the perennial mysteries of philosophy involve holistic concepts that cannot be reduced. In his words, "The I is not a combination of body parts or brain states or bits of information, but a unity of selfness over time, a single locus that is nowhere in particular" (p. 564). Our vivid awareness of a self, like awareness more generally, may not be explicable in terms of the mechanistic workings of the brain.

However, even if our subjective sense of self cannot be understood within the framework of empirical science, all of the aspects of the self reviewed here are represented in our brains and play important roles in human information processing, from guiding bodily movement to providing an organizing schema for memory. The self thus remains a central topic for psychology and cognitive neuroscience. Although our review suggests that the brain and cognitive sciences have yet to overcome certain methodological difficulties in studying the self, we are optimistic that they soon will.

References

Adolphs, R. (2001). The neurobiology of social cognition. *Current Opinion in Neurobiology, 11*, 231–239.

Adolphs, R., Tranel, D., & Damasio, A.R. (2003). Dissociable neural systems for recognizing emotions. *Brain and Cognition, 52*, 61–69.

Aguirre, G.K. (2003). Functional imaging in behavioral neurology and cognitive neuropsychology. In: T.E. Feinberg & M.J. Farah (Eds.), *Behavioral Neurology and Cognitive Neuropsychology* (2nd ed., pp. 85–96). New York: McGraw Hill.

Blakemore, S.-J. & Frith, C. (2003). Self-awareness and action. *Current Opinion in Neurobiology, 13*, 219–224.

Bush, G., Luu, P., & Posner, M.I. (2000). Cognitive and emotional influences in anterior cingulate cortex. *Trends in Cognitive Sciences, 4*, 215–222.

Conway, M.A., Turk, D.J., Miller, S.L., Logan, J., Nebes, R.D., Meltzer, C.C., & Becker, J.T. (1999). A positron emission tomography (PET) study of autobiographical memory retrieval. *Memory, 7*, 679–702.

Craik, F.I.M., Moroz, T.M., Moscovitch, M., Stuss, D.T., Winocur, G., Tulving, E., & Kapur, S. (1999). In search of the self: A positron emission tomography study. *Psychological Science, 10*, 26–34.

Davidson, R.J. & Irwin, W. (1999). The functional neuroanatomy of emotion and affective style. *Trends in Cognitive Sciences, 3*, 11–21.

Drevets, W.C. & Raichle, M.E. (1998). Reciprocal suppression of regional cerebral blood flow during emotional versus higher cognitive processes: Implications for interactions between emotion and cognition. *Cognition and Emotion, 12*, 353–385.

Farrer, C. & Frith, C.D. (2002). Experiencing oneself vs. another person as being the cause of an action: The neural correlates of the experience of agency. *NeuroImage, 15*, 596–603.

Fink, G.R., Markowitsch, H.J., Reinkemeier, M., Bruckbauer, T., Kessler, J., & Heiss, W.-D. (1996). Cerebral representations of one's own past: Neural networks involved in autobiographical memory. *Journal of Neuroscience, 16*, 4275–4282.

Forster, K.I. (1992). Memory-addressing mechanisms and lexical access. In: R. Frost & L. Katz (Eds.), *Orthography, Phonology, Morphology and Meaning* (pp. 413–434). Amsterdam: Elsevier.

Fossati, P., Hevenor, S.J., Graham, S.J., Grady, C., Keightley, M.L., Craik, F., & Mayberg, H. (2003). In search of the emotional self: An fMRI study using positive and negative emotional words. *American Journal of Psychiatry, 160,* 1938–1945.

Gillihan, S.J. & Farah, M.J. (in press). Is self special? A critical review of evidence from experimental psychology and cognitive neuroscience. *Psychological Bulletin.*

Gusnard, D.A., Akbudak, E., Shulman, G.L., & Raichle, M.E. (2001). Medial prefrontal cortex and self-referential mental activity: Relation to a default mode of brain function. *Proceedings of the National Academy of Sciences, 98,* 4259–4264.

Hildebrand, D. (1986). *Statistical Thinking for Behavioral Scientists.* Boston: Duxbury Press.

Jeannerod, M., Farrer, C., Franck, N., Fourneret, P., Posada, A., Daprati, E., & Georgieff, N. (2003). Action recognition in normal and schizophrenic subjects. In: T. Kircher & A. David (Eds.), *The Self in Neuroscience and Psychiatry* (pp. 380–406). Cambridge: Cambridge University Press.

Johnson, S. C., Baxter, L. C., Wilder, L. S., Pipe, J. G., Heiserman, J. E., & Prigatano, G. P. (2002). Neural correlates of self-reflection. *Brain, 125,* 1808–1814.

Jones, R. A., Sensenig, J., & Haley, J.V. (1974). Self-descriptions: Configurations of content and order effects. *Journal of Personality and Social Psychology, 30,* 36–45.

Kelley, W.M., Macrae, C.N., Wyland, C.L., Caglar, S., Inati, S., & Heatherton, T.F. (2002). Finding the self? An event-related fMRI study. *Journal of Cognitive Neuroscience, 14,* 785–794.

Kircher, T.T.J., Brammer, M., Bullmore, E., Simmons, A., Bartels, M., & David, A.S. (2002). The neural correlates of intentional and incidental self processing. *Neuropsychologia, 40,* 683–692.

Kircher, T.T.J. & David, A. (Eds.). (2003). *The Self in Neuroscience and Psychiatry.* Cambridge: Cambridge University Press.

Kircher, T.T.J., Senior, C., Phillips, M.L., Benson, P.J., Bullmore, E.T., Brammer, M., Simmons, A., Williams, S.C.R., Bartels, M., & David, A.S. (2000). Towards a functional neuroanatomy of self processing: Effects of faces and words. *Cognitive Brain Research, 10,* 133–144.

Kjaer, T.W., Nowak, M., & Lou, H.C. (2002). Reflective self-awareness and conscious states: PET evidence for a common midline parietofrontal core. *NeuroImage, 17,* 1080–1086.

Lane, R.D., Fink, G.R., Chau, P.M.-L., & Dolan, R.J. (1997). Neural activation during selective attention to subjective emotional responses. *Neuroreport, 8,* 3969–3972.

Leube, D., Knoblich, G., Erb, M., & Kircher, T.T.J. (2003). Observing one's hand become anarchic: An fMRI study of action identification. *Consciousness and Cognition, 12,* 597–608.

Lou, H.C., Luber, B., Crupain, M., Keenan, J.P., Nowak, M., Kjaer, T.W., Sackeim, H.A., & Lisanby, S. H. (2004). Parietal cortex and representation of the mental self. *Proceedings of the National Academy of Sciences, 101,* 6827–6832.

Macrae, C.N., Moran, J.M., Heatherton, T.F., Banfield, J.F., & Kelley, W.M. (2004). Medial prefrontal activity predicts memory for self. *Cerebral Cortex, 14,* 647–654.

Maguire, E.A. & Mummery, C.J. (1999). Differential modulation of a common memory retrieval network revealed by positron emission tomography. *Hippocampus, 9,* 54–61.

McGuire, P.K., Silbersweig, D.A., & Frith, C.D. (1996). Functional neuroanatomy of verbal self-monitoring. *Brain, 119,* 907–917.

Mitchell, J.P., Heatherton, T.F., & Macrae, C.N. (2002). Distinct neural systems subserve person and object knowledge. *Proceedings of the National Academy of Sciences, 99,* 15238–15243.

Nyberg, L., Cabeza, R., & Tulving, E. (1996). PET studies of encoding and retrieval: The HERA model. *Psychonomic Bulletin and Review, 3,* 135–148.

Pinker, S. (1997). *How the Mind Works.* New York: Norton.

Rogers, T.B., Kuiper, N.A., & Kirker, W.S. (1977). Self-reference and the encoding of personal information. *Journal of Personality and Social Psychology, 35,* 677–688.

Ruby, P. & Decety, J. (2001). Effect of subjective perspective taking during simulation of action: A PET investigation of agency. *Nature Neuroscience, 4,* 546–550.

Slamecka, N.J. & Graf, P. (1978). The generation effect: Delineation of a phenomenon. *Journal of Experimental Psychology: Human Learning and Memory, 4,* 592–604.

Spence, S.A., Brooks, D.J., Hirsch, S.R., Liddle, P.F., Meehan, J., & Grasby, P.M. (1997). A PET study of voluntary movement in schizophrenic patients experiencing passivity phenomena (delusions of alien control). *Brain, 120,* 1997–2011.

Symons, C.S. & Johnson, B.T. (1997). The self-reference effect in memory: A meta-analysis. *Psychological Bulletin, 121,* 371–394.

Tulving, E., Kapur, S., Craik, F.I.M., Moscovitch, M., & Houle, S. (1994). Hemispheric encoding/retrieval asymmetry in episodic memory: Positron emission tomography findings. *Proceedings of the National Academy of Science, 91,* 2016–2020.

Vogeley, K., Bussfeld, P., Newen, A., Hermann, S., Happé, F., Falkai, P., Maier, W., Shah, N.J., Fink, G.R., & Zilles, K. (2001). Mind reading: Neural mechanisms of theory of mind and self-perspective. *NeuroImage, 14,* 170–181.

Zysset, S., Huber, O., Ferstl, E., & von Cramon, D.Y. (2002). The anterior frontomedian cortex and evaluative judgment: An fMRI study. *NeuroImage, 15,* 983–991.

4

Neural Hierarchies and the Self

TODD E. FEINBERG

Not everyone agrees that selves exist. Kant (1781) was a firm believer in the existence and unity of the self and placed the primordial, unified "I" at the center of his philosophy. He claimed there was a "transcendental unity of apperception" that existed a priori to all mental activity. In sharp contrast to this opinion, William James argued in his *The Principles of Psychology* that the "ego" was nothing but "a 'cheap and nasty' edition of the soul" (1890; reprinted 1983, p. 345). Although James conceded that there is something that could be appropriately referred to as the self, he denied that there is any single entity that could be called an "I" or "ego" at its center. James maintained that there are only "passing states of consciousness," and our experience of mental unity is simply due to the fact that we as individuals experience successive mental states in our stream of consciousness that are uniquely our own. If one could combine all these experiences in a single mind one could create a self without any inner "I" pulling it all together. James even believed that if several independent minds shared a common experience and past, one could produce the same mental unity among minds that we as single minds experience:

> Successive thinkers, numerically distinct, but all aware of the same past in the same way, form an adequate vehicle for all the experience of personal unity and sameness which we actually have. And just such a train of successive thinkers is the stream of mental states . . . which psychology treated as a natural science has to assume. . . . The logical conclusion seems then to be that *the states of consciousness are all that psychology needs to do her work with. Metaphysics or theology may prove the Soul to exist; but for psychology the hypothesis of such a substantial principle of unity is superfluous.* (1892; reprinted 1985, p. 70)

James's misgivings about the existence of the self highlights an important point: *if there is something that can be referred to as a "self," it must exist as a unified entity.* Neurophysiologist Charles Sherrington was a firm believer in the unified self. Sherrington, in his book *Man on His Nature* (1941), eloquently explained why he believed in the existence of the self:

> The self is a unity. The continuity of its presence in time, sometimes hardly broken by sleep, its inalienable "interiority" in (sensual) space, its consistency of view-point,

the privacy of its experience, combine to give it status as a unique existence. . . . It regards itself as one, others treat it as one. It is addressed as one, by a name to which it answers. The Law and the State schedule it as one. It and they identify it with a body which is considered by it and them to belong to it integrally. In short, unchallenged and unargued conviction assumes it to be one. The logic of grammer endorses this by a pronoun in the singular. All its diversity is merged into oneness. (Sherrington, 1941)

Prior to all these writers, Descartes was perhaps the first to consider how the divisible brain creates the unification of the mind and self. He reasoned that a single midline structure, the pineal gland, could serve as the physical locus of unification of the individual "soul":

The reason that persuades me that the soul cannot have any other place in the whole body than this gland, where it immediately exercises its functions, is that I consider that the other parts of our brain are all double so that we have two eyes, two hands, two ears, and, finally all the organs of our external senses are double; and that inasmuch as we have only one solitary and simple thought of one single thing during the same moment, it must necessarily be that there is some place where the two images which come from the two eyes, or the two other impressions which come from a single object by way of the double organs of the other senses, may unite before they reach the soul, so that they do not present to it two objects instead of one. It can easily be conceived how these images or other impressions could unite in this gland through the mediation of the spirits that fill the cavities of the brain. There is no other place in the body where they could be thus united unless it be in the gland. (Descartes, 1649; reprinted 1996)

We now know that there is no single place in the nervous system where neural activity "all comes together" to create unification of perception. We also know that although we subjectively feel there is a single unified self that is the source of our actions, there is no centralized "ghost in the machine" (Ryle, 1949) from which actions originate. When one looks within the brain to find the *source* of one's "will," one finds that there is no central, integrated, and unified physical source nor "pontifical neurons" (Barlow, 1995) in the brain that "command" one's actions

Since there is no unified place where perception, action, or the self are materially integrated, other solutions to the problem of the unity of mind and self have been offered. One way to explain the unity of visual consciousness identifies synchronized oscillations as the source of mental unity. Neurons coding for different perceptual attributes of a single object are all firing at the same frequency, and the attributes of a different object are firing at another frequency. In this way a particular object is represented coherently in the brain and can be distinguished from other objects (Crick & Koch, 1990; Crick, 1994; Engel et al., 1991; Gray et al., 1989a; 1989b; 1992; Konig & Engel 1995; Newman, 1999; von der Malsburg,1995;).

In another theory Edelman (1989) suggested that reentrant cortical integration (RCI) represents the major integrative factor in the brain's construction of a unified consciousness. According to Edelman, it is RCI, the back-and-forth signaling from multiple brain areas, that allows segregated and distributed brain areas to "pull together" integrated representations. Within this framework Edelman proposed that this mechanism would enable visual consciousness to be unified without there being any particular place where all the brain's inputs are *physically* integrated.

Emergence, the Mind, and the Self

A different approach to the problem of mental unity emphasizes the *hierarchical* nature of the nervous system and posits that the self and mind *emerge* in unified fashion from the diverse parts of the brain at the highest levels of the neural hierarchy. There are many different versions of the concept of emergence (for general reviews see Beckermann, Flohr & Kim, 1992; Van Gulick, 2001; Morowitz, 2002). According to philosopher Jaegwon Kim, the concept of emergence holds that

> . . . although the fundamental entities of this world and their properties are material, when material processes reach a certain level of complexity, genuinely novel and unpredictable properties emerge, and this process of emergence is cumulative, generating a hierarchy of increasingly more complex novel properties. Thus, emergentism presents the world not only as an evolutionary process but also as a *layered structure*—a hierarchically organized system of levels of properties, each level emergent from and dependent on the one below. (Kim, 1992)

Emergent properties are generally viewed as the result of *hierarchically* ordered entities (Allen & Starr, 1982; Ayala & Dobzhansky, 1974; Pattee, 1970; 1973; Salthe, 1985; Whyte, Wilson, & Wilson, 1969;). According to most concepts of emergence (see, for example, Morowitz, 2002) and in line with Kim's definition above, emergence in living things is said to occur as the result of a hierarchically organized systems in which each level of complexity produces *novel* emergent features from the levels below it. C. Lloyd Morgan, a leader of the school of emergentism, explained the emergence of mental phenomenan in terms of a hierarchical biological model in which the unified mind emerges at the "peak of the pyramid" of the biological hierarchy:

> In the foregoing lecture the notion of a pyramid with ascending levels was put forward. Near its base is a swarm of atoms with relational structure and the quality we may call atomicity. Above this level, atoms combine to form new units, the distinguishing quality of which is molecularity; higher up, on one line of advance, are, let us say, crystals wherein atoms and molecules are grouped in new relations of which the expression is crystalline form; on another line of advance are organisms with a different kind of natural relations which give the quality of vitality; yet higher, a new kind of natural relatedness supervenes and to its expression the word "mentality" may be applied. (Morgan, 1923, p. 35)

The Nobel Laureate psychologist Roger Sperry viewed the mind, subjectivity, and "psychic forces" as emergent features of the brain that in turn control the brain from whence they came. Like Morgan, Sperry viewed the mind–brain relationship in hierarchical terms and supposed that the neural elements of the brain combine in increasingly complex configurations until at the summit of organization the mind emerges:

> . . . consciousness was conceived to be a dynamic emergent of brain activity, neither identical with, nor reducible to, the neural events of which it is mainly composed. Further, consciousness was not conceived as an epiphenomenon, inner aspect, or other passive correlate of brain processing, but rather to be an active integral part of the cerebral process itself, exerting potent causal effects in the interplay of cere-

bral operations. In a position of top command at the highest levels in the hierarchy of brain organization, the subjective properties were seen to exert control over the biophysical and chemical activities at subordinate levels. It was described initially as a brain model that puts "conscious mind back into the brain of objective science in a position of top command . . . a brain model in which conscious, mental, psychic forces are recognized to be the crowning achievement . . . of evolution." (Sperry, 1977; reprinted in Trevarthen, 1990, p. 382)

Sperry believed that the unified self and consciousness were the highest emergent features of the neural hierarchy:

We do not look for conscious awareness in the nerve cells of the brain, nor in the molecules or atoms of brain processing. Along with the larger as well as lesser building blocks of brain function, these elements are common as well to unconscious, automatic and reflex activity. For the subjective qualities we look higher in the system at organizational properties that are select and special to operations at top levels of the brain hierarchy and which are seen to supersede in brain causation the powers of their neuronal, molecular, atomic, and subatomic infrastructure. (Sperry, 1984, p. 671)

According to Sperry, the subjective self emerges at the "top levels of the brain hierarchy" where it occupies "a position of top command." Sperry's account posits that the mind is a radically emergent feature of the brain and therefore is "more than the sum of the parts" of the brain (see also Sperry, 1966) and can emerge *unified* from the brain—like the eye that emerges from the top of the pyramid on a dollar bill (Fig. 4–1).

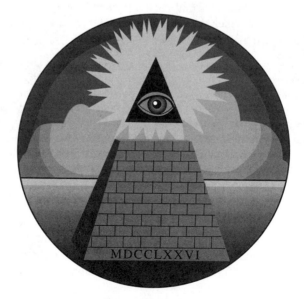

Figure 4–1. A pyramidal hierarchical model of the brain and self. A model of this type envisions the neural hierarchy in the shape of a pyramid. According to this view, the levels of the neural hierarchy are part of a non-nested hierarchy in which the unified self and mind emerge at the summit of the pyramid.

Emergence and Neural Hierarchies

The idea that the self emerges unified at the pinnacle of the neural hierarchy, if correct, would provide a solution for the problem of mental unity. This hypothesis is appealing for several reasons. The integrated mind and the unified self entail the "highest" and most advanced forms of cognitive processing, and the phylogenetically most advanced regions of the nervous system, for example the prefrontal cortices, are indeed situated "higher" on the neuroaxis when compared with regions, such as the midbrain, that subserve more automatic behaviors. As noted by Sanides (1975), evolutionary processes fostered the rostral migration of functions and made the forebrain and eventually the cerebral cortex the leading structure in the mammalian brain. It therefore seems reasonable to suppose that "higher cortical functions" requiring the involvement of the most highly evolved forms of consciousness might *emerge* within the most advanced and evolved brain regions.

It is also the case that, in general, neurons located in anatomically "higher" positions (downstream) on the neuroaxis possess "higher," or more abstract, response characteristics than neurons positioned earlier (upstream) in perceptual pathways. For example, the receptive fields of retinal cells early in the visual processing respond to simple and small points of light, but in cortical area V1, a line of adjacent firing cells, each responsive to an individual point of light, converges upon a single simple cortical cell further along the processing stream. This allows a single higher-order cell to respond to a line (Hubel & Wiesel, 1962; 1965; 1977; 1968; 1979; Hubel, 1988). In like fashion, multiple simple cortical cells converge upon single higher-order cells further along the processing stream to create what Hubel and Wiesel (1962; 1965; 1977; 1968; 1979) called *complex* cortical cells, and complex cells in turn converge upon single neurons to create *hypercomplex* cells. Each hierarchical level higher up the processing stream codes for increasingly specific, complex, and abstract response properties. The progression from simple to increasingly complex cells is an example of what Zeki (1993) terms "topical convergence." This hierarchical process ultimately produces advanced "higher-order" cells that possess amazingly specific response properties. For example, there are neurons in the inferior temporal cortex far "downstream" from the simple cells found early in the primary visual region that respond preferentially to highly specific and complex stimuli such as hands or faces. Neurons of this type are sometimes referred to as "grandmother" cells, a cell so specific that it fires only to the face of one's own grandmother (Barlow, 1995). While cells of that degree of specificity do not exist, it is in general the case that cells that are located farther along in a sensory processing stream have more specific response characteristics than do cells earlier in that stream.

Theoretical Obstacles to the Hierarchical Emergence of the Self

While the processing streams of perceptual systems are hierarchical and allow for the emergence of higher-order perceptual features, the idea that the mind or the self could emerge at the pinnacle of the neural hierarchy cannot be correct. In both perception and action, there is no emergence of a unified self, or mind, or consciousness at the top of the neural hierarchy. Returning to the visual processing described above, a retinal cell early in the perceptual stream monitors a small and specific point in the visual field, while a hypercomplex cell such as a face cell will react to a face that appears almost *anywhere* in the visual field. Cells early in the visual stream with small receptive fields "know" where each line of the face is, but these early cells do not "know" that a given line is part of a face. Conversely, face cells "know" there is a face, but due to the process of topical convergence, these cells do not know where the face is located in space. Therefore, while it is true that cells of the brain project to successive levels in a hierarchical fashion in order to code for increasingly specific complex and abstract properties, the information coded by cells earlier in the process is not and cannot be lost in awareness (for one form of experimental proof of this principle, see the aperture experiment by Movshon and coworkers [1985]). As Zeki observes, cells comprising *both* the early and the late stages of the visual processing stream must make a unique contribution to consciousness (see, for example, Beckers & Zeki, 1995).

In the same way the analysis of action demonstrates that *intention,* or *will,* does not emerge at the peak of the neural hierarchy. For instance, when we speak we do not consciously send a command to the tongue to move up and down or left and right in a particular sequence. Indeed, we could not do this if we tried. The average speaker has no idea which particular muscles to move when speaking. And even if we did have this knowledge, we do not possess the fine motor control to specifically move a given muscle fiber to produce a certain sound. Finally, even if we were to possess the knowledge and the requisite control to consciously move each muscle of speech into action, if we were required to do so when speaking, we would lose the overall integration of the speech act. We need to focus on the abstract purpose of speaking, the idea we wish to convey, rather than on the way our lips are moving or the way a single fiber in the tongue is firing. Therefore, the control of action is not entirely at the highest, most explicitly conscious, levels of the neural hierarchy but is distributed across multiple hierarchical levels.

The Nested Hierarchy of the Self

I have argued previously (Feinberg, 1997; 2000; 2001a; 2001b) that the principle problem with prior accounts of the neural hierarchy with reference to the self and the mind is that the brain is not organized like a pyramid. In Sperry's model the brain and the mind are envisioned as aspects of a particular type of hierarchy known as a *non-nested hierarchy.* A non-nested hierarchy has a pyramidal structure with a clear-cut top and bottom in which higher levels control the operation of lower levels (Allen & Starr, 1982; Salthe, 1985). An example of a non-nested hierarchy is a military command, with its general at the top and successively lower levels of command below. This conforms to what Sperry had in mind when he spoke of a "top command" that subordinated lower levels of a hierarchy. However, as I have tried to demonstrate, the neural substrate of the self spans multiple hierarchical levels without a material "summit" or final common pathway at the top.

An alternative framework for viewing the mind–brain relationship is a type of hierarchy known as a *compositional* or *nested hierarchy*. All living things operate as nested hierarchies. At the lower levels of an organism are organelles that are combined to produce single cells that are in turn organized to produce tissues, which are then combined to produce organs that are ultimately organized to produce an entire living organism.

There are at least two significant differences between non-nested and nested hierarchies with reference to the relationship between lower and higher levels. First, in a non-nested hierarchy the lower and higher levels of the hierarchy are physically independent entities. In an army the general is not composed of his staff or his troops. In contrast, in a nested hierarchy such as an organism, the elements composing the lower levels of the hierarchy are physically combined, or *nested,* within higher levels to create increasingly complex wholes.

The second difference between non-nested and nested hierarchies pertains to hierarchical control. The control that higher levels impose on lower levels is referred to as *constraint* (Pattee, 1970; 1973). In a non-nested hierarchy the constraint of the hierarchy comes from the top. In an army a general issues orders that are communicated down the chain of command until the orders are executed. In a nested hierarchy, in contrast, the constraint of the system is embodied within the entire hierarchical system. In organisms individual cells constrain the organelles to perform cellular metabolism, the organs of the body constrain the cells so that they, for example, secrete enzymes, and at the highest level the entire organism constrains the individual organs to perform all the functions necessary for its survival. Therefore, there is no "general" within the organism directing its operation; rather, the constraint of the organism's operation is generated from within the entire nested system of the organism. In the nested hierarchy of a living thing, all parts make a contribution to the life and activity of the organism, and in the nested hierarchy of a person, many parts of the living brain make a contribution to the self. Consider again the face and responsive "grandmother" cells. The existence of such cells makes it appear that a single "grandmother" cell, at the top of the perceptual hierarchy, in and of itself embodies the representation of an entire face. But while a "grandmother" cell might respond quite selectively to a face, the conscious representation of the face of one's actual grandmother requires contributions from diverse and widely separated brain regions. Just like each organelle makes a contribution to the life of a cell, in the nested hierarchy of a mind all the lower-order elements that make up total awareness of the face make a contribution to consciousness. Lower-order features combine in the mind as "part of"—or *nested* within—higher-order features. Therefore, to say an element is "bound" to another is simply another way of saying that they are represented in awareness *dependently* and are *nested* together.

A Neuroanatomical Model of the Nested Hierarchy of the Self

What is required is an alternative approach to the neural hierarchy that avoids the aforementioned pitfalls of a pyramidal model and is consistent with the nested nature of the neural hierarchy. John Hughlings Jackson (1884) provided what was perhaps the first hierarchical approach to the nervous system. According to his account, the nervous system evolved from simple *automatic* reflexes controlled by the lowest hierarchical levels of the nervous system to *voluntary* forms of action that are produced by the highest cortical levels of the brain. For Jackson, while higher-order aspects of the self and the mind are associated with higher-order neural structures, mind and self do not emerge at the summit of the neural hierarchy. Rather, as one progresses up the neural hierarchy there is a gradual transition from primitive to increasingly abstract aspects of the mind and self.

Swash (1989), in an extensive reevaluation of Jackson's views on the hierarchical nature of the nervous system, provides the following summary.

> Evolution of function within the nervous system was conceived by Jackson as a passage from the most to the least organised, from the most simple to the most complex, and from the most automatic to the most voluntary (Taylor 1931/32). Dissolution was understood to be the reverse of the process of evolution. From the lowest to the highest centres there was increasing complexity *(differentiation),* increasing definiteness *(specialization),* and increasing *integration* (of function). In general, the higher the centres the more numerous the interconnections of the units *(cooperation).*

As noted by Meares (1999), Jackson identified the self with the highest levels of the nervous system:

> . . . Jackson conceived of the CNS as having a hierarchical organization that reflects evolutionary history. He used "the terms lowest, middle, and highest centres . . . as proper names . . . to indicate evolutionary levels" (Taylor, 1931/32). Ascending levels show increasing integration and coordination of sensorimotor representations. The highest-level coordination, which allows the greatest volunatary control, depends on prefrontal activity. Self is a manifestation of this highest level of consciousness. (Meares, 1999, p. 1851)

Therefore, a Jacksonian model of neural functioning requires that the highest and most abstract properties of mind and intention, and therefore the most integrated aspects of the self, require the contribution of the highest levels of the neural hierarchy. But we also must recognize that the self does not "emerge" at the top of a neural hierarchy. How can we reconcile the hierarchical attributes of perception and intention as outlined above with our knowledge of the anatomy of the nervous system?

In an effort to produce a neuroanatomical model of the self that is consistent with the anatomical and functional features enumerated above, I offer the following tentative model of the self (Fig. 4–2):

Beginning at the lowest levels of the neural hierarchy relevant to the self, Strehler (1991) argues that there is sufficient neural complexity for a primordial self at the level of the upper brainstem. According to this point of view, the paired superior colliculi are the most primitive brain structures that receive the perquisite information necessary for the development of a self. The paired colliculi receive information from the visual system in addition to information derived from memory and other inputs to produce a "coherent sense of selfness." The colliculi receive a highly precise retinotopic visual representation, in addition to auditory, vestibular, and affective inputs sufficient to generate a coherent sense of selfness. Panksepp

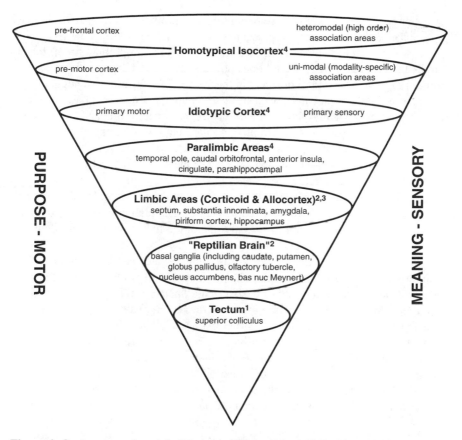

Figure 4–2. A proposed model of the neural basis of the self. In this model lower levels of the neural hierarchy are viewed as nested within higher levels, and all levels of the neural hierarchy make a contribution to the self. For the tectal level see Strehler (1991). The concept and anatomy of the "reptilian brain" is derived from MacLean (1973; 1990; see Fig. 4–3). The limbic level is based in part on MacLean's paleomammalian brain. The anatomy of this level is derived from Mesulum (2000; see Fig. 4–4); however, the paleomammalian brain of MacLean would include structures from Mesulum's limbic and paralimbic levels. Subsequent levels and their anatomy are derived and adapted from Mesulum (2000; see Fig. 4–4) and Fuster (2002; 2003). When these levels are considered as parts of a nested hierarchy, the sensory-perceptual systems are constrained by the highest levels of *meaning,* and the motor-intentional systems are constrained by the highest levels of *purpose* achieved by the brain (Feinberg, 2001a). Note that in contrast to Figure 4–1, this model has an inverted pyramidal, or cone-shaped, configuration.

(1998) points out that the superior colliculi receive visual, auditory, and somatosensory afferent information and also control certain primitive motor functions, and therefore might provide the substrate for a primordial amphibian self. He adds that the mesencephalic central gray, situated just below the colliculi, contains the basic neural substrate for many emotional processes including fear, anger, pleasure, pain, and sexual responses. He suggests, "The superior colliculus is especially in-

teresting because it is here that we begin to get a glimmer of the first evolutionary
appearance of a sophisticated representation of the self (Panksepp, 1998, p. 77).

I have argued previously (Feinberg, 2001a) that the amphibian brain, for example the brain of a frog, indeed does possess a rudimentary consciousness and
mind. Frogs can respond to objects "in the world" in a fashion that suggests that
even these simple organisms have a sufficiently complex neural apparatus to produce behaviors that can rightfully be described as "meaningful" and "conscious."
Based on these considerations, I think one interpretation of Strehler's argument is
that the lowest level of the primordial self exists at the level of the midbrain and
colliculi, and this represents the lowest level of the neural hierarchy of the self.

To determine the next highest level of the neural hierarchy relevant to the self, I
suggest we look to the work of Paul MacLean (see, for example, MacLean, 1973;
1990; see Panksepp, 1998, for an excellent review and elaboration of this theory.).
MacLean's model of the brain is actually one of the few explicitly nested and hierarchical models of the neural axis (Fig. 4–3).

According to MacLean, the neuroaxis of vertebrates can be roughly divided
into three nested hierarchical levels. The phylogenetically oldest level of the brain
he called the *reptilian brain,* and it consists of the "matrix of the upper brainstem and
comprising much of the reticular system, midbrain, and basal ganglia." MacLean
referred to the basal ganglia and the structures associated with it at this level of the
neuroaxis as the R-complex, or reptilian brain. Animals with a reptilian brain, as
enumerated by MacLean, are capable of a wide array of complex and diverse behaviors, including establishment of a territory, trail making and patrolling, ritual-
istic displays of defense, triumph, greeting, courtship, and the formation of social
groups. The next-higher level he called the *paleomammalian brain,* and this level

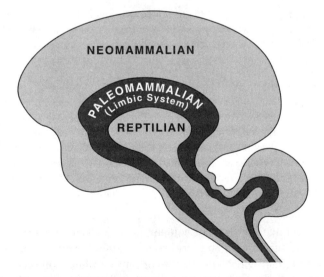

Figure 4–3. MacLean's (1973; 1990) diagram of the hierarchical organization of the three
basic brain types (*reptilian, paleomammalian,* and *neomammalian*). MacLean referred to
this as the "triune brain."

is essentially comprised of the limbic system that is superimposed upon the reptilian brain. Animals with a paleomammalian brains display, in addition to many of the aforementioned behaviors, more sophisticated social behaviors including maternal nurturing behaviors, separation distress calls, play behaviors, and a wider range of social displays and behaviors. The highest level of the neuroaxis, comprised of the neocortex, he called the *neomammalian brain.* The neomammallian brain sits atop the other two levels and is responsible, in its highest development, for the advanced forms of thought and behavior that culminate in the mind of primates and humans.

Although the margins of these levels are not clear-cut and are the subject of ongoing debate, the appeal of MacLean's approach is the manner in which he lays out a hierarchical approach to the nervous system that can be roughly correlated with a corresponding hierarchy of behaviors. I find this approach particularly useful when determining the nested levels of the neural hierarchy of the self. I suggest that we can assign to MacLean's reptilian brain the next-highest level of the neural hierarchy of the self.

MacLean's designations of the paleomammalian and neomammalian brain are quite broad and general and cover a wide range of behavioral features and neural structures. Mesulum (2000) provides a more fine-tuned hierarchical model of these levels (Fig. 4–4).

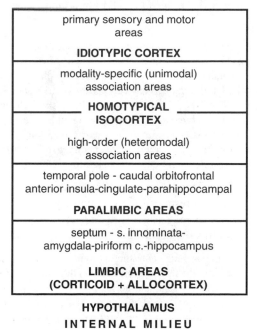

Figure 4–4. The cortical zones of the human brain according to Mesulum. (*Source:* Mesulum, M.-M. [2000]. *Principles of Behavioral and Cognitive Neurology,* 2nd ed. New York: Oxford University Press, p. 8, with permission.)

Mesulum proposes that the cerebral cortex can be organized into five hierarchically arranged subtypes—*limbic, paralimbic, heteromodal association, unimodal association,* and *primary sensory-motor regions.* The rationale for this arrangement is based on anatomical, physiological, and behavioral experiments in the macaque monkey.

In this ordering, limbic areas that are in the most direct contact with the "internal milieu" and responsible for behaviors that are phylogentically relatively ancient are hierarchically situated at the base of his model. This level corresponds to MacLean's paleomammalian brain and therefore can be viewed as the next major hierarchical level of the neural axis. By the same logic, paralimbic regions, the next hierarchical level on Mesulum's scheme, can be placed one level higher than the limbic regions.

The next-highest level in Mesulum's scheme, however, is a bit more problematic. As indicated above, after limbic and paralimbic regions, Mesulum provides the following sequence of brain levels: heteromodal association, unimodal association, and primary sensory-motor regions. A somewhat paradoxical feature of this approach is that primary sensory and motor regions, which subserve basic sensory and motor functions, are at the highest level of the hierarchy, and heteromodal association cortices, regions that are generally viewed as subserving phylogenetically advanced integrative and associative functions, are considered to be mid-level in the hierarchy.

As Mesulum himself points out, however, there is controversy in regard to what cortical regions represent the most advanced hierarchical levels of the nervous system:

> There are two divergent opinions about the primary areas. One is to consider them as the most elementary (even rudimentary) component of the cerebral cortex; the other is to consider them as its most advanced and highly differentiated component (Sanides, (1970). The latter point of view can be supported from the vantage point of cytoarchitectonics. Thus, the primary visual, somatosensory, and auditory cortices display a "koniocortical" architecture representing the highest level of development with respect to granualization and lamination, whereas the primary motor cortex displays a unique "macropyramidal" architecture characterized by highly specialized giant pyramidal neurons known as betz cells. (Mesulum, 2000, p. 11)

Sanides (1969;1970;1975) was the most prominent advocate of the point of view that the cortical regions responsible for simple sensory and motor functions are hierarchically more advanced and evolved than tertiary multimodal frontal and parietal zones. He based this opinion for the most part on architectonic features:

> This conclusion, of course, is quite contradictory to the assumption that the primary sensory and motor areas are the first in evolution. On the contrary: the koniocortical areas which are the heaviest myelinated cortical areas within the sensory regions present the most recent stage in sensory cortex evolution and the area gigantopyramidalis which is the heaviest myelinated motor area presents the most recent stage in motor cortex evolution, an inference which is also suggested by the highest architectonic specialization of these areas and is paralleld by the highest functional specialization. (Sanides, 1969)

This arrangement runs into problems, however. As already noted above, the prefrontal cortices and polymodal "higher-order" association cortices are the brain regions responsible for the highest-order, most abstract mental processes. These are also the brain areas that undergo the greatest degree of expansion during brain evolution. Furthermore, there is an explicitly hierarchical pattern within the primate visual system based on patterns of cortical connectivity. V1 (primary visual cortex) is the lowest level of the neural hierarchy, and association cortical areas are considered to be hierarchically higher (DeYoe & Van Essen, 1988; Felleman & Van Essen, 1991;Van Essen et al., 1992). Finally, Kass (1989) points out evolutionary patterns that indicate that unimodal association and heteromodal brain regions, interposed between sensory and motor functions, are the areas that display the greatest development in evolution. Development of these "middle stages" of sensory processing allows a greater amount of sensory processing prior to a motor response:

> The simple hierarchies of visual areas, with little more than beginning and end stations, that characterize the brains of mice and hedgehogs become complex hierarchies, like those of monkeys and cats, by the addition of new visual areas in the middle stages of processing. As a result, a change occurs from the situation where the first cortical station, area 17, directly accesses some of the end or near end cortical stations in the frontal and limbic cortex, as in rats and mice . . . to where area 17 relates to only early stages of a lengthy hierarchy, as in monkeys. (Kass, 1989, p. 130)

Therefore, there is concordance between Jacksonian hierarchical principles and known patterns of cortical connectivity. The brain regions that are the least reflexive, the least organized (hard wired), the most voluntary, the most complex, and the most integrated with other brain areas are the heteromodal association regions. And while koniocortical primary motor and sensory areas may be highly evolved and specialized, the heteromodal brain regions are the hierarchically highest levels of the nervous system. Mesulum in a later work (2002) supports this point of view when he opines that the "prefrontal cortex appears to sit at the apex of behavioral hierarchies." Fuster (2002; 2003) emphatically affirms that polymodal association and prefrontal cortices represent, respectively, the highest levels of the sensory and motor hierarchies. Therefore, I suggest that in succession, the next three levels of the neural hierarchy are the idiotypical primary sensory and motor regions, the homotypical unimodal association and premotor areas, and finally the heteromodal association areas and the prefrontal regions representing the uppermost levels of the hierarchy. It is of interest to note that in contrast to Figure 4−1, the overall configuration of the nested hierarchy of the self as envisaged in Figure 4−2 has an upside down pyramidal, or conical, configuration.

Meaning, Purpose, and the Nested Hierarchy of the Self

The unified self is created by a nested system of hierarchically arranged structures that create our perceptions and actions. With no single unified pontifical region or neuron at the top of the hierarchy and no inner homunculus bringing coherence and unity to our actions, how does the entire system of the self function in an organized fashion? How do the higher levels of the neural hierarchy control, or *constrain,* lower levels?

I have argued (Feinberg, 2001a, 2001b) that when one considers the sensory system, *meaning* provides the constraint that "pulls" the mind together to form the "inner I" of the self. Mental representations created at different hierarchical levels do not "physically" merge. Rather, *meanings* that are produced at successive hierarchical levels are conjointly represented in awareness to produce *higher levels of meaning,* and it is the successively higher levels of meaning that produce the "topdown" constraint upon the individual elements. In this process the constraint of the whole upon the parts does not result in the elimination of these individual parts. Rather, constraint leads to the elimination of the *independence* of each part from the others when operating within the framework of the nested hierarchy of the mind and the self. These parts are represented dependently, and therefore they are represented *meaningfully* in consciousness. Thus, the *unified subjective experience* that we experience as the integrated self is the result of the *nested hierarchy of meaning* created by the brain.

When one considers the motor system, the *purpose* or *intention* of action sits at the highest level of the action hierarchy, brings unity to action, and constrains all the lower-level neuronal elements that are part of the action (Fig. 4–2). The activity of neurons at lower levels of the hierarchy are nested within the higher levels of the motor hierarchy, and the purpose of the act provides the *constraint* of higher levels upon lower levels.

Conclusion

In summary, I have proposed a tentative theoretical model of the self that takes into account functional, neuroanatomical, and behavioral features. The model proposes that we view the higher nervous system as a nested hierarchy of levels. In contrast to earlier models that view the self as emerging from the brain like the eye atop a pyramid, this model views the neural architecture of the self as an upside down pyramid, or a cone. While the hierarchically highest levels of the neural axis make the highest and most abstract aspects of the self possible, all levels make a contribution to the integrated self. We experience a unified and single self, as opposed to multiple selves from multiple hierarchical levels, because lower-order as well as higher-order elements are part of the nested hierarchy of the self. The highest levels of the perceptual hierarchy are constrained by the highest levels of meaning, and the highest levels of the motor system are constrained by the highest possible level of purpose. In this manner many brain regions are coordinated into a single nested entity that constitutes the unified self, and the self is ultimately a *nested hierarchy of meaning and purpose created by the brain.*

References

Allen,T.F.H & Starr, T.B. (1982). *Hierarchy. Perspectives for Ecological Complexity*. Chicago: University of Chicago Press.

Ayala, F.J. & Dobzhansky, T. (1974). *Studies in the Philosophy of Biology. Reduction and Related Problems*. London: Macmillan Press.

Barlow, H. (1995). The neuron doctrine in perception. In: M.S. Gazzaniga, (Ed.), *The Cognitive Neurosciences* (pp. 415–435). Cambridge, MA: MIT Press.

Beckermann, A., Flohr, H., & Kim, J. (Eds). (1992). *Emergence or Reduction? Essays on the Prospects of Nonreductive Physicalism*. New York: Walter de Gruyter.

Beckers, G. & Zeki, S. (1995). The consequences of inactivating areas V1 and V5 on visual motion perception. *Brain, 118:* 49–60.

Campbell, D.T. (1974). Downward causation in hierarchically organized biological systems. In: F.J. Ayala & T. Dobzhansky (Eds.). *Studies in the Philosophy of Biology,* (pp. 179–186). Berkeley and Los Angeles: University of California Press.

Crick, F.H.C. (1994). *The Astonishing Hypothesis*. New York: Basic Books.

Crick, F. & Koch, C. (1990). Towards a neurobiological theory of consciousness. *Seminars in Neuroscience, 2,* 263–275.

Descartes, R. *Les passions de l'ame*. 1649, pt. I, article 32. In: E. Clarke and C.D. O'Malley, *The Human Brain and Spinal Cord*, 2nd ed. (p. 471). San Francisco: Norman, 1996.

DeYoe, E.A. & Van Essen, D.C. (1988). Concurrent processing streams in monkey visual cortex. *Trends in Neuroscience, 11,* 219–226.

Edelman, G.M. (1989). *The Remembered Present. A Biological Theory of Consciousness*. New York: Basic Books.

Engel, A.K., König, P., Kreiter, A.K., & Singer, W. (1991). Interhemispheric synchronization of oscillatory neuronal responses in cat visual cortex. *Science, 252,* 1177–1179.

Feinberg, T.E. (1997). The irreducible perspectives of consciousness. *Seminars in Neurology, 17,* 85–93.

Feinberg, T.E. (2000).The nested hierarchy of consciousness: A neurobiological solution to the problem of mental unity. *Neurocase, 6,* 75–81.

Feinberg, T.E. (2001a). *Altered Egos: How the Brain Creates the Self*. New York: Oxford University Press.

Feinberg, T.E. (2001b). Why the mind is not a radically emergent feature of the brain. *Journal of Consciousness Studies, 8 (no. 9–10),* 123–145.

Felleman, D.J. & Van Essen, D.C. (1991). Distributed hierarchical processing in the primate cerebral cortex. *Cerebral Cortex, 1,*1–47.

Fuster, J.M. (2002). Physiology of executive functions: The perception-action cycle. In: D.T. Stuss & R.T. Knight (Eds.). *Principles of Frontal Lobe Function* (pp. 96–108). New York: Oxford University Press.

Fuster, J.M. (2003). *Cortex and Mind: Unifying Cognition*. New York: Oxford University Press.

Gray, C.M. & Singer, W. (1989a). Stimulus-specific neuronal oscillations in orientation columns of cat visual cortex. *Proceedings of the National Academy of Science, 86,* 1698–1702.

Gray, C.M., König, P.A., Engel, A.K., & Singer, W. (1989b). Oscillatory responses in cat visual cortex exhibit inter-columnar synchronization which reflects global stimulus properties. *Nature, 338,* 334–337.

Gray, C.M., Engel, A.K., König, P., & Singer, W. (1992). Synchronization of oscillatory neuronal responses in cat striate cortex: Temporal properties. *Visual Neuroscience, 8,* 337–347.

Hubel, D.H. (1988). *Eye, Brain, and Vision.* New York: Scientific American Library.

Hubel, D.H. & Wiesel, T.N. (1962). Receptive fields, binocular interaction and functional architecture in the cat's visual cortex. *Journal of Physiology (London), 160,* 106–154.

Hubel, D.H. & Wiesel, T.N. (1965). Receptive fields and functional architecture in two non striate visual areas (18 and 19) of the cat. *Journal of Neurophysiology, 28,* 229–289.

Hubel, D.H. & Wiesel, T.N. (1968). Receptive fields and functional architecture of monkey striate cortex. *Journal of Physiology (London), 195,* 215–243.

Hubel, D. H. & Wiesel, T.N. (1977). The Ferrier Lecture: Functional architecture of macaque monkey visual cortex. *Proceedings of the Royal Society of London B, 198,* 1–59.

Hubel, D.H. & Wiesel, T.N. (1979). Brain mechanisms of vision. *Scientific American, 241, 3,* 150–162.

Jackson, J.H. (1884). Evolution and dissolution of the nervous system. Croonian Lectures delivered at the Royal College of Physicians. In: J. Taylor (Ed.) *Selected Writings of John Hughlings Jackson, vol. 2,* (pp. 45–75). New York: Basic Books, 1958.

James, W. (1892). *Psychology: The Briefer Course.* In: G. Allport (Ed.), *Psychology: The Briefer Course.* Notre Dame, IN: University of Notre Dame Press, 1985.

James, W. (1890). *The Principles of Psychology.* Cambridge, MA: Harvard University Press, 1983.

Kant, I. (1781). *Critique of Pure Reason,* trans. J.M.D. Meiklejohn (1934). London: J.M. Dent & Sons.

Kass, J.H. (1989). Why does the brain have so many visual areas? *Journal of Cognitive Neuroscience, 1,* 121–135.

Kim, J. (1992). Downward causation in emergentism and nonreductive physicalism. In: A. Beckermann, H. Flohr, & J. Kim (Eds.) *Emergence or Reduction? Essays on the Prospects of Nonreductive Physicalism* (pp. 119–138). New York: Walter de Gruyter.

Konig, P. & Engel, A.K. (1995). Correlated firing in sensory-motor systems. *Current Opinion in Neurobiology, 5,* 511–519.

MacLean, P.D. (1973). A triune concept of the brain and behavior. In: T. Boag & D. Campbell (Eds.) *The Hincks Memorial Lectures* (pp. 6–66).Toronto: University of Toronto Press.

MacLean, P.D. (1990). *The Triune Brain in Evolution: Role in Paleocerebral Functions.* New York: Plenum.

Meares, R. (1999). The contribution of Hughlings Jackson to an understanding of dissociation. *American Journal of Psychiatry, 156,* 1850–1855.

Mesulum, M.-M. (2000). *Principles of Behavioral and Cognitive Neurology,* 2nd ed. New York: Oxford University Press.

Mesulum, M.-M. (2002). The human frontal lobes: Transcending the default mode through contingent encoding. In: D.T. Stuss & R.T. Knight (Eds.) *Principles of Frontal Lobe Function* (p. 24). New York: Oxford University Press.

Morgan, C.L. (1923). *Emergent Evolution.* London: Williams & Norgate.

Morowitz, H. (2002). *The Emergence of Everything: How the World Became Complex.* New York: Oxford University Press.

Movshon, J.A., Adelson, E.H., Gizzi, M.S., & Newsome, W.T. (1985). The analysis of moving visual pattern. In: C. Chagas, R. Gattass, & V. Gross (Eds.), *Pattern Recognition Mechanisms* (pp. 117-151). New York: Springer.

Newman, J. (Ed.). Special Issue: Temporal binding and consciousness. *Consciousness and Cognition, 8* (2), 1999.

Panksepp, J.(1998). *Affective Neuroscience: The Foundations of Human and Animal Emotions.* New York: Oxford University Press.

Pattee, H.H. (1970). The problem of biological hierarchy. In: C.H. Waddington (Ed.) *Towards a Theoretical Biology 3.* Chicago: Aldine.

Pattee, H.H. (1973). *Hierarchy Theory. The Challenge of Complex Systems.* New York: George Braziller.

Ryle, G. (1949). *The Concept Of Mind.* London: Hutchinson & Company.

Salthe, S.N. (1985). *Evolving Hierarchical Systems: Their Structure and Representation.* New York: Columbia University Press.

Sanides, F. (1969). Comparative architectonics of the neocortex of mammals and their evolutionary interpretation. *Annals of the New York Academy of Sciences, 167,* 404–423.

Sanides, F. (1970). Functional architecture of motor and sensory cortices in primates in the light of a new concept of neorcortex evolution. In: C.R. Noback & W. Montagna (Eds.) *The Primate Brain* (pp. 137–208). New York: Appleton-Century-Crofts.

Sanides, F. (1975). Comparative neurology of the temporal lobe in primates including man with reference to speech. *Brain and Language, 2,* 396–419.

Sherrington, C. (1941). *Man on His Nature.* New York: Macmillan.

Sperry, R.W. (1966). Brain bisection and mechanisms of consciousness. In: J.C. Eccles, (Ed.) *Brain and Conscious Experience* (pp. 298–313). New York: Springer-Verlag.

Sperry, R.W. (1977). Forebrain commissurotomy and conscious awareness. *Journal of Medical Philosophy, 2,* (no. 2), 101–26. Reprinted in: C. Trevarthen (Ed.) *Brain Circuits and Functions of the Mind* (pp. 371–388). New York: Cambridge University Press, 1990.

Sperry, R.W. (1984). Consciousness, personal identity and the divided brain. *Neuropsychologia, 22,* 661–673.

Strehler, B.L. (1991). Where is the self? A neuroanatomical theory of consciousness. *Synapse, 7,* 44–91.

Swash, M. (1989). John Hughlings Jackson: A historical introduction. In: C. Kennard & M. Swash (Eds.) *Hierarchies in Neurology. A Reappraisal of a Jacksonian Concept* (p. 9). New York: Springer-Verlag.

Van Essen, D.C., Anderson, C.H., & Felleman, D.J. (1992). Information processing in the primate visual system: An integrated system perspective. *Science, 255,* 419–1423.

Van Gulick, R. (2001). Reduction, emergence, and other recent options on the mind/body problem. A philosophical overview. *Journal of Consciousness Studies, 8* (no. 9–10), 1–34.

von der Malsburg, C. (1995). Binding in models of perception and brain function. *Current Opinion in Neurobiology, 5,* 520–526.

Whyte, L.L., A.G., Wilson & Wilson, D. (1969). *Hierarchical Structures.* New York: American Elsevier.

Zeki, S.A (1993). *A Vision of the Brain.* Oxford: Blackwell Scientific Publications.

5

The Frontal Lobes and Self-Awareness

DONALD T. STUSS, R. SHAYNA ROSENBAUM,
SARAH MALCOLM, WILLIAM CHRISTIANA,
AND JULIAN PAUL KEENAN

Concepts of disorders of awareness and the "self" have evolved over time, with speculation about the self–brain relation extending back likely thousands of years (see Chapter 15, this volume). More than a century ago William James (1891–1952) proposed a unified theory surrounding the concept of self and consciousness. In subsequent years psychologists, neurologists, and neuroscientists have discovered that a significant number of characteristics that James attributed to the self are similar to those functions that are disrupted following frontal lobe damage. Critchley (1953) discussed specific syndromes such as denial of illness and autotopagnosia as disorders of awareness. In the 1960 and 1970s, common neurological thought considered denial, unawareness of deficit, and unconcern as the same phenomenon, with a continuum of severity being the key factor. More detailed behavioral and neuropsychological analysis, finer-grained anatomical specificity, and the advent of functional imaging made evident two important facts in the study of awareness and the brain: there are different types of disordered awareness, which are dissociable anatomically and functionally, and the frontal lobes play a very key role in certain disorders of awareness. This bears resemblance to the way in which more "executive–cognitive" functions of the frontal lobes became differentiated over time, with greater understanding of the integrated organization within the entire brain.

In this chapter we summarize a hierarchical framework proposed by Stuss, Picton, and Alexander (2001) that suggests different levels of awareness of self (see also Stuss, 1991a; 1991b) to account for the variations in attributions of awareness to different brain regions. This awareness of self, or autonoetic (self-knowing) consciousness, has been linked to theory of mind, meta-cognition, episodic autobiographical memory, and the continuity of the self from the past into the future (Stuss & Benson, 1984, 1986; Stuss, Gallup, & Alexander, 2001; Wheeler, Stuss, & Tulving, 1997). These proposals have a direct connection to James's idea of continuity and the importance of certain memories in the formation of the self.

More recently, Endel Tulving noted the relation of the self to the future as critical for the concept of self. Tulving's term *chronesthesia* has been introduced to investigate an individual's ability to mentally travel into the future (Tulving, 2002; see also Keenan, Gallup, & Falk, 2003).

This chapter also serves to challenge current thinking on the relationship among theory of mind, autobiographical memory, and the frontal lobes, which is too global. Further distinctions, both anatomical and theoretical–functional, are likely to be unveiled. We conclude by reformulating the hierarchical framework of self-awareness and prescribe novel approaches for guiding future research.

The Framework

At its simplest level, being aware requires being conscious, as opposed to being "unconscious," with an adequate level of arousal. This state is measured by tools such as the Glasgow Coma Scale (Teasdale & Jennet, 1974). This arousal and general awareness of one's environment are related to the integrity of the brainstem reticular formation, specific brainstem nuclei, and thalamo-cortical projections. Depending on which of these regions are involved, damage can result in coma, stupor, obtundation, wandering attention, or phasic inattention (Benson & Geschwind, 1975; Plum & Posner, 1966). Lipowski (1990) used the terms *hypoactive* and *hyperactive delirium*, states similar in description to stupor (drifting attention) and wandering attention, respectively.

Higher levels of the nervous system assume ample arousal to develop and function adequately. The organization of information in the higher levels occurs via construction of models (see Craik, 1943; Johnson-Laird, 1983; Miller, Galanter, & Pribram, 1960; Picton & Stuss, 2000; Yates, 1985, for other modeling frameworks). That is, to simplify life by facilitating future analysis of incoming information, the brain constructs a model of what has been experienced. This modeling construction is accomplished iteratively, with feedback interaction between the model and the experience, until there is a reasonable fit with the incoming information. It is assumed that the model is experienced as a way to understand information, rather than experiencing the information directly; this simplifies, regulates, and facilitates different responses and actions to the internal and external environment. The framework proposes that the building blocks of experience (the constructed models) are organized in hierarchical levels. This creates a highly interactive integrated "system of systems," with top-down and bottom-up exchanges. While extremely efficient, a potential problem is that once established, the constructed model may be difficult to modify. The limbic reinforcement of the existing model (e.g., continual reinforcement of the way the world is seen and the responses that are selected) may also resist change (Stuss & Alexander, 1999). Thus, while being effective in terms of processing stimuli, the system can remain rigid in terms of ontogeny, which detracts from its adaptability.

The level above that of basic arousal is one comprised of processing the basic contents and/or knowledge of the world. The models at this level are generally accepted to be in the more posterior cortical regions responsible for sensory–perceptual processes, as well as posterior motor areas of the brain. At this level information is separately organized into domain-, or knowledge-, specific modules (e.g., vision, audition, visual–perceptual, etc.) that are anatomically distinct, though interactive (Fodor, 1983; Moscovitch, 1992). Construction of different knowledge categories helps automatize interpretation and response in different situations, thus creating an organism that has a high temporal responsiveness. Disorders of awareness at this level are related to the independent modules, depending on which brain region is damaged. Thus, patients with Wernicke's aphasia secondary to left temporal lobe damage often lack awareness of their comprehension difficulties. However, their sensitivity to and awareness of other aspects of the world (and self) often lead families to assume that these patients somehow have intact comprehension with deficits of expression (Benson, 1979). Patients with right parietal lobe damage have been reported to have different disorders of awareness (e.g., neglect, paralysis) dependent on lesion location or transcranial magnetic stimulation (TMS) administration site (Fierro et al., 2000). That is, where there is damage to more posterior regions, the resulting disturbed awareness is domain-specific. This can result in a disorder of awareness specific to the content of that module (i.e., a true anosagnosia, or lack of knowledge of the disorder).

A separate third level of disturbed awareness was suggested by a case study of a patient with bilateral frontal lobe damage, more extensive on the right (Alexander, Stuss, & Benson, 1979). Several months into the recovery process after weekend visits home to his family, this patient reported having a new family, different but similar to the family he had had before his accident. This duplication of the family represents a case of Capgras syndrome, or reduplicative paramnesia. This patient's claim was interpreted as being secondary to his deficient frontal lobe executive dysfunction, because at the time of testing, his general neuropsychological abilities such as intelligence, memory, and visual–perceptual functioning (including facial recognition) were normal. When asked what he would say if someone else made a similar claim, he could provide a rational explanation of why this would not be possible. This self-referential versus other-referential judgment suggested that the models of the external world (level two) were intact, but that the self model was impaired because of a deficit in judgment in reconciling incongruent factual knowledge; it was a deficit in top-down judgment based on frontal lobe executive dysfunction. This interpretation made sense in light of one of James's criteria for "self": a person's identity ultimately arises from personal judgments of his or her identity, with a sameness and continuity (James, 1952).

Although this made anatomical and theoretical sense, what was not originally explained was the patient's strength of conviction that this was a different family—the patient could never be swayed from his belief in a second family, despite his knowledge that this was not correct (knowledge is not necessarily insight). James again presented a potential solution. When an individual's knowledge presents in the form of memories that possess the feelings of warmth, intimacy, and immediacy, the knowledge then becomes a fundamental part of one's self. These feelings of warmth and intimacy are linked to memories (episodic, autobiographical), which lead to quite a number of other aspects of self. Judgment of one's self through these remembrances provides a feeling of continuity of consciousness as well as a sense of unity. Personal memories are essential for a sense of self, as they are used to evaluate one's self in a greater context. James theorized that continuity plays a large role in the concept of self. The self is not disrupted by time gaps in consciousness such as sleep; there is a steady, continuous feeling of the self that remains across time. Memories of events contribute to the stability of the self, and such memories are part of the core of the self. However, while an individual's sense of "I" comes from having the same memories over time, the self can also be (and perhaps *should* be?) altered slowly over time through the modeling process. That is, maturation is a natural occurrence in the development of the self.

A review of the published reports of Capgras syndrome revealed that what was duplicated was indeed relevant and important to the individual (Alexander et al., 1979). A patient had two warm and salient memories of families, one from before the injury and one that evolved during the period of recovery (when still confused) of a family that was similar but not quite the same. When he recovered, the patient was left with two emotionally salient memories that had been "affectively burnt in" (Stuss & Alexander, 1999). However, these two separate constructed experiential models could not be reconciled because of higher-level deficits in planning, judgment, and monitoring of the patient's own situation—the level related to the executive functions of the frontal lobes, whereby the content of one's own world is sculpted by decisions. Without the ability to make a decision, the models become locked in and cannot be changed.

A fourth level has also been postulated, one that views all information in light of a personal history, from the past and projecting into the future. James also commented on this aspect of self. Individuals not only have the ability to be aware of something, they also have the ability to be aware of this awareness. The apparently highest level of self-reflectiveness or self-consciousness is the ability of our mind not only to know something, but also to be aware that it knows it. It is at this level that the self is related not only to past time, but also to the future. A person is not restricted to what has happened in the past or what is happening in the present. A self-possessing individual is able to think about future events, set future goals, and generate future outcomes. Individuals can use memories of the past to make decisions about the future.

The evidence for this level derives from the experiences of two patients with right frontal damage (Stuss, 1991a, b; Stuss & Alexander, 1999) who had superior intelligence, excellent performance on neuropsychological assessment, including tests of executive functioning, but who could not use this information to guide their own lives. They had adequate knowledge of their problems, could even identify the steps necessary to rectify the problems, but did not follow up on or use this knowledge. These patients were hypothesized to have deficits in the mental model of themselves. They had adequate knowledge (models at the level of modular knowledge), intact ability to make appropriate judgments (frontal lobe executive functioning level), but did not have a clear purpose to organize and guide the use of these lower levels. There is strong evidence to suggest that this level is also related to the frontal lobes, with likely preeminence of the right frontal lobe (Craik et al., 1999; Stuss & Alexander, 1999; Stuss & Anderson, 2004).

The framework of levels of "self" assists in understanding the previous efforts that described disturbances of self after brain damage. It turns out that Critchley was correct in his hypothesis that there are disturbances of self following posterior brain damage. However, such disturbances appear to be somewhat limited and domain-specific. James also was likely correct in many of his assumptions, including the idea that the "self" is central in terms of cognitive processing. James's ideas can be related to the notion that disorders of self-awareness can be viewed as a continuum from denial to unconcern and that the levels are not isolated, but are part of integrated anatomical and functional systems.

The framework has extended James's concept by suggesting that there may be a separation between a more "executive" level of self, where decisions are made, and a higher level of self, which is more central and overarching. In the rest of this chapter, we examine more evidence for this division, investigate the relation of the "central" self to theory of mind, and deliberate on the possibility of a more refined definition of the fourth level of self-awareness.

Application of the Framework to Theory of Mind

Now that we have laid down a broad framework, we will explore in greater detail the highest level of awareness as it relates to "theory of mind," an ability or collection of abilities that enables perhaps only humans to infer the mental states of others (Premack & Woodruff, 1978; Frith & Frith, 2003). Our capacity for cooperation, deception, compassion, and humor rests on this ability to recognize in others a set of beliefs that might not correspond to our own beliefs or to reality. The concept of theory of mind (also known as "mentalizing"; Frith, Morton, & Leslie, 1991) has gained theoretical prominence over the past two decades largely as a result of its application to autism to better characterize the disorder (Baron-Cohen, Leslie, & Frith, 1985; Baron-Cohen, 1995). Findings that theory of mind is virtually nonexistent in autistic children helped encourage investigators to uncover the neural basis of this deficit using complementary neuropsychological and neuroimaging approaches.

Initial efforts to understand the biological basis of theory of mind yielded evidence that the frontal lobes play a key part in a presumably widespread network of brain regions. However, the frontal lobes constitute a large part of the brain, and describing the exact anatomical correlates within the frontal region is difficult. It is less clear what the necessary and unique contributions of separable regions within the frontal lobes to theory of mind are, let alone how one might parcel theory of mind into component cognitive-emotional processes. By starting with the known roles of the frontal lobes and their theoretical-functional correlates, we will be in a better position to revisit the more central theme of self-awareness and its affiliates.

Case and group studies have informed localization as precise as that between cognition and emotion within dorsal lateral (DL) and ventral medial (VM) sectors of prefrontal cortex (PFC), respectively (for a review, see Stuss & Levine, 2002). Strong DLPFC-hippocampal connections may account for difficulties in online manipulation of information in working memory, selective attention, inhibition of a prepotent response, strategic retrieval from memory, and conceptual reasoning (those functions often considered "executive") observed in patients with lesions restricted to DLPFC (e.g., Goldman-Rakic, 1996; Petrides, 1996). By contrast, given its strong reciprocal connections with emotion-related limbic areas (Nauta, 1971; Pandya & Barnes, 1987), patients with lesions to VMPFC show disturbed emotional processing, adherence to social norms, and assignment of reward-value to decision-making (Damasio, 1994; Eslinger & Damasio, 1985; Rolls, 2000). This region is further differentiated from a more superior aspect of medial PFC involved in initiation and motivation, such that damage to this division can result in an apathetic syndrome (Cummings, 1993; Stuss & Benson, 1986; Stuss et al., 2002).

This knowledge of functional-anatomical specificity of the frontal lobes should be considered in understanding the relationship of theory of mind to the brain. Does theory of mind figure into the functional domain of either DLPFC; that is, is theory of mind related to the executive functions of the frontal lobes? Do the emotional–self-regulatory functions associated with VMPFC make it well suited for theory of mind? Or does it require the simultaneous recruitment of both centers? Perhaps there is an additional region dedicated exclusively to its function? In order to answer these questions, one must review definitions of, and even redefine, theory of mind. At the very least, we must agree on what theory of mind is not.

There is suggestion in the literature that theory of mind impairment may be reduced to executive dysfunction, which is most associated with damage to DLPFC and its connections with domain-specific regions. For example, conceptual reasoning is necessary for deciphering the contents of another person's mind based on facial expressions processed by the amygdala (e.g., Baron-Cohen et al., 1994, 1999; Fine, Lumsden, & Blair, 2001; Shaw et al., 2004) and actions processed by the temporoparietal junction (Frith & Frith, 1999). Response inhibition is also employed when one is faced with having to ignore one's own privileged knowledge of reality in favor of another person's false belief[1] (e.g., Perner & Lang, 1999). Associations between executive function and theory of mind ability have been documented in studies of normally developing children (Flynn, O'Malley, & Wood, 2004; Frye, Zelazo, & Palfai, 1995; Ozonoff, Pennington, & Rogers, 1991), children with autism (Zelazo et al., 2002), and patients with adult-onset frontal lobe damage (Channon & Crawford, 2000).

However, the association may be questioned. This pattern of results may be a function of nonspecific pathology in the patient studies that invade DLPFC, such that the role of different regions could not be well differentiated. Moreover, certain theory of mind tasks have processing demands that load heavily on executive function. In addition, the actual patient data point to an anatomical relationship that does not support the executive function hypothesis. Of the handful of large group studies of adults with relatively focal frontal lesions (Rowe et al., 2001; Shamay-Tsoory et al., 2003; Stone, Baron-Cohen, & Knight, 1998; Stuss, Gallup, & Alexander, 2001), all except one (Rowe et al., 2001) showed significantly greater mentalizing impairment in patients with selective lesions to orbital or medial PFC than to DLPFC. In the one exception, even though there was no greater deficit in one group than the other, the problems in mentalizing were independent of any executive difficulties. Findings across neuroimaging investigations are likewise mixed, though the invariable area of overlap in the frontal lobes across a wide range of paradigms is again medial and not lateral (Baron-Cohen et al., 1999; Castelli et al., 2000; Fletcher et al., 1995; Gallagher et al., 2000, 2002; Goel et al., 1995; McCabe et al., 2001; Saxe & Kanwisher, 2003; see also Gallagher & Frith, 2003, for a detailed review). In fact, theory of mind is preserved in patients with DLPFC lesions when tasks are modified in a way that reduces or eliminates demands on executive function (Fine et al., 2001; Rowe et al., 2001; Varley, Siegal, & Want, 2001). While the executive functions are primarily related to dorsolateral frontal regions, the neuropsychological and neuroimaging literatures converge on orbital–ventral and medial aspects of PFC as necessary for constructing a theory of mind.

The problem in associating theory of mind with executive function is also apparent in other populations. When the need to inhibit an overriding response is reduced, healthy children perform better on false belief tests (Wellman, Cross, & Watson, 2001). Conversely, autistic children are impaired on theory of mind tests that have no executive component (Baron-Cohen, 1995; Baron-Cohen et al., 1994, 1999) and succeed on nonsocial reasoning tests that are equivalent to typical mentalizing tests in terms of inhibitory demands (see also Pickup & Frith, 2001, for similar findings in schizophrenic patients). Recently, we found that children with both autism and Asperger's syndrome present deficits of self-awareness as measured by the self-recognition test (Keenan, et al., 2004). In this study children with mental retardation significantly outperformed the autism and Asperger's groups, suggesting that self-awareness, similar to theory of mind, is not tied to executive function. Of note is the fact that the autism and Asperger's groups scored similarly despite very different verbal abilities. This finding suggests that language is not tied to self-awareness.

There is other support to suggest that the regions found to correlate with the self and theory of mind are not tied directly to executive processes. To determine the role of these regions, we (Keenan, data under preparation) have used TMS to disrupt processing. When TMS was applied to the right medial ventral regions (Fp2–10/20 international system), self-judgments were disrupted. TMS delivered to this region is thought to influence activity in the superior frontal and medial frontal gyrus. Therefore, the manipulation of self-awareness can be achieved in the absence of disruption of classic executive regions. Similar to our experience with clinical populations (e.g., Asperger), we have found, in fact, little to no evidence to support the claim that executive functioning is related to self or theory of mind.

Thus, there is ample evidence to suggest that executive functions are not necessary for theory of mind and possibly self-recognition, and it is not surprising that these functions might occupy distinct neural regions. This tentatively supports our distinctions between levels three and four of the framework.

Although there is a strong relationship between theory of mind and the medial PFC, finer specialization within the expanse of medial PFC is still possible and may reveal a more distinct region that defies functional segregation. It may be here that cognition and emotion are fully integrated and inseparable. Work in a number of laboratories has indicated that the frontal pole, within the region of BA 10 and supplied by branches of the anterior cerebral artery, is a candidate convergence site for cognitive–emotional processing. Interestingly, proximity of lesion to the frontal pole in stroke patients strongly predicts depression (Narushima, Kosier, & Robinson, 2003), a disorder that, by itself, has implications for affective–cognitive processing. The polar area, though simple architectonically in terms of cell body density, is complex in terms of dendritic spine density and in its predominant interconnections with other higher-order PFC regions (Petrides & Pandya, 1994). Several authors have proposed a potentially unique role for this region (Burgess, in press; Stuss et al., 2001).

In a recent review of the topic, Ramnani and Owen (2004) suggested that these regions are particularly well-suited for transmodal coordination of inputs, which could be modeled within the context of executive functioning. Integration of two or more discrete solutions to cognitive "problems" would then allow for the pursuit of a more widespread behavioral goal. Inherent in this model is the idea that frontal "functioning" focuses on information processing rather than the tasks at hand.

We take this proposal one step further to account for the even more elusive social cognitive phenomenon of theory of mind. The ability to reflect on one's own mental state and apply this self-inference to appreciate the mental states of others is often compromised in patients with lesions to VMPFC, with a trend toward the frontal pole as the critical region of overlap (Shammi & Stuss, 1999; Stuss et al., 2001). This group as a whole fails to appreciate humor and expresses particular difficulty realizing that they are being engaged in a task of deception in which they must point to a location opposite to one that an experimenter chooses.

This proposal leads to another question of the functional basis of theory of mind. The polar area has also been ascribed a role in another uniquely human capacity, autobiographical episodic memory, which has to do with awareness of the self as a continuous entity. Tulving (1985) suggested that episodic memories are related to self-awareness through autonoetic consciousness. Autonoetic consciousness, in turn, is the ability to mentally represent and become aware of subjective experiences in the past, present, and future (Wheeler, Stuss, & Tulving, 1997). Ingvar (1985) suggested that the frontal lobes generate "memories of the future." Based in part on the work of Ingvar, Tulving suggested that autonoetic consciousness is related to the frontal lobes. Wheeler and coworkers proposed that episodic memory might rely on mental models and imagery function of the right frontal lobe, which are also involved in self-awareness (Keenan, Gallup, & Falk, 2003). Wheeler and his colleagues suggested that the prefrontal regions, particularly on the right, provide the necessary organization for episodic memory to guide the recall of memories that are associated with emotions. Following this, the memories recalled are connected with plans and expectations for the future. The prefrontal regions transfer these episodic memories into self-reflective consciousness. This is a highly personalized consciousness that allows for the creation and execution of future plans.

Tulving, Risberg, and Ingvar (1988) measured regional cerebral blood flow during the recall of personal events and found evidence that supports the idea that the frontal lobes are involved with the recall of past events. Based on PET studies, Tulving and colleagues (1994) proposed that left frontal lobe activation is associated with memory encoding, whereas right frontal lobe activation is associated with the retrieval of episodic memories. Further evidence of frontal lobe involvement was reported by Levine and colleagues (1998). They reported a patient who had lost all personal past memories due to trauma. MRI revealed a ventrolateral right frontal lesion involving damage to the ventral pathways to and from the right temporal lobe. This patient later relearned life's memories. However, these memories were recalled without affect, such that they were not "burnt in." A PET investigation of this patient revealed that these new memories were not truly episodic and, instead, were learned through the semantic memory system. This pattern of dissociation was established with the "remember–know" paradigm, in which an event is assigned a "remember" response only if it evokes the recollection of the specific time and place defining the event's occurrence and a "know" response if familiarity goes only as far as recognizing that an event had occurred in the past (Tulving, 1985). Due to this patient's injuries, the "new" memories did not contain feelings of warmth, intimacy, and immediacy. These feelings are believed to be necessary for the memory to be incorporated into one's sense of self.

A number of imaging studies have examined both self and other perspectives. An initial fMRI study by Vogeley and colleagues (2001) used narrative stories that involved both first- and third-person perspective-taking. The areas of activation for the combination of self and theory of mind (or first- and third-person perspective) involved regions consistent with our theory. Both medial regions of the prefrontal cortex and right lateral prefrontal cortex were activated (Fig. 5–1a).

These data were followed up by Platek and colleagues (2004). Similar to the Vogeley and coworkers study, both self and other perspectives were examined in the same participants. The tasks, however, were quite different. In the self task participants were asked to view their own face, which was contrasted with viewing other people's faces (see Keenan, Gallup, & Falk, 2003, for a review of self-face and brain correlates). It was found that self-faces activated regions of the right prefrontal cortex, including polar regions (Fig. 5–1b). These data are similar to those found in mirror sign patients (see Chapter 9, this volume).

There are additional reasons to suspect a close link between theory of mind and autonoetic consciousness as indexed by autobiographical memory. Theory of mind tasks demand "putting yourself in someone else's shoes," which may be similar to putting yourself in your own shoes but at a different time and place when reexperiencing a personal episode. Both emerge close in time in ontogenetic development (Howe & Courage, 1997; Welch-Ross, 1997). Both require the abstraction or imagining of imperceptible mental states that do not lend themselves to physical inspection. In other words, stripped of our ability to mentalize, we are at the mercy of what is currently being experienced and perceived in the external world. Others have espoused that "experiential awareness" is a necessary condition for the development of theory of mind (Welch-Ross, 1995), with evidence that at least free recall predates theory of mind (Perner & Ruffman, 1995).

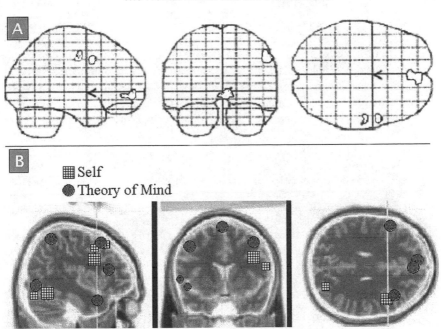

Figure 5–1. An adaptation of Vogeley and colleagues (2001) and Platek and colleagues (2004). Presented in the upper section (A) are the results of Vogeley, where self and theory of mind are coplotted. Note the regions of activation include the medial and right frontal cortex. Below, the data of Platek are represented (B). The regions active for self (squares) and theory of mind (circles) correspond to the regions found by Vogeley. These data suggest that medial prefrontal areas, along with right-hemisphere frontal regions, are involved in higher levels of self.

This long list of coincidences, however, does not inevitably translate into a causal relationship. For example, the well-studied amnesiac patient K.C., who has informed theories of autonoetic consciousness and chronosthesia as a result of an extremely impoverished autobiographical episodic memory, shows clear appreciation of humor and can easily reflect on his current state of mind and that of others (Rosenbaum et al., 2005). It may be safe to say that a critical feature of these two abilities is a sense of self that is free of time rather than a sense of continuity over time. It remains for future research to assess, in a manner similar to that for executive function, whether autobiographical memory is essential for theory of mind.

Future Directions and Extension of the Framework: Implications of the Model

Inherent in Stuss and colleagues' (2001) original formulation of awareness is a largely bottom-up structure in which lower levels in the hierarchy feed forward into higher levels, with any exchange in the opposite direction occurring with an immediately adjacent subordinate. In extending this framework we now emphasize two other features. First, we adopt a more flexible top-down approach, one in which the highest levels have the capacity to work with all levels below that are relevant to the task or process at hand. Second, there may be additional dissociations that have been hidden by this flexible top-down functioning. The frontal lobes have the ability to make theory of mind and self-awareness appear seamless, concealing their true multicomponent nature. By taking a network perspective, it is possible to hypothesize and test for the missing links in this multicomponent central ability.

Acknowledgments

Research reported in this chapter was possible because of research or personnel funding by the Medical Research Council of Canada/Canadian Institutes of Health Research (CIHR), the Ontario Mental Health Foundation, and the Reva James Leeds Chair in Neuroscience and Research Leadership to D. Stuss, a Heart and Stroke Foundation of Canada/CIHR postdoctoral fellowship to R. S. Rosenbaum, the Posluns Centre for Stroke and Cognition at Baycrest Centre, and the Heart and Stroke Foundation of Ontario Centre for Stroke Recovery.

Note

1. The typical false belief test assesses a subject's ability to represent a character's mistaken belief about the location of an object that differs from the subject's own belief (first-order) or another character's belief about the first character's belief about the location of an object (second-order; Perner & Wimmer, 1988).

References

Alexander, M.P., Stuss, D.T., & Benson, D.F. (1979). Capgras syndrome: A reduplicative phenomenon. *Neurology, 29*(3), 334–339.

Baron-Cohen, S. (1995). *Mindblindness: An Essay on Autism and Theory of Mind.* Cambridge, MA: MIT Press.

Baron-Cohen, S., Leslie, A.M., & Frith, U. (1985). Does the autistic child have a "theory of mind?" *Cognition, 21,* 37–46.

Baron-Cohen, S., Ring, H., Moriarty, J., Shmitz, P., Costa, D., & Ell, P. (1994). Recognition of mental state terms: A clinical study of autism, and a functional neuroimaging study of normal adults. *British Journal of Psychiatry, 165,* 640–649.

Baron-Cohen, S., Ring, H. A., Wheelwright, S., Bullmore, E.T., Brammer, M.J., Simmons, A., & Williams, S.C.R. (1999). Social intelligence in the normal and autistic brain: An fMRI study. *European Journal of Neuroscience, 11,* 1891–1898.

Benson, D.F. (1979). *Aphasia, Alexia, and Agraphia.* New York: Churchill Livingstone.

Benson, D.F. & Geschwind, N. (1975). Psychiatric conditions associated with focal lesions of the central nervous system. In: S. Arieti & M. Reiser (Eds.) *American Handbook of Psychiatry: Vol. 4. Organic Disorders and Psychosomatic Medicine* (2nd ed., pp. 208–243). New York: Basic Books.

Burgess, P.W., Simons, J.S., Dumontheil, I., & Gilbert, S.J. (in press). The gateway hypothesis of rostral prefrontal cortex (area 10) function. In: J. Duncan, L. Phillips, & P. McLeod (Eds.) *Speed, Control and Age: In Honour of Patrick Rabbitt.* Oxford: Oxford University Press.

Castelli, F., Happé, F., Frith, U., & Frith, C. (2000). Movement and mind: A functional imaging study of perception and interpretation of complex intentional movement patterns. *Neuroimage, 12,* 314–325.

Channon, S. & Crawford, S. (2000). The effects of anterior lesions on performance on a story comprehension test: Left anterior impairment on a theory of mind-type task. *Neuropsychologia, 38,* 1006–1017.

Craik, F.I.M., Moroz, T.M., Moscovitch, M., Stuss, D.T., Winocur, G., Tulving, E., & Kapur, S. (1999). In search of the self: A positron emission tomography study. *Psychological Science, 10,* 27–35.

Craik, K. (1943). *The Nature of Explanation.* Cambridge: Cambridge University Press.

Critchley, M. (1953). *The Parietal Lobes.* Oxford: Williams & Wilkins.

Cummings, J. (1993). Frontal-subcortical circuits and human behavior. *Archives of Neurology, 50,* 873–880.

Damasio, A.R. (1994). *Descartes' Error: Emotion, Reason, and the Human Brain.* New York: Avon Books.

Eslinger, P.J. & Damasio, A.R. (1985). Severe disturbance of higher cognition after bilateral frontal lobe ablation: Patient EVR. *Neurology, 35,* 1731–1741.

Fierro, B., Brighina, F., Oliveri, M., Piazza, A., La Bua, V., Buffa, D., & Bisiach, E. (2000). Contralateral neglect induced by right posterior parietal rTMS in healthy subjects. *Neuroreport, 11,* 1519–1521.

Fine, C., Lumsden, J., & Blair, R.J. (2001). Dissociation between "theory of mind" and executive functions in a patient with early left amygdala damage. *Brain, 124* (pt 2), 287–298.

Fletcher, P.C., Happe, F., Frith, U., Baker, S.C., Dolan, R.J., Frackowiak, R.S.J., & Frith, C.D. (1995). Other minds in the brain: A functional imaging study of "theory of mind" in story comprehension. *Cognition, 57* (2), 109–128.

Flynn, E., O'Malley, C., & Wood, D. (2004). A longitudinal, microgenetic study of the emergence of false belief understanding and inhibition skills. *Developmental Science, 7,* 103–115.

Fodor, J.A. (1983). *The Modularity of Mind.* Cambridge, MA: MIT Press.

Frith, C. & Frith, U. (1999). Interacting minds: A biological basis. *Science, 286,* 1692–1695.

Frith, U. & Frith, C.D. (2003). Development and neurophysiology of mentalising (Special Issue: Mechanisms of Social Interaction), *Philosophical Transactions of the Royal Society of London Series B, 358,* 459–473.

Frith, U., Morton, J., & Leslie, A.M. (1991). The cognitive basis of a biological disorder: Autism. *Trends in Neurosciences, 14,* 433–443.

Frye, D., Zelazo, .D., & Palfai, T. (1995). Theory of mind and rule-based reasoning. *Cognitive Development, 10,* 483–527.

Gallagher, H.L. & Frith, C.D. (2003). Functional imaging of 'theory of mind'. *Trends in Cognitive Sciences, 7,* 77–83.

Gallagher, H.L., Happe, F., Brunswick, N., Fletcher, P.C., Frith, U., & Frith, C.D. (2000). Reading the mind in cartoons and stories: An FMRi study of "theory of mind" in verbal and non-verbal tasks. *Neuropsychologia, 38,* 11–21.

Gallagher, H.L., Jack, A.I., Roepstorff, A., & Frith, C.D. (2002). Imaging the intentional stance in a competitive game. *Neuroimage, 16,* 814–821.

Goel, V., Grafman, J., Sadato, N., & Hallet, M. (1995). Modeling other minds. *Neuroreport: An International Journal for the Rapid Communication of Research in Neuroscience, 33,* 623–642.

Goldman-Rakic, P.S. (1996). The prefrontal landscape: Implications of functional architecture for understanding human mentation and the central executive. *Philosophical Transactions of the Royal Society of London Series B, 351,* 1445–1453.

Howe, M.L. & Courage, M.L. (1997). The emergence and early development of autobiographical memory. *Psychological Review, 104,* 499–523.

Ingvar, D.H. (1985). "Memory of the future": An essay on the temporal organization of conscious awareness. *Human Neurobiology, 4,* 127–136.

James, W. (1952). Principles of psychology. In: R.M. Hutchins (Series Ed.), M.J. Adler, & W. Brockway (Vol. Eds.), Great Books of the Western World: vol. 53. *William James.* Chicago: Encyclopedia Britannica. (Original work published 1890).

Johnson-Laird, P.N. (1983). *Mental Models: Towards a Cognitive Science of Language, Inference, and Consciousness.* Cambridge, MA: Harvard University Press.

Keenan, J.P., Christiana, W., Malcolm, S., & Johnson, A. (2004, April). Mirror-self recognition in autism and Asperger's syndrome: Implications for neurological correlates. Poster presented at the Eleventh Annual Cognitive Neuroscience Society Meeting, San Francisco, CA.

Keenan, J.P., Gallup G.G., Jr., & Falk, D. (2003). *The Face in the Mirror: The Search for the Origins of Consciousness.* New York: Harper Collins.

Levine, B., Black, S. E., Cabeza, R., Sinden, M., McIntosh, A.R., Toth, J.P., Tulving, E., & Stuss, D.T. (1998). Episodic memory and the self in a case of isolated retrograde amnesia. *Brain, 121,* 1951–1973.

Lipowski, Z.J. (1990). *Delirium: Acute Confusional States.* New York: Oxford University Press.

McCabe, K., Houser, D., Ryan, L., Smith, V., & Trouard, T. (2001). A functional imaging study of cooperation in two-person reciprocal exchange. *Proceedings of the National Academy of Sciences, 98,* 11832–11835.

Miller, G.A., Galanter, E.H., & Pribram, K.H. (1960). *Plans and the Structure of Behavior.* New York: Holt, Rinehart & Winston.

Moscovitch, M. (1992). Memory and working with memory: A component process model based on modules. *Journal of Cognitive Neuroscience, 4,* 257–267.

Narushima K., Kosier J.T., & Robinson R.G. (2003). A reappraisal of poststroke depression, intra- and inter-hemispheric lesion location using meta-analysis. *Journal of Neuropsychiatry and Clinical Neuroscience, 15,* 422–430.

Nauta, W.J.H. (1971). The problem of the frontal lobe: A reinterpretation. *Journal of Psychiatry Research, 8,* 167–187.

Ozonoff, S., Pennington, B.F., & Rogers, S.J. (1991). Executive function deficits in high functioning autistic children: Relationship to theory of mind. *Journal of Child Psychology and Psychiatry, 32,* 1081–1105.

Pandya, D.N. & Barnes, C.L. (1987). Architecture and connections of the frontal lobe. In: E. Perecman (Ed.), *The Frontal Lobes Revisited* (pp. 41–72). New York: IRBN Press.

Perner, J. & Lang, B. (1999). Development of theory of mind and executive control. *Trends in Cognitive Science, 3,* 337–344.

Perner, J. & Ruffman, T. (1995). Episodic memory and autonoetic consciousness: Developmental evidence and a theory of childhood amnesia. *Journal of Experimental Child Psychology, 59* (*3*), 516–548.

Perner, J.E. & Winner, H. (1988). Misinformation and unexpected change: testing the development of epistemic-state attribution. *Psychological Research, 50,* 191–197.

Petrides, M. (1996). Specialized systems for the processing of mnemonic information within the primate frontal cortex. *Philosophical Transactions of the Royal Society of London Series B, 351,* 1455–1461.

Petrides, M. & Pandya, D.N. (1994). Comparative architectonic analysis of the human and the macaque frontal cortex. In: F. Boller & J. Grafman (Eds.) *Handbook of Neuropsychology,* vol. 9 (pp. 17–58). Amsterdam: Elsevier.

Pickup, G.J. & Frith, C.D. (2001). Theory of mind impairments in schizophrenia: symptomatology, severity and specificity. *Psychological Medicine, 31,* 207–220.

Picton, T.W. & Stuss, D.T. (2000). Consciousness. In: E.E. Bittar & N. Bittar (Eds.), *Biological Psychiatry* (pp. 1–25). Stamford, CT: JAI Press.

Platek, S., Keenan, J.P., Gallup, G.G., & Mohamed, F. (2004). Where am I? The neurological correlates of self and other. *Cognitive Brain Research, 19,* 114–122.

Plum, F. & Posner, J.B. (1966). *The Diagnosis of Stupor and Coma,* 3rd ed. Philadelphia: FA Davis Co.

Premack, D. & Woodruff, G. (1978). Does the chimpanzee have a theory of mind? *Behavioral & Brain Sciences, 1,* 515–526.

Ramnani, N. & Owen A.M. (2004). Anterior prefrontal cortex (BA 10): What can anatomy and functional neuroimaging tell us about function? *Nature Reviews Neuroscience, 5,* 184–194.

Rolls, E.T. (2000). The orbitofrontal cortex and reward. *Cerebral Cortex, 10,* 284–294.

Rosenbaum, R.S., Köhler, S., Schacter, D.L., Moscovitch, M., Westmacott, R., Black, S.E., Gao, F., & Tulving, E. (2005). The case of K.C.: Contributions of a memory-impaired person to memory theory. *Neuropsychologia,* in press.

Rowe, A.D., Bullock, P.R., Polkey, C.E., & Morris, R.G. (2001). "Theory of mind" impairments and their relationship to executive functioning following frontal lobe excisions. *Brain, 124,* 600–616.

Saxe, R. & Kanwisher, N. (2003). People thinking about thinking people. The role of the temporo-parietal junction in "theory of mind." *Neuroimage, 19,* 1835–1842.

Shamay-Tsoory, S.G., Tomer, R., Berger, B.D., & Aharon-Peretz, J. (2003). Characterization of empathy deficits following prefrontal brain damage: The role of the right ventromedial prefrontal cortex. *Journal of Cognitive Neuroscience, 15,* 324–337.

Shammi, P. & Stuss, D.T. (1999). Humour appreciation: A role of the right frontal lobe. *Brain, 122,* 657–666.

Shaw, P., Lawrence, E.J., Radbourne, C., Bramham, J., Polkey, C.E., & David, A.S. (2004). The impact of early and late damage to the human amygdala on 'theory of mind' reasoning. *Brain, 127,* 1535–1548.

Stone, V.E., Baron-Cohen, S. & Knight, R.T. (1998). Frontal lobe contributions to theory of mind. *Journal of Cognitive Neuroscience, 10* (5), 640–656.

Stuss, D.T. (1991a). Disturbance of self-awareness after frontal system damage. In: G.P. Prigatano & D.L. Schacter (Eds.) *Awareness of Deficit after Brain Injury: Clinical and Theoretical Issues* (pp. 63–83). New York: Oxford University Press.

Stuss, D.T. (1991b). Self, awareness, and the frontal lobes: A neuropsychological perspective. In: J. Strauss & G.R. Goethals (Eds.) *The Self: Interdisciplinary Approaches* (pp. 255–278). New York: Springer-Verlag.

Stuss, D.T. & Alexander, M.P. (1999). Affectively burnt in: A proposed role of the right frontal lobe. In: E. Tulving (Ed.) *Memory, Consciousness and the Brain: The Tallinn Conference* (pp. 215–227). Philadelphia: Psychology Press.

Stuss, D.T., Alexander, M.P., Floden, D., Binns, M.A., Levine, B., McIntosh, A.R., Rajah, N., & Hevenor, S.J. (2002). Fractionation and localization of distinct frontal lobe processes: Evidence from focal lesions in humans. In: D.T. Stuss & R.T. Knight (Eds.) *Principles of Frontal Lobe Function* (pp. 392–407). London: Oxford University Press.

Stuss, D.T. & Anderson, V. (2004). The frontal lobes and theory of mind: Developmental concepts from adult focal lesion research. *Brain and Cognition, 55,* 69–83.

Stuss, D.T. & Benson, D.F. (1984). Neuropsychological studies of the frontal lobes. *Psychological Bulletin, 95,* 3–28.

Stuss, D.T. & Benson, D. F. (1986). *The Frontal Lobes.* New York: Raven.

Stuss, D.T., Gallup, G.G., & Alexander, M.P. (2001). The frontal lobes are necessary for "theory of mind." *Brain, 124,* 279–286.

Stuss, D.T. & Levine, B. (2002). Adult clinical neuropsychology: Lessons from studies of the frontal lobes. *Annual Review of Psychology, 53,* 401–433.

Stuss, D.T., Picton, T.W., & Alexander, M.P. (2001). Consciousness, self-awareness and the frontal lobes. In: S.P. Salloway, & P.F. Malloy (Eds.) *The Frontal Lobes and Neuropsychiatric Illness* (pp. 101–109). Washington, DC: American Psychiatric Publishing.

Teasdale, G. & Jennett, B. (1974). Assessment of coma and impaired consciousness: A practical scale. *Lancet, 2,* 81–84.

Tulving, E. (1985). Memory and consciousness. *Canadian Psychology, 26,* 1–12.

Tulving, E. (2002). Chronesthesia: Awareness of subjective time. In: D.T. Stuss & R.C. Knight (Eds.) *Principles of Frontal Lobe Functions* (pp. 311–325). New York: Oxford University Press.

Tulving, E., Kapur, S., Craik, F.I.M., Moscovitsch, M., & Houle, S. (1994). Hemispheric encoding/retrieval asymmetry in episodic memory: Positron emission tomography findings. *Proceedings of National Academy of Sciences, 91,* 2016–2020.

Tulving, E., Risberg, J., & Ingvar, D.H. (1988). Regional cerebral blood flow and episodic memory retrieval. *Bulletin of the Psychonomic Society, 26,* 522.

Varley, R., Siegal, M., & Want, S.C. (2001). Severe impairment in grammar does not preclude theory of mind. *Neurocase, 7,* 489–493.

Vogeley, K., Bussfeld, P., Newen, A., Herrmann, S., Happé, F., & Falkai, P. (2001). Mind reading: Neural mechanisms of theory of mind and self-perspective. *Neuroimage, 14,* 170–181.

Welch-Ross, M.K. (1995). An integrative model of the development of autobiographical memory. *Developmental Review, 15,* 338–365.

Welch-Ross, M.K. (1997). Mother-child participation in conversation about the past: Relationships to preschoolers' theory of mind. *Developmental Psychology, 33,* 618–629.

Wellman, H.M., Cross, D., & Watson, J. (2001). Meta-analysis of theory-of-mind development: The truth about false belief. *Child Development, 72,* 655–684.

Wheeler, M.A., Stuss, D.T., & Tulving, E. (1997). Toward a theory of episodic memory: The frontal lobes and autonoetic consciousness. *Psychological Bulletin, 121,* 331–354.

Yates, J. (1985). The content of awareness is a model of the world. *Psychological Review, 92,* 249–284.

Zelazo, P.D., Jacques, S., Burack, J.A., & Frye, D. (2002). The relation between theory of mind and rule use: Evidence from persons with autism-spectrum disorders. *Infant & Child Development, 11,* 171–195.

6

Autobiographical Disorders

ESTHER FUJIWARA AND HANS J. MARKOWITSCH

Disturbances of autobiographical memory can result from organic pathologies such as focal brain lesions and neurodegenerative diseases that affect brain areas critical for autobiographical memory processing. Likewise, autobiographical memory can be severely affected in psychiatric syndromes associated with metabolic brain changes in similar brain regions as in neurological diseases. In this chapter, after presenting an overview of memory systems and their associated brain regions, we give examples of autobiographical memory disorders in neurological and psychiatric diseases. Furthermore, we show the similarity of both to the condition of psychogenic amnesia.

Memory Systems

Memory can be divided according to aspects of time and content. The traditional time-oriented classification refers to the concepts of ultra-short-term, short-term, and long-term memory. Whereas ultra-short-term memory lasts for up to hundreds of milliseconds (Cowan, 1984), short-term memory covers seconds to minutes or includes 4 to 10 bits of information (Miller, 1956; Yoshino, 1993). As a special form of short-term memory, working memory allows active holding and manipulation of information over a limited time range and provides the possibility of processing information online (Baddeley, 2000). Any information that is not forgotten and exceeds the limited capacity of short-term and working memory is assigned to long-term memory stores. Especially in patients with memory disorders, a further time-oriented categorization is of importance, namely the distinction between old and new memories. In organic amnesia the time of a brain injury or onset of brain pathology can distinguish old from new memories, whereas in psychiatric diseases this turning point can be the experience of a psychological trauma or stressful event (Kopelman, 2002). The inability to access information that happened before the incident is called retrograde amnesia, whereas anterograde amnesia is the incapacity to acquire new information after the incident.

It has long been known that in amnesic patients memory is not evenly affected by deteriorations. Content-based classifications of memory may be the best way to describe the pattern of memory loss seen in amnesia. Hierarchically arranged from the most complex to the simplest, one can distinguish five separate but interdependent systems (Fig. 6–1). Episodic memory requires conscious and self-related reflection, or autonoëtic consciousness, it is the conjunction of subjective time, autonoëtic consciousness and the experiencing self, allowing mental time travel to the past and containing context-embedded, specific, and distinctive events. Semantic memory refers to present-oriented general knowledge and contains context-free facts. Retrieval of semantic information is conscious, though one does not have to employ self-related processing. Therefore, it is thought to be associated with noëtic consciousness. Perceptual memory refers to feelings of familiarity on the basis of presemantic (sensory) information only. Priming facilitates the nonconscious processing of previously perceived information. Finally, procedural memory refers to highly automated sensorimotor skills (Markowitsch, 2003; Tulving, 2001).

The terms *episodic memory* and *autobiographical memory* are often used interchangeably. However, some autobiographical information such as one's own name or date of birth has a context-free character. This type of autobiographical information is also known as personal semantic memory (Kopelman & Kapur, 2001).

The hierarchical organization of the memory systems may result from their ontogenetic and phylogenetic development, whereby episodic memory evolves latest (Tulving, 2002). According to some authors, episodic memory is largely re-

Episodic memory	Semantic memory	Perceptual memory	Priming	Procedural memory
"When I found that starfish during my last holiday in Greece"	The Atlantic Ocean is west of Europe			

Figure 6–1. Memory systems arranged by complexity from left to right (modified from Markowitsch, 2003); Examples illustrate remembering a holiday trip (episodic memory), knowing geographical facts (semantic memory), recognizing a spider from its perceptual features only (perceptual memory), easier and faster recognizing a melody from its parts following a previous presentation (priming), and executing motor procedures such as riding a bike and eating with a fork and knife (procedural memory).

stricted to humans (Suddendorf & Busby, 2003), whereas others suggest that some animals also exhibit "episodic-like memory" (Clayton, Bussey, & Dickinson, 2003). Lower memory systems can operate without higher systems. This assumption is confirmed in species that exhibit only lower memory systems such as perceptual memory, which can be tested by visual or auditory recognition paradigms (Aggleton & Pearce, 2001). Another example of the independent functioning of lower memory systems relates to human ontogenesis. Children by the age of about four years can acquire semantic knowledge about the world without, however, displaying episodic memory abilities. They are not yet able to retrieve temporally and contextually specific events from their personal past (Reese, 2002). Moreover, loss of episodic memory with spared semantic knowledge and perceptual memory is usually seen in patients with acquired brain lesions or neurodegenerative diseases (Vargha-Khadem, Gadian, & Mishkin, 2001).

Memory and the Brain

Stable long-term memory formation requires several steps of information processing. Prior to permanent storage, information first has to be registered at the sensory organs (*registration*) and initially preprocessed (*encoding*). Then, preprocessed information is embedded into existing information networks and associated with previous contents (*consolidation*). Once information is successfully consolidated, memory engrams are permanently stored (*storage*) and can, in principle, be retrieved later on (*retrieval*). Every time stored information is retrieved again, it will be altered (*re-encoding*). Thus, the initial memory trace undergoes considerable change through repeated retrieval (Tulving, 2001). Depending on the memory system in question, these processes rely on different brain regions. We focus on the higher-level episodic and semantic memory systems here.

Encoding and consolidation of episodic and semantic memory primarily rely on the integrity of so-called bottleneck structures of the limbic system (Brand & Markowitsch, 2003). Damage or dysfunction within these structures can strongly impair the acquisition of new memories (Corkin et al., 1997; Scotville & Milner, 1957; von Cramon, Markowitsch, & Schuri, 1993). Furthermore, prefrontal brain regions contribute to episodic (Köhler et al., 2004) and semantic memory encoding (Maguire & Frith, 2004). There is considerable debate about the duration of the consolidation process, ranging from minutes and days in animal experiments up to years and decades in human studies with healthy and brain damaged individuals (Dudai, 2004). The majority of information is stored in posterior cortical networks from which information can be retrieved. Damage to the posterior association cortex can lead to irreversible loss of formerly stored memory contents, as is seen in patients with dementia and hypoxia (Caine & Watson, 2000; Meguro et al., 2001). In these patients the amnesia has to be understood as resulting from permanent loss of the original memory engrams (see below). Memory retrieval heavily relies on (pre) frontal brain regions as is seen in functional neuroimaging studies with healthy subjects (Fletcher & Henson, 2001) as well as patients with frontal

lobe damage. Regions of the temporofrontal junction might be particularly important, as patients with combined lesions to frontal and anterior temporal lobes
have memory retrieval deficits (Kroll et al., 1997). Interconnected via the uncinate
fascicle, these regions may act as trigger structures to activate cortical storage networks (Markowitsch, in press). Analogous to the idea of reencoding, there is controversy about whether memories become labile and have to repeatedly consoli-
date every time they are activated (Dudai, 2004).

One of the most prominent features of autobiographical–episodic memory is
its emotional nature. The role of emotions in memory is of particular importance
since emotional connotation, if within certain limits (see below), usually enhances
subsequent memory processes (Ochsner & Schacter, 2000). Brain areas associated
with emotional processing and emotional memory include the amygdala, prefrontal
cortex (especially ventromedial prefrontal and orbitofrontal cortex), anterior cingulate gyrus, ventral striatum, septum/basal forebrain, and insula (Davidson &
Irwin, 1999). How do emotions modulate memories? It has been suggested that
the key brain region for this modulation is the amygdala, which possesses numerous systemic-hormonal afferents whose input is combined and distributed via
efferents to subcortical and cortical memory-relevant brain structures (e.g., the
hippocampal formation; Aggleton, 2000). Possibly, stress hormones or glucocorticoids mediate this memory modulation (McGaugh & Roozendaal, 2002). Glucocorticoids can selectively enhance amygdala-dependent emotional learning and
simultaneously impair hippocampus-dependent nonemotional learning (Buchanan
& Lovallo, 2001; McGaugh & Roozendaal, 2002). If stress hormone levels are
moderately elevated, one can observe memory-enhancing effects, whereas massive and long-lasting exhibition to glucocorticoids disturbs memory processes
(Kim & Yoon, 1998).

Though stress and glucocorticoids affect various kinds of memories, emotional autobiographical episodic memory is particularly vulnerable to stress-related
deteriorations. As will be described later in this chapter, effects of stress on autobiographical episodic memory are observed in several psychiatric disorders (e.g.,
posttraumatic stress disorder, [PTSD]). First, we will turn to autobiographical memory itself and to the question of how it can be disturbed in neurological disorders.

Autobiographical Disturbances: Memory, Emotion, and the Self

Though autobiographical memory comprises episodic and semantic aspects, the
term *autobiographical memory* most often denotes retrieval of personal past experiences. The vivid recollection of those memories is, at least partly, related to the
evocation of the formerly experienced emotional states (Dolan et al., 2000). To assign events to autobiographical memory, episodic memory contents have to be integrated with a sense of self-coherence and self-continuity across the individual
time axis reaching to the past as well as to the future (Larsen, Thompson, & Hansen,
1996). Due to its complex nature, autobiographical episodic memory involves broad
networks of interacting brain regions. In functional neuroimaging studies with

healthy subjects corresponding brain activation comprised a bilateral but predominantly left-hemispheric network of ventrolateral, dorsolateral and ventromedial prefrontal cortex, temporal pole, lateral and medial temporal cortex including hippocampal and parahippocampal complex, temporoparietal junction area as well as posterior cingulate retrosplenial cortex, and cerebellar regions (Maguire, 2001). Though some parts of this network may act centrally on memory processes (medial temporal cortex, hippocampal formation), others may integrate (poly)sensory, emotional, and memory-related information in a conjoint manner (posterior cingulate gyrus, posterior association cortex; Maddock, Garrett, & Buonocore, 2003). Further areas such as the ventromedial prefrontal cortex are most likely involved in self-referential processes (Johnson et al., 2002) during autobiographical retrieval.

The relationship between autobiographical memory and self is considered powerful, if not inseparable. According to Conway and Pleydell-Pearce (2000), autobiographical knowledge defines the range of goals of the self by which the construction of new autobiographical memories is reciprocally modulated. In their view, autobiographical memories are derived from experiences of previous goal attainment or failure, and retrieval or forgetting of personal events may serve to reduce perceived discrepancies in self. Wilson and Ross (2003) propose similar interdependencies. Their temporal self-appraisal theory claims a bidirectional relation between autobiographical memory and current identity. It suggests that autobiographical memory serves to enhance feelings of personal identity and consistency through time. The authors give evidence for self- and time-dependent memory biases and demonstrate how a tendency of perceived self-improvement over a lifetime can distort autobiographical recall (Karney & Frye, 2002). On the other hand, current self-views can be changed by the emotional connotation and temporal remoteness of retrieved autobiographical memories (Ross & Wilson, 2002).

We suggest that autobiographical disturbances can result from deficits in temporally integrated and contextually accurate recollection of former episodic memories, emotional disturbances, or self-related problems. Most often, however, they arise from combined deficits in the realms of memory, emotion, and self.

Autobiographical Disorders in Neurological Diseases

In neurological diseases autobiographical disorders are most often reported in the context of other memory deteriorations such as generally impaired episodic and semantic memory. In brain damaged patients the inability to acquire and retain new information is more frequently and consistently reported than is loss of remote memories (Kopelman, 2002). Therefore, neurologically caused deficits in remote autobiographical memory are usually accompanied by anterograde learning impairment. Discrete lesions to diencephalic and limbic regions can cause anterograde memory deficits, whereas retrograde amnesia mostly results from significant involvement of subcortical and cortical brain areas (Kapur, 1999). Accordingly, the majority of neurological patients suffering from combined retrograde and anterograde amnesia exhibit bilateral diencephalic, limbic, and/or neocortical brain damage. Examples for this condition are patients with neurodegenerative diseases such as patients with Alzheimer dementia (Greene & Hodges, 1996). Alzheimer dementia (AD) is usually accompanied by gradual loss of autobiographical memories, with retrieval deteriorations starting in more recent time periods and sparing childhood memories (Piolino et al., 2003). This amnesic pattern, also described as Ribot's law (Ribot, 1881), may be associated with accumulating damage to medial temporal cortical and other limbic areas, critical regions for acquiring new episodic memories (Braak & Braak, 1997). AD patients' pronounced autobiographical memory loss in more recent time periods might therefore reflect retrieval disruptions and accumulated anterograde episodic memory deficits (Greene & Hodges, 1996). Patients with so-called semantic dementia (SD) exhibit more anterior and lateral frontotemporal damage, predominantly in the left hemisphere. In contrast to AD patients, they show a reverse temporal gradient in that their autobiographical memory for very recent time periods is usually better preserved than is that for more remote memories (Graham et al., 2003). This sparing of recently acquired autobiographical memories might be due to the relative preservation of the hippocampal complex in SD allowing the encoding and—within a brief time window— the retrieval of new events, whereas language deterioration and deconstruction of more remote cortical memory stores abolish access to old memories (Hodges & Graham, 2001). Beyond core memory processes, deteriorations to other and probably more vital components of autobiographical memory such as visual imagery might lead to autobiographical disorders (Ogden, 1993). As was pointed out by Greenberg and Rubin (2003), memory-relevant brain structures such as anterior and medial temporal and (pre) frontal cortex may be necessary though not sufficient for the retrieval of remote memories. Instead Greenberg and Rubin (2003) suggested that only a combined lesion could cause autobiographical memory deficits. According to their metaanalysis of autobiographical memory loss following brain damage, the most consistently observed lesion pattern comprised lateral temporal brain regions storing semantic knowledge and posterior association cortices (e.g., occipital lobes) processing sensory features of episodic long-term memory information. The latter finding is in good accordance with Conway's notion of episodic memory, which he suggested relies primarily on retrieval of sensory perceptual details of previous events (Conway, 2001).

Instances of focal retrograde amnesia affecting autobiographical memory without additional anterograde amnesia are rare, and previous cases' associated brain damage differed largely. Some patients showed lesions to core memory structures such as thalamic nuclei (Miller et al., 2001), temporal lobes (Fujii et al., 1999), or temporo-frontal junction area (Markowitsch et al., 1993). In other patients brain damage mainly affected bilateral posterior association cortex (Carlesimo et al., 1998).

Confabulation, the production of fictitious narratives, can be understood as a specific form of autobiographical disorder. In neurological conditions, spontaneous confabulations are associated with memory deficits resulting from posterior orbitofrontal, basal forebrain, or limbic damage (Schnider et al., 2000). Confabulations might be based on a combination of amnesia and executive dysfunctions so that problems in source monitoring enhance the probability of these drastic memory errors (Johnson & Raye, 1998). However, these and related hypotheses about mechanisms of confabulation and false memories (Schacter, Norman, & Koutstaal, 1998) do not directly address one of the most striking features of confabulated narratives: their reference to actual autobiographical events in the patients' past. It has been reported that confabulating patients erroneously act with overlearned, stereotyped behaviors from their personal past (e.g., leaving the house at 8 o'clock in the morning to go to work) as though they were still functional in their current situational context (e.g., in the hospital) (Dalla Barba et al., 1997). These symptoms were described as an impaired awareness of the flow of time in memory or disintegration of the individual time axis resulting in autobiographical mistakes (Dalla Barba et al., 1997). Furthermore, confabulating patients have a subjective feeling of reality for their narrations (Schnider, 2003). As suggested by Schnider, these feelings might result from dysfunctional monitoring for ongoing reality, in that currently irrelevant memory traces are insufficiently suppressed so that memories are experienced with a sense of salience and current personal relevance. These emotional distortions correspond to the implicated lesions in confabulation (i.e., posterior orbitofrontal cortex, basal forebrain, and limbic and paralimbic structures), which also form part of the brain's intrinsic reward system (Pihan et al., 2004).

Taken together, in neurological diseases extensive loss of former autobiographical memories is usually accompanied by additional learning impairments. Corresponding brain damage most consistently points to bilateral implication of the posterior association cortex. Though this lesion pattern was also observed in a few single cases with selective retrograde amnesia, others had damage to the temporofrontal junction area. Mimicking autobiographical memory, confabulation may result from actual but temporally confused memory traces experienced with a feeling of reality. This deterioration is most consistently associated with posterior orbitofrontal cortex damage (see also Chapter 8 for a discussion of confabulations and the self).

Autobiographical Disorders in Psychiatric Diseases

Complete and irreversible loss of the entire autobiography is similarly rare in psychiatric diseases as it is in neurological disorders. However, autobiographical memory loss in psychiatric patients has been known for a long time (Ganser, 1898; Pick, 1884). Also more recently, dissociative disorders and psychogenic amnesia are characterized by this type of retrieval disruption (Markowitsch, 2003). Less global autobiographical disturbances are observed in schizophrenia, depression, and PTSD.

Schizophrenia is usually not associated with primary autobiographical memory loss. Characterized by a profound disorder of thought and reasoning accompanied by delusions and eventually hallucinations (American Psychiatric Association, 1994), the disorder is associated with structural or functional disturbances in prefrontal brain regions (Broadbelt, Byne, & Jones, 2002; Byne & Davis, 1999).

These pathologies correspond to frontal lobe-associated cognitive dysfunctions, which in the context of memory can affect autonoëtic remembering while sparing noëtic knowing (Sonntag et al., 2003). Autobiographical memory can as well be implicated (Elvevåg et al., 2003). Schizophrenic patients' recall of autobiographical memories lacks specific temporal and contextual details (Riutort et al., 2003). This kind of overgeneralized autobiographical memory is also observed in depression (see below). Deficient autobiographical memory in schizophrenia may further be related to theory of mind (ToM) abilities. As was investigated by Corcoran and Frith (2003), schizophrenic patients' autobiographical event memory was corre-lated with their ToM performance, that is, the capacity to infer one's own or other people's mental states, intentions, and attitudes, and is considered crucial for so-cial skills (Baron-Cohen, 1995). Corcoran and Frith suggested that schizophrenic patients may be unable to apply the necessary context for retrieval of specific so-cial information, be it explicitly autobiographical, as in personal events, or not, as in ToM situations. Thus, in schizophrenia autobiographical episodic memory may lack the contextual and emotional details of healthy subjects' memories.

Overgeneralization of autobiographical events is also observed in depressive patients. Instead of reporting temporally and contextually distinctive episodes, they tend to give categoric descriptions of summarized repeated occasions (Barnhofer et al., 2002; de Decker et al., 2003). This retrieval style is further associated with poor recovery from the disease (Brittlebank et al., 1993). A possible underlying mechanism is described by Williams (1996) and referred to as "mnemonic inter-lock." He suggests that over-general autobiographical retrieval is encouraged by a ruminative self-focus that reciprocally fosters over-general retrieval. In depression this style is assumed to develop early in life so that avoidance of conscious re-collection becomes an automated habit. Furthermore, according to Williams, de-pressive patients show a tendency to retrieve negative self-referential categoric descriptions (e.g., "I have always failed"). If potentially negative retrieval cues are encountered, these categoric descriptions are triggered in an automated way. Re-lated and frequently used self-descriptions are elicited only within this level of de-scription stage (e.g., "I used to fail at school," "I never had friends," etc.), meaning that retrieval moves across the hierarchy rather than down to more specific levels. Thus, over-general memory emerges from a blockade or truncation (mnemonic in-terlock) of the search for specific events and instead results in an over-elaboration of self-related general categories. Emotionally motivated over-stable self-views may prevent autonoëtic remembering of autobiographical episodes and instead fa-cilitate noëtic retrieval of categoric events. How does this tendency develop in child-hood and later on? One of the most likely triggers is the experience of trauma.

A large body of evidence emphasizes the close relationship between stress and depression (Holsboer, 2001), and PTSD patients show a heightened prevalence of comorbid depression (Breslau et al., 2000; Franklin & Zimmerman, 2001). On the neurological level the mediating factor between both diseases may be a dysregula-tion of glucocorticoid signaling. As glucocorticoids are required for reliable mem-ory formation and retrieval, especially if the memory contents are of an emotional nature (see above), hypersecretion of glucocorticoids and reduced responsiveness to glucocorticoids as seen in depression or hypocortisolism as in PTSD (Raison & Miller, 2003) may correspond to deficits in encoding and retrieving specific autobiographical events. Directly comparing the impacts of traumatic experiences versus depressive symptoms on over-general autobiographical retrieval, some studies suggest a major influence of trauma (de Decker et al., 2003; Harvey, Bryant, & Dang, 1998). Recently, Hermans and colleagues (2004) found that autobiographical memory specificity in depressed patients was unrelated to depression severity but significantly correlated to the presence and severity of physical abuse. Given the high comorbidity of PTSD with depression it can therefore be reasoned that experience of trauma might be the primary mediator of over-generalized autobiographical memory, at least in depression (but see Wessel et al., 2001).

Trauma and depression have both been identified as possible triggers of more global autobiographical memory loss, as is seen in dissociative disorders and psychogenic amnesia (Markowitsch, 1999). Dissociative amnesia, dissociative fugue, and dissociative identity disorder occur after the experience of severe psychological trauma or extremely stressful situations and time periods (American Psychiatric Association, 1994). Following van der Kolk (1994) the mechanism of dissociation enables an individual to fragment, de-realize, and depersonalize traumatic experiences from current self-awareness. This can be the case during extremely traumatic experiences. However, in patients with dissociative disorders this pattern of separating certain experiences from ongoing self-awareness remains stable in everyday life. Acute dissociative reactions to a trauma, as, for example, in acute stress disorder, are predictive of later development of PTSD (Birmes et al., 2003; Marshall & Schell, 2002). Therefore, dissociation—though a powerful psychological protection in the acute situation—is disadvantageous as a long-term stress coping strategy. Not all cases of global autobiographical memory loss without structural brain damage can be classified as dissociative disorders. However, as in other psychogenic amnesias, recent or childhood trauma and/or concurrent depression have been reported (Markowitsch, 1999, 2003).

Convergence of Organic and Psychological Mechanisms in Psychogenic Amnesia

Psychogenic amnesia, more neutrally labeled as functional amnesia, is characterized by loss of autobiographical memory, sometimes also extending to impersonal semantic and procedural memory. Retrieval deficits can extend to the entire previous life or consist of only specific, often trauma-related information and time periods (Markowitsch, 1999). The unequivocal distinction between organic or psychogenic etiology for psychogenic amnesia can be doubted for several reasons. As was pointed out by Kopelman (2002) and Markowitsch (1996), somatic and psychiatric problems commonly co-occur in all forms of selective retrograde amnesia. For instance, some previous cases of psychogenic amnesia had detectable brain pathology, which, however, was insufficient to account for the severity of the retrieval deficits (Costello et al., 1998; Kapur, 2000). Thus, even in the presence of brain pathology, psychological processes may influence onset of, severity of, and recovery from amnesic symptoms. Second, in the absence of structural brain damage, resting state functional brain disturbances were reported in some patients implicating the temporal lobes (Nakamura et al., 2002; Sellal et al., 2002), frontotemporal junction (Markowitsch, Calabrese et al., 1997), or wider damage including frontal and/or posterior association cortex (Lucchelli, Muggia, & Spinnler, 1995; Markowitsch et al., 1998). In all these cases a part of the distributed network of brain areas relevant for autobiographical memory retrieval (see above) was implicated despite the fact that they did not show structural brain damage. What happens if these patients attempt to access their forgotten past? A few functional neuroimaging studies have addressed this question. In this regard, brain activation of patient N.N. (Markowitsch, Fink et al., 1997), who suffered from autobiographical episodic retrograde amnesia following a fugue, was studied with water positron emission tomography (^{15}O-PET) while he attempted to retrieve autobiographical episodes. N.N. showed a largely left-lateralized activation pattern of frontotemporal regions compared to primarily right-hemispheric activity seen in healthy control subjects (Fink et al., 1996). In the healthy subjects a lateralization to the left hemisphere was detected during retrieval of semantic information. It was therefore suggested that N.N. processed his autobiography as if it was personally irrelevant semantic information. This corresponded to an emotional detachment from personal memories that were obvious on the behavioral level (Markowitsch, Fink et al., 1997). On the other hand, an overly emotional processing of remote memories was hypothesized in the psychogenic amnesia patient of Yasuno et al. (2000). In ^{15}O-PET, their patient processed semantic remote information (famous faces) with enhanced activation in the right prefrontal cortex and right anterior medial temporal regions including the amygdala as well as decreased activity in the right anterior cingulate. In contrast, healthy control subjects showed bilateral hippocampal activity and, corresponding to the semantic nature of the stimuli, more left lateralised prefrontal activation. Due to the enhanced amygdala activity, the authors assumed an overly emotional and especially negatively valenced processing of semantic remote information in their patient. Moreover, after recovery from psychogenic amnesia, the patient's right hemispheric limbic and cortical hyperactivity during this task resolved to normal at a one-year follow-up examination (see also case A.M.N. of Markowitsch et al., 1998; Markowitsch et al., 2000). One further patient, studied by Costello and coworkers (1998), could be considered as well. This case is somewhat different from the aforementioned patients, since the onset of his amnesia was clearly an organic disease (stroke) and he sustained hemorrhage to the left dorsolateral prefrontal cortex. However, the patient also presented with signs of psychogenic rather than organic retrograde retrograde amnesia. During retrieval attempt of remote versus newly acquired autobiographical episodes or impersonal information, he showed increased activity in precuneus and decreased activity in right posterior ventrolateral frontal cortex and left superior frontal cortex in the region of the structural damage. Costello and colleagues suggested that the retrieval deficit had been caused by a lack of activation in the right ventral frontal cortex, corresponding with deficient recursive self-cueing during autobiographical retrieval. Levine and coworkers (1998) gave corresponding evidence for this region to be critical in a neurologically caused autobiographical disorder. Their patient M.L. had sustained severe head trauma resulting in a focal brain lesion restricted to right ventral prefrontal cortex and underlying white matter connecting frontal inferior frontal cortex and anterior temporal pole. Patient M.L. showed selective impairment of self-monitoring functions and autonoëtic memory retrieval.

Conclusion

Autobiographical memory is one of the most complex functions to be investigated with functional neuroimaging techniques. This complexity is embodied in the large network of activated brain regions during autobiographical memory retrieval, which involves core memory regions (the hippocampal formation), areas of self-related processing (medial prefrontal cortex), and those of sensory-emotional integration (posterior association cortex and posterior cingulate gyrus). Given that effective recollection of autobiographical memories requires all of these areas, autobiographical disorders in neurological and psychiatric populations rarely correspond to circumscribed regions in the brain. Instead, autobiographical disorders can result from lesions or functional disturbances that disrupt information processing within this distributed network of brain areas. Dramatic cases of autobiographical memory loss, as in psychogenic amnesia, provide evidence of how severe emotional stress or self-related problems can correspond to a total blockade of memory contents. A few previous cases of psychogenic and focal amnesia showed that—in neurological and in psychiatric conditions—key regions for autobiographical retrieval may overlap (e.g., right ventral frontal cortex). Moreover, a functional impairment of those and other emotion- and self-related regions was observed during the retrieval attempt of irretrievable autobiographical memories. Though this evidence remains correlational, these single cases provide the best support for the assumption that autobiographical memory, emotion, and self-related processing are intricately connected, both behaviorally and neurologically.

References

Aggleton, J.P. (2000). *The Amygdala: A Functional Analysis.* Oxford: Oxford University Press.

Aggleton, J.P. & Pearce, J.M. (2001). Neural systems underlying episodic memory: insights from animal research. *Philosophical Transactions of the Royal Society of London—Series B: Biological Sciences, 356,* 1467–1482.

American Psychiatric Association (1994). *Diagnostic and Statistical Manual of Mental Disorders,* 4th ed. Washington DC: American Psychiatric Association.

Baddeley, A. (2000). Short-term and working memory. In: E. Tulving & F.I.M. Craik (Eds.) *The Oxford Handbook of Memory* (pp. 77–92). New York: Oxford University Press.

Barnhofer, T., de Jong-Meyer, R., Kleinpass, A., & Nikesch, S. (2002). Specificity of auto-biographical memories in depression: An analysis of retrieval processes in a think-aloud task. *British Journal of Clinical Psychology, 41,* 411–416.

Baron-Cohen, S. (1995). *Mindblindness.* Cambridge, MA: MIT Press.

Birmes, P., Brunet, A., Carreras, D., Ducasse, J.L., Charlet, J.P., Lauque, D., Sztulman, H., & Schmitt, L. (2003). The predictive power of peritraumatic dissociation and acute stress symptoms for posttraumatic stress symptoms: A three-month prospective study. *American Journal of Psychiatry, 160,* 1337–1339.

Braak, H. & Braak, E. (1997). Frequency of stages of Alzheimer-related lesions in different age categories. *Neurobiology of Aging, 18,* 351–357.

Brand, M. & Markowitsch, H.J. (2003). The principle of bottleneck structures. In: R.H. Kluwe, G. Lüer & F. Rösler (Eds.) *Principles of Learning and Memory* (pp. 172–184). Basel: Birkhäuser.

Breslau, N., Davis, G.C., Peterson, E.L., & Schultz, L.R. (2000). A second look at co-morbidity in victims of trauma: The posttraumatic stress disorder-major depression connection. *Biological Psychiatry, 48,* 902–909.

Brittlebank, A.D., Scott, J., Williams, J.M., & Ferrier, I.N. (1993). Autobiographical memory in depression: State or trait marker? *British Journal of Psychiatry, 162,* 118–121.

Broadbelt, K., Byne, W., & Jones, L.B. (2002). Evidence for a decrease in basilar dendrites of pyramidal cells in schizophrenic medial prefrontal cortex. *Schizophrenia Research, 58,* 75–81.

Buchanan, T.W. & Lovallo, W.R. (2001). Enhanced memory for emotional material following stress-level cortisol treatment in humans. *Psychoneuroendocrinology, 26,* 307–317.

Byne, W. & Davis, K.L. (1999). The role of prefrontal cortex in the dopaminergic dysregulation of schizophrenia. *Biological Psychiatry, 45,* 657–659.

Caine, D. & Watson, J.D. (2000). Neuropsychological and neuropathological sequelae of cerebral anoxia: A critical review. *Journal of the International Neuropsychological Society, 6,* 86–99.

Carlesimo, G.A., Sabbadini, M., Loasses, A., & Caltagirone, C. (1998). Analysis of the memory impairment in a post-encephalitic patient with focal retrograde amnesia. *Cortex, 34,* 449–460.

Clayton, N.S., Bussey, T.J., & Dickinson, A. (2003). Can animals recall the past and plan for the future? *Nature Neuroscience Reviews, 4,* 685–691.

Conway, M.A. (2001). Sensory-perceptual episodic memory and its context: Autobiographical memory. *Philosophical Transactions of the Royal Society of London-Series B: Biological Sciences, 356,* 1375–1384.

Conway, M.A. & Pleydell-Pearce, C.W. (2000). The construction of autobiographical memories in the self-memory system. *Psychological Review, 107,* 261–288.

Corcoran, R. & Frith, C.D. (2003). Autobiographical memory and theory of mind: Evidence of a relationship in schizophrenia. *Psychological Medicine, 33,* 897–905.

Corkin, S., Amaral, D.G., Gonzalez, R.G., Johnson, K.A., & Hyman, B.T. (1997). H.M.'s medial temporal lobe lesion: Findings from magnetic resonance imaging. *Journal of Neuroscience, 17,* 3964–3979.

Costello, A., Fletcher, P.C., Dolan, R.J., Frith, C.D., & Shallice, T. (1998). The origins of forgetting in a case of isolated retrograde amnesia following a hemorrhage: Evidence from functional imaging. *Neurocase, 4,* 437–446.

Cowan, N. (1984). On short and long auditory stores. *Psychological Bulletin, 96,* 341–370.

Dalla Barba, G.F., Cappelletti, J.Y., Signorini, M., & Denes, G. (1997). Confabulation: Remembering 'another' past, planning 'another' future. *Neurocase, 3,* 425–436.

Davidson, R.J. & Irwin, W. (1999). The functional neuroanatomy of emotion and affective style. *Trends in Cognitive Sciences, 3,* 11–21.

de Decker, A., Hermans, D., Raes, F., & Eelen, P. (2003). Autobiographical memory specificity and trauma in inpatient adolescents. *Journal of Clinical Child and Adolescent Psychology, 32,* 22–31.

Dolan, R.J., Lane, R., Chua, P., & Fletcher, P. (2000). Dissociable temporal lobe activations during emotional episodic memory retrieval. *Neuroimage, 11,* 203–209.

Dudai, Y. (2004). The neurobiology of consolidations, or, how stable is the engram? *Annual Review of Psychology, 55,* 51–86.

Elvevåg, B., Kerbs, K.M., Malley, J.D., Seeley, E., & Goldberg, T.E. (2003). Autobiographical memory in schizophrenia: An examination of the distribution of memories. *Neuropsychology, 17,* 402–409.

Fink, G.R., Markowitsch, H.J., Reinkemeier, M., Bruckbauer, T., Kessler, J., & Heiss, W.-D. (1996). Cerebral representation of one's own past: Neural networks involved in autobiographical memory. *Journal of Neuroscience, 16,* 4275–4282.

Fletcher, P.C. & Henson, R.N.A. (2001). Frontal lobes and human memory: Insights from functional imaging. *Brain, 124,* 849–881.

Franklin, C.L. & Zimmerman, M. (2001). Posttraumatic stress disorder and major depressive disorder: Investigating the role of overlapping symptoms in diagnostic comorbidity. *Journal of Nervous & Mental Disease, 189,* 548–551.

Fujii, T., Yamadori, A., Endo, K., Suzuki, K., & Fukatsu, R. (1999). Disproportionate retrograde amnesia in a patient with herpes simplex encephalitis. *Cortex, 35,* 599–614.

Ganser, S.J. (1898). Ueber einen eigenartigen hysterischen Dämmerzustand. *Archiv für Psychiatrie und Nervenkrankheiten, 30,* 633–640.

Graham, K.S., Kropelnicki, A., Goldman, W.P., & Hodges, J.R. (2003). Two further investigations of autobiographical memory in semantic dementia. *Cortex, 39,* 729–750.

Greenberg, D.L. & Rubin, D.C. (2003). The neuropsychology of autobiographical memory. *Cortex, 39,* 687–728.

Greene, J.D. & Hodges, J.R. (1996). The fractionation of remote memory. Evidence from a longitudinal study of dementia of Alzheimer type. *Brain, 119,* 129–142.

Harvey, A.G., Bryant, R.A., & Dang, S.T. (1998). Autobiographical memory in acute stress disorder. *Journal of Consulting and Clinical Psychology, 66,* 500–506.

Hermans, D., Van Den Broeck, K., Belis, G., Raes, F., Pieters, G., & Eelen, P. (2004). Trauma and autobiographical memory specificity in depressed inpatients. *Behaviour Research and Therapy, 42,* 775–789.

Hodges, J.R. & Graham, K.S. (2001). Episodic memory: Insights from semantic dementia. *Philosophical Transactions of the Royal Society of London-Series B: Biological Sciences, 356,* 1423–1434.

Holsboer, F. (2001). Stress, hypercortisolism and corticosteroid receptors in depression: Implications for therapy. *Journal of Affective Disorders, 62,* 77–91.

Johnson, M.K. & Raye, C.L. (1998). False memories and confabulation. *Trends in Cognitive Sciences, 4,* 137–145.

Johnson, S.C., Baxter, L.C., Wilder, L.S., Pipe, J.G., Heiserman, J.E., & Prigatano, G.P. (2002). Neural correlates of self-reflection. *Brain, 125,* (1808–1814).

Kapur, N. (1999). Syndromes of retrograde amnesia: A conceptual and empirical synthesis. *Psychological Bulletin, 6,* 800–825.

Kapur, N. (2000). Focal retrograde amnesia and the attribution of causality: An exceptionally benign commentary. *Cognitive Neuropsychology, 17,* 623–637.

Karney, B.R. & Frye, N.E. (2002). "But we've been getting better lately": Comparing

prospective and retrospective views of relationship development. *Journal of Personality and Social Psychology, 82,* 222–238.

Kim, J.J. & Yoon, K.S. (1998). Stress: Metaplastic effects in the hippocampus. *Trends in
Neurosciences, 21,* 505–509.

Köhler, S., Paus, T., Buckner, R.L., & Milner, B. (2004). Effects of left inferior prefrontal
stimulation on episodic memory formation: A two-stage fMRI-rTMS study. *Journal of
Cognitive Neuroscience, 16,* 178–188.

Kopelman, M.D. (2002). Disorders of memory. *Brain, 125,* 2152–2190.

Kopelman, M.D. & Kapur, N. (2001). The loss of episodic memories in retrograde amnesia:
Single-case and group studies. *Philosophical Transactions of the Royal Society of London-
Series B: Biological Sciences, 356,* 1409–1421.

Kroll, N.E., Markowitsch, H.J., Knight, R.T., & von Cramon, D.Y. (1997). Retrieval of old
memories: The temporofrontal hypothesis. *Brain, 120,* 1377–1399.

Larsen, S.F., Thompson, C.P., & Hansen, T. (1996). Time in autobiographical memory. In:
D.C. Rubin (Ed.) *Remembering Our Past* (pp. 129–156). New York: Cambridge University Press.

Levine, B., Black, S.E., Cabeza, R., Sinden, M., Mcintosh, A.R., Toth, J.P., Tulving, E., &
Stuss, D.T. (1998). Episodic memory and the self in a case of isolated retrograde amnesia. *Brain, 121,* 1951–1973.

Lucchelli, F., Muggia, S., & Spinnler, H. (1995). The "Petites Madeleines" phenomenon in
two amnesic patients: Sudden recovery of forgotten memories. *Brain, 118,* 167–183.

Maddock, R.J., Garrett, A.S., & Buonocore, M.H. (2003). Posterior cingulate cortex activation by emotional words: fMRI evidence from a valence decision task. *Human Brain
Mapping, 18,* 30–41.

Maguire, E.A. (2001). Neuroimaging studies of autobiographical event memory. *Philosophical Transactions of the Royal Society of London, Biological Sciences, 356,* 1441–1451.

Maguire, E.A. & Frith, C.D. (2004). The brain network associated with acquiring semantic
knowledge. *Neuroimage, 22,* 171–178.

Markowitsch, H.J. (1996). Organic and psychogenic retrograde amnesia: Two sides of the
same coin? *Neurocase, 2,* 357–371.

Markowitsch, H.J. (1999). Functional neuroimaging correlates of functional amnesia. *Memory, 5/6,* 561–583.

Markowitsch, H.J. (2003). Psychogenic amnesia. *Neuroimage, 20,* S132–S138.

Markowitsch, H.J. (in press). The neuroanatomy of memory. In: P.W. Halligan & D.T. Wade
(Eds.) *The Effectiveness of Rehabilitation for Cognitive Deficits.* Oxford: Oxford University Press.

Markowitsch, H.J., Calabrese, P., Fink, G.R., Durwen, H.F., Kessler, J., Härting, C., König,
M., Mirzaian, E.B., Heiss, W.-D., Heuser, L., & Gehlen, W. (1997). Impaired episodic
memory retrieval in a case of probable psychogenic amnesia. *Psychiatry Research:
Neuroimaging, 74,* 119–126.

Markowitsch, H.J., Calabrese, P., Liess, J., Haupts, M., Durwen, H.F., & Gehlen, W. (1993).
Retrograde amnesia after traumatic injury of the fronto-temporal cortex. *Journal of
Neurology, Neurosurgery, and Psychiatry, 56,* 988–992.

Markowitsch, H.J., Fink, G.R., Thöne, A., Kessler, J., & Heiss, W.-D. (1997). A PET study
of persistent psychogenic amnesia covering the whole life span. *Cognitive Neuropsychiatry, 2,* 135–158.

Markowitsch, H.J., Kessler, J., Van der Ven, C., Weber-Luxenburger, G., Albers, M., &
Heiss, W.D. (1998). Psychic trauma causing grossly reduced brain metabolism and cognitive deterioration. *Neuropsychologia, 36,* 77–82.

Markowitsch, H.J., Kessler, J., Weber-Luxenburger, G., Van der Ven, C., Albers, M., & Heiss, W.D. (2000). Neuroimaging and behavioral correlates of recovery from mnestic block syndrome and other cognitive deteriorations. *Neuropsychiatry, Neuropsychology & Behavioral Neurology, 13,* 60–66.

Marshall, G.N. & Schell, T.L. (2002). Reappraising the link between peritraumatic dissociation and PTSD symptom severity: Evidence from a longitudinal study of community violence survivors. *Journal of Abnormal Psychology, 111,* 626–636.

McGaugh, J.L. & Roozendaal, B. (2002). Role of adrenal stress hormones in forming lasting memories in the brain. *Current Opinion in Neurobiology, 12,* 205–210.

Meguro, K., LeMestric, C., Landeau, B., Desgranges, B., Eustache, F., & Baron, J.C. (2001). Relations between hypometabolism in the posterior association neocortex and hippocampal atrophy in Alzheimer's disease: A PET/MRI correlative study. *Journal of Neurology, Neurosurgery, & Psychiatry, 71,* 315–321.

Miller, G.A. (1956). The magical number seven plus minus two. Some limits on our capacity for processing information. *Psychological Review, 63,* 244–257.

Miller, L.A., Caine, D., Harding, A., Thompson, E.J., Large, M., & Watson, J.D. (2001). Right medial thalamic lesion causes isolated retrograde amnesia. *Neuropsychologia, 39,* 1037–1046.

Nakamura, H., Kunori, Y., Mori, K., Nakaaki, S., Yoshida, S., & Hamanaka, T. (2002). Two cases of functional focal retrograde amnesia with impairment of object use. *Cortex, 38,* 613–622.

Ochsner, K.N. & Schacter, D.L. (2000). A social cognitive neuroscience approach to emotion and memory. In: J.C. Borod (Ed.) *The Neuropsychology of Emotion. Series in Affective Science* (pp. 163–193). Oxford: Oxford University Press.

Ogden, J.A. (1993). Visual object agnosia, prosopagnosia, achromatopsia, loss of visual imagery, and autobiographical amnesia following recovery from cortical blindness: Case M.H. *Neuropsychologia, 31,* 571–589.

Pick, A. (1884). Vom Bewusstsein in Zuständen sogenannter Bewusstlosigkeit. *Archiv für Psychiatrie und Nervenkrankheiten, 15,* 202–223.

Pihan, H., Gutbrod, K., Baas, U., & Schnider, A. (2004). Dopamine inhibition and the adaptation of behavior to ongoing reality. *Neuroreport, 15,* 709–712.

Piolino, P., Desgranges, B., Belliard, S., Matuszewski, V., Lalevee, C., De la Sayette, V., & Eustache, F. (2003). Autobiographical memory and autonoetic consciousness: Triple dissociation in neurodegenerative diseases. *Brain, 126,* 2203–2219.

Raison, C.L. & Miller, A.H. (2003). When not enough is too much: The role of insufficient glucocorticoid signaling in the pathophysiology of stress-related disorders. *American Journal of Psychiatry, 160,* 1554–1565.

Reese, E. (2002). Social factors in the development of autobiographical memory: The state of the art. *Social Development, 11,* 124–142.

Ribot, T. (1881). *Les maladies de la memoire.* Paris: Baillière.

Riutort, M., Cuervo, C., Danion, J.M., Peretti, C.S., & Salame, P. (2003). Reduced levels of specific autobiographical memories in schizophrenia. *Psychiatry Research, 117,* 35–45.

Ross, M. & Wilson, A. E. (2002). It feels like yesterday: Self-esteem, valence of personal past experiences, and judgments of subjective distance. *Journal of Personality and Social Psychology, 82,* 792–803.

Schacter, D.L., Norman, K.A., & Koutstaal, W. (1998). The cognitive neuroscience of constructive memory. *Annual Review of Psychology, 49,* 289–318.

Schnider, A. (2003). Spontaneous confabulation and the adaptation of thought to ongoing reality. *Nature Neuroscience Reviews, 4,* 662–671.

Schnider, A., Ptak, R., von Daniken, C., & Remonda, L. (2000). Recovery from spontaneous confabulations parallels recovery of temporal confusion in memory. *Neurology,*
55, 74–83.

Scoville, W.B. & Milner, B. (1957). Loss of recent memory after bilateral hippocampal lesions. *Journal of Neurology, Neurosurgery, and Psychiatry, 20,* 11–21.

Sellal, F., Manning, L., Seegmuller, C., Scheiber, C., & Schoenfelder, F. (2002). Pure retrograde amnesia following mild head trauma: A neuropsychological and metabolic
study. *Cortex, 38,* 499–509.

Sonntag, P., Gokalsing, E., Olivier, C., Robert, P., Burglen, F., Kauffmann-Muller, F.,
Huron, C., Salame, P., & Danion, J.M. (2003). Impaired strategic regulation of contents
of conscious awareness in schizophrenia. *Consciousness and Cognition, 12,* 190–200.

Suddendorf, T. & Busby, J. (2003). Mental time travel in animals? *Trends in Cognitive Sci-*
ences, 7, 391–396.

Tulving, E. (2001). Episodic memory and common sense: How far apart? *Philosophical*
Transactions of the Royal Society of London, Biological Sciences, 356, 1505–1515.

Tulving, E. (2002). Episodic memory: From mind to brain. *Annual Review of Psychology,*
53, 1–25.

van der Kolk, B.A. (1994). The body keeps the score: Memory and the evolving psychobiology of posttraumatic stress. *Harvard Review of Psychiatry, 1,* 253–265.

Vargha-Khadem, F., Gadian, D.G., & Mishkin, M. (2001). Dissociations in cognitive memory: The syndrome of developmental amnesia. *Philosophical Transactions of the Royal*
Society of London-Series B: Biological Sciences, 356, 1435–1440.

von Cramon, D.Y., Markowitsch, H.J., & Schuri, U. (1993). The possible contribution of
the septal region to memory. *Neuropsychologia, 31,* 159–180.

Wessel, I., Meeren, M., Peeters, F., Arntz, A., & Merckelbach, H. (2001). Correlates of autobiographical memory specificity: The role of depression, anxiety and childhood trauma.
Behaviour Research and Therapy, 39, 409–421.

Williams, J.M.G. (1996). Depression and the specificity of autobiographcial memory. In:
D.C. Rubin (Ed.) *Remembering Our Past* (pp. 244–267). New York: Cambridge University Press.

Wilson, A.E. & Ross, M. (2003). The identity function of autobiographical memory: Time
is on our side. *Memory, 11,* 137–149.

Yasuno, F., Nishikawa, T., Nakagawa, Y., Ikejiri, Y., Tokunaga, H., Mizuta, I., Shinozaki,
K., Hashikawa, K., Sugita, Y., Nishimura, T., & Takeda, M. (2000). Functional anatomical study of psychogenic amnesia. *Psychiatry Research: Neuroimaging, 99,* 43–57.

Yoshino, R. (1993). Magical numbers of human short-term memory: Efficient designs of
biological memory systems? *Behaviormetrika, 20,* 171–186.

7

Body Image and the Self

GEORG GOLDENBERG

Intuitively an intimate link exists between knowing oneself and knowing one's body. Two central aspects of the self are mirrored by the image of one's body: one's body is an indivisible entity that remains constant when the outer world changes, and one's body shares basic features with the bodies of other human beings. Thus, the body image reflects two essential properties of the self: it is a unique entity different from the external world, and it is one instance of universal human nature.

The uniqueness and universality of one's body are recognized by most persons without a need for inference or reasoning. The immediacy of their recognition makes them candidates for being rooted in dedicated, perhaps even innately predetermined, neural structures (Melzack, 1990). In this chapter I will call into doubt this conclusion by demonstrating that the body image is the fragile result of fleeting integration of current perceptual inputs, prior experience, and culturally acquired knowledge. The argument will be based on disorders of the body image resulting from either experimental manipulations or brain damage.

The chapter focuses on two topics relevant to the two basic properties outlined above: Awareness of the current configuration and permanent structure of one's own body and knowledge of the structure of human bodies in general. Both of these topics concern the conscious perception of one's body. Creation of a conscious image of one's body does not exhaust the ways in which the brain receives and processes information about the structure of the body: The brain needs constant monitoring and computation of the current body configuration for the control of goal-directed motor actions. The body representations needed for motor control are embedded in the mechanisms of sensorimotor coordination and usually do not enter consciousness as an explicit image. In this chapter dissociations between implicit processing of body-related information and the conscious body image will be repeatedly discussed for clarification of the purposes and limits of the conscious body image.

The the concept of the body image has a long and controversial history in clinical neurology and neuropsychology. It has been invoked to explain a wide array of neurological, psychiatric, and psychosomatic symptoms (Schilder, 1935; Critchley, 1950; Poeck & Orgass, 1971; Denes, 1990). As a step toward classification of the bewilderingly manifold manifestations of body-related symptoms, it has been proposed to retain the term *body image* for the conscious image of one's body and to use *body schema* for representations implicit in motor coordination (Gallagher, 1986). I will use *body image* and *image of one's body* only for the conscious mental image of one's body.

Knowing One's Own Body

Disorders of sensing and knowing one's own body can concern three aspects of the body image: the current configuration of the body parts, the permanent structure of the body, and the distinction between one's own body and external objects.

The Current Configuration of One's Body

The neurological term for perception of one's own body is *proprioception.* Proprioception derives from coordination of multiple sensory channels, most of which are also employed for perceiving external objects:

For persons with intact vision, visual experience is the predominant sense for perceiving the spatial structure of external objects, whereas direct sight of one's own body is limited to the limbs and the lower front portion of the trunk. However, mirrors, photography, and electronic recording provide ample opportunities for seeing one's own body as completely as it can be seen by anyone else.

Somatosensory input from cutaneous surface receptors subserves primarily recognition of external stimuli but can also be analyzed with respect to their localization on the body. One can also touch oneself. Tactual exploration of one's own body differs from exploration of external objects by the coincidence of tactile sensations from touching and touched body parts. This coincidence can serve as a clue for recognizing one's own body as being the object of touch.

Somatosensory information from mechanoreceptors in deep skin layers, joint capsules, tendons, and muscles are exclusively proprioceptive. Data from the physiology of motor control and perception suggest that in addition to this feedback from moving body parts, "efference copies" of motor commands are monitored (van Holst & Mittelstaedt, 1950; Wolpert, Ghahramani, & Jordan, 1995). In routine behavior we do not become aware of motor commands as differing from actual movement, but motor commands may rise to consciousness when there is discrepancy between motor command and execution (Gandevia, 1982; Jeannerod, 1997). Further proprioceptive input is provided by vestibular sensations. They signal the force and direction of gravity and hence the static position of the body as well as accelerations of the body in any axis of space.

There is thus a rank order of the specifity of different sensory channels for body perception. According to this order one might expect awareness of the current configuration of one's own body to rely most heavily on afferences from joints and muscles, less on tactile, and least on visual information, but it seems that our brains use other heuristics for creating the body image.

Visual Capture

Seeing the touch of a rubber or plaster hand simultaneously with feeling touch of the subject's own hand hidden from view leads to the illusion that the external hand is the subject's own. The illusion is contingent upon strict synchrony between seen and felt touch and upon placement of the external hand in a position that the subject's own hand could possibly assume without violating anatomical constraints (Tastevin, 1937; Botvinick & Cohen, 1998; Pavani, Spence, & Driver, 2000).

The dominance of visual over proprioceptive location of sensations has been termed *visual capture* (Tastevin, 1937; Rock & Harris, 1967). Its power has been demonstrated impressively in patients with left-side hemineglect. These patients correctly report isolated touch of the left side of their body but ignore it when there is simultaneous touch of the right side, a phenomenon known as tactile extinction. Vision of left-sided touch alleviates and vision of right-sided touch augments the degree of left-sided extinction. This effect is not simply due to an attraction of attention to the side where the visual stimulus appears, because a visual stimulus presented nearby, but unequivocally external to, the touched limb has no effect. The effect can, however, be obtained by seeing the touch of a rubber hand (Farnè et al., 2000; Ladavas et al., 2000).

Before accepting the counterintuitive conclusion that the brain gives more weight to vision than to proprioception for determining the configuration of the body, one must consider an apparently minor detail of these experiments: The subjects's hands remained in a static position, whereas the illusions depended on a strict synchrony between the temporal course of seen and felt touch. This constellation poses a double disadvantage for proprioceptive information: First, this information comes from muscles, tendons, joints and, in the case of motor intentions, efference copies, all tuned to detect and control limb movements. Presumably, when the limbs rest in a static position, input from these sources is at a minimal resting level and does not attract much attention. Second, even if such information arrives, it does not change over time and hence neither corresponds with nor overtly conflicts with the synchrony of vision and touch.

Indeed, visual capture does meet resistance when the limb is moving, at least when movements are active and hence accompanied by efference copies of motor intentions. Using a mirror makes it possible to explore the conflicts between active movement and visual feedback. If the mirror is placed sagitally (perpendicular to the front of the body) at body midline and one looks into it from one side, vision of the opposite hand is replaced by the reflected image of the hand on that side. If this hand is moved, a symmetrical movement of the hidden opposite hand will be shown regardless of what it is actually doing. A compelling feeling of moving the hidden hand in accordance with its pretended image can arise when it is immobile, particularly when both hands hold movable objects of the same shape (e. g., rings hanging on a horizontal stick), removing discrepancies in the temporal modulation of tactile sensations by contact of the moving or resting hand with the table. If the hidden hand performs active movements incompatible with the mirror image, one feels a conflict between intention and execution rather than an uncontradicted feeling of moving the hand in accordance with its visual appearance (Gregory, 1997; Fink et al., 1999), presumably because visual capture cannot override the discrepancy between the time courses of seen and executed movements. The principle of synchrony beteween sensations emanating from the same source weighs heavier than the dominance of vision over proprioception.

Proprioception for Motor Control
Dominance of vision over proprioception is reversed when the purpose of body perception is automatized motor control rather than creation of a conscious body image. An impressive illustration of the importance of somatosensory proprioception for motor control has been provided by two patients who lost all proprioceptive afferences from the body up to the neck as a result of peripheral nerve diseases (Cole & Paillard, 1995; Cole, 1995). The most dramatic symptom of complete sensory loss was an inability to make purposeful movements. Lacking somatosensory information about the actual position of moving limbs, the patients produced poorly oriented and ineffective movements of inappropriate strength. Eventually they learned to replace proprioceptive afferences with visual control of moving body parts. One of them even succeeded in learning to walk again, whereas the other patient remained wheelchair bound. However, movement control remained highly abnormal in both patients. Coordinated movements required constant visual monitoring and allocation of attention. Even the ambitious patient who remastered walking could not entertain a discussion nor admire the beauties of the landscape while walking.

There are two conclusions to be drawn from these exceptional patients. The first is that processing of body configuration for routine motor control and for conscious awareness of one's body rely on sensory channels differently: Whereas motor control is based heavily on proprioception, awareness of one's body gives more weight to vision. The second conclusion is that the conscious image of one's body can replace implicit processing for motor coordination only to a very limited degree and with great effort. The awkwardness of conscious control of motor actions is experienced by persons whose nervous system is perfectly intact when they try to assume an explicitly given body configuration or perform an explicitly defined movement pattern in acquiring new skills in sports, dancing, or miming.

The Permanent Structure of One's Body

The experiments considered up to this point concerned the current configuration but not the permanent structure of the body image. For example, the rubber hand illusions worked only as long as the rubber hands were placed in anatomically plausible positions compatible with knowledge about the permanent structure of the body. Other experiments, however, suggest that established knowledge about the permanent structure of one's body is not safe from illusions.

External vibration of a muscle stimulates deep receptors in much the same way as extending that muscle. It therefore gives rise to an illusory feeling of limb movement. This feeling is strong enough to create strange sensations of impossible body configurations (Lackner, 1988). For example, vibration of the biceps brachii while the fingers are holding the nose leads to a "Pinocchio effect" of apparent lengthening of one's nose. Conversely, vibrating the triceps brachii creates a sensation of the head being pushed backward and downward into the body be- yond all limits of anatomical possiblity. Ramchandran and Hirstein (1998) pro- duced a Pinnochio effect by seating blindfolded subjects behind another person facing the same direction. The experimenter's left hand took the blindfolded sub- ject's left index finger and used it to repeatedly tap and stroke the other person's nose while his right hand tapped and stroked the subject's own nose in synchrony. After a few seconds, the subjects developed the illusion that their own noses had either been dislocated or stretched out to occupy the place of the other person's nose.

Illusions of impossible body configurations demonstrate that conscious body perception sacrifices the permanence of body shape if it comes into conflict with the temporal dynamics of ongoing sensations. The synchrony between holding the nose and stretching the arm or, respectively, between touching a nose and feeling touch on the nose is most parsimonously accounted for by lengthening of the nose. Synchrony among current sensations is weighted more heavily than is fidelity to lifelong experience.

Phantom Limbs
Whereas illusory distortions of body shape testify to the fragility of the body image, phantoms of missing body parts seem to demonstrate its obstinacy in main- taining the image of an intact body against compelling evidence of mutilation. The occurrence of body part phantoms was among the first (Pick, 1915) and continues to be among the most impressive arguments for the contention that a permanent body image underlies and modifies the way we experience our own bodies (Mel- zack, 1990). I have previously discussed body part phantoms (Goldenberg, 2002; Goldenberg, 2003). Here discussion will concentrate on the questions of whether they can be considered a true reflection of a premorbid or even innate image of a complete body, and whether their shape can be altered by experience or experi- mentally induced illusions.

After amputation of a limb nearly all the victims continue to have the propri- oceptive sensation of its presence in spite of visual and tactile evidence of its ab- sence. Over the course of weeks and months, however, the input from external senses molds the experience. In patients fitted with protheses phantoms frequently adapt to their shape (Poeck, 1969; Melzack et al., 1997). Some amputatees inte- grate the prothesis into their body image and identify it with the phantom. They feel touch directly at the surface of the prothesis rather than deducing it from the prothe- sis's pressure on the stump (Poeck, 1969). Presumably, the repeated experience of synchrony between seeing touch on the prosthesis and feeling pressure on the stump has been accomodated by dislocating the tactile sensation to the prothesis.

Upper-limb protheses have less influence on shape and size of phantoms than do lower-limb protheses (Haber, 1956), but visual capture of upper-limb phantoms has been convincingly demonstrated in a series of experiments by Ramachandran and coworkers (Ramachandran & Hirstein, 1998). They created illusory vision of the amputated arm by means of a mirror reflecting the patient's opposite arm or the gloved arm of another person. Movement of the mirror image induced a feeling of phantom movement, regardless of whether the patient's or the experimenter's arm had induced the illusion. When the patient's intact arm was touched, patients felt touch at the mirror location on the phantom. This illusion was contingent on the actual application of touch to the intact arm. Seeing touch of the experimenter's hand mirrored to the phantom did not induce a feeling of touch on the phantom. A synchrony between any feeling of touch and vision of phantom touch was necessary for inducing a feeling of touch on the phantom.

Plasticity of phantom experience is not conditional upon the Influence of prostheses or experimental interventions. Over time the proximal portion of limb phantoms tends to fade in most patients (Haber, 1956; Poeck, 1969; Frederiks, 1985; Ramachandran & Hirstein, 1998). This can lead to the strange sensation of the distal limb being disconnected from, but still belonging to, the body (Haber, 1956; Poeck, 1969; Frederiks, 1985) or to telescoping of the limb, resulting eventually in the anatomically impossible location of fingers inside the stump (Pick, 1915; Poeck, 1969; Frederiks, 1985). Full-sized phantoms may be in unnatural positions that violate anatomical constraints. For example, the hand of a phantom arm may penetrate intro the chest (Bornstein, 1949). There is a report of one girl who after amputation of her congenitally deformed right leg developed one phantom adapted to the prothesis, one reproducing the original deformation, and one consisting of toes fixed to the stump, thus experiencing a coexistence of three right legs (Lacroix et al., 1992).

Plasticity of phantoms after amputation calls into doubt the power of premorbid experience for fixating the body image. The occurrence of phantoms in children with congenital absence of limbs challenges the importance of premorbid experience from another perspective. As these children never had the experience of an intact body, their phantoms seem to be manifestations of an innately predetermined body image that unfolds even without any support from experience.

The possibility of phantom limbs in persons with congenital absence or very early amputation of limbs has been reliably established (Weinstein, Sersen, & Vetter, 1964; Poeck, 1969; Saadah & Melzack, 1994; Melzack et al., 1997; Brugger et al., 2000), but their frequency is substantially lower than after later amputation. Permanent phantoms are reported by some 10% of persons with congenital absence or very early amputation of limbs as compared to about 90% of persons amputated after the age of 10 years (Poeck, 1969; Saadah & Melzack, 1994). They are more frequent in children who had been fitted with protheses than in those without, and they usually adapt their size and shape to the prothesis (Weinstein, Sersen, & Vetter, 1964; Poeck, 1964; Lacroix et al., 1992; Saadah & Melzack, 1994). Some persons report they have had phantoms as long as they can remember (Poeck, 1964; Brugger et al., 2000), but in the majority phantoms occur only in later childhood. The mean age for the appearance of phantoms in congenital absence of limbs is 9 years (Melzack et al., 1997). This latency cannot be exhaustively explained by younger childrens' inability to distinguish their legs and arms as distinct body parts, because already at 5 years of age children perform virtually errorlessly when asked to point to their legs, knees, arms, and hands (Poeck & Orgass, 1964).

Although the affected children never had proprioceptive experience of an intact limb, they did, of course, see the normal bodies of other persons. Depending on whether one emphasizes that phantoms occur at all, or whether one emphasizes that they occur in only a minority of persons and only after years without them, one may draw very different conclusions concerning the neural and cognitive mechanisms underlying phantoms of congenitally absent limbs. The first emphasis endorses the existence of a genetically determined "neuromatrix" ready to support the image of a complete body even against conflicting evidence from the senses (Melzack, 1990). The second emphasis, however, suggests that the brain has enough plasticity to transform knowledge about the universal structure of human bodies into a convincing proprioceptive sensation of having a complete body conforming wtih this universal structure.

Distinguishing One's Own Body from an External Object

Integrating a prosthesis or a rubber hand into the image of one's own body dissolves the border between one's body and external objects, but as these external objects are situated in continuity with the body the dissolution preserves at least the unity of the body. In this section I will discuss evidence that even the apparently unequivocal distinction between a spatially continuous body and distant external objects may be subject to modifications and distortions.

Motor Control for Tool and Object Use

Integration of manipulated objects into the configuration of one's own body is a common feature of skilled tool use. The motor commands for using a computer mouse react to visual feedback from the cursor on the screen rather than from the hand moving the mouse. When a car driver presses down the gas pedal the motor command is tuned to feedback from the velocity of the car rather than from the position of the foot, and when navigating into a parking slot the driver reacts to imminent touch of the car as if the surface of the car were the limit of her or his own body. This unity with the car does not apply to the passengers within the vehicle (Critchley, 1950). It is conditional upon active manipulation and may thus be another manifestation of the central nervous system's propensity to exploit synchrony—in this case between motor commands and the action of external objects—for unification of information from different modalities (McClelland, Rumelhart, & Hinton, 1986; Singer & Gray, 1995).

Of course, if the user of a computer and the driver of a car were asked to indicate the limits of their own bodies, they would include neither the screen nor the car. The integration of external objects into the extension of one's body concerns motor coordination but does not alter the conscious body image.

Personal versus Extrapersonal Hemineglect

Patients with hemineglect may neglect not only one half of external space but also one half of their own body (see Chapter 8). Whether hemineglect of one's own body and of external objects can dissociate has implications for understanding the neural substrate of the body image. If local brain damage could selectively affect or spare the mental representation of only the small sector of space occupied by one's own body, this would be a strong argument in favor of a specialized body image based on a dedicated neural substrate.

Studies that examined the possibility that neglect of one half of the body may dissociate from neglect of one half of external space yielded inconsistent results (Bisiach et al., 1986; Beschin & Robertson, 1997; Cocchini, Beschin, & Jehkonen, 2001). Although the possiblity of selective hemineglect of either extrapersonal or personal space was recognized by all, the frequency of such dissociations varies widely depending on the criteria for defining presence or absence of hemineglect. Interpretation of dissociations is further complicated by differences in the modalities involved in testing personal and extrapersonal hemineglect: Whereas hemineglect of external objects is mostly assessed by tests of visual exploration, tactile exploration is the predominant modality for testing personal neglect. This is problematic, however, because hemineglect in tactile and visual exploration can dissociate even when both are assessed only for external objects (Vallar et al., 1994).

Another approach to investigating the specifity of body centered hemineglect is variation of the position of limbs with respect to external space. In patients with left hemineglect blindfolded detection of touch of the left hand improves when the hand is placed across the body midline into the right hemispace (Aglioti et al., 1996), and touch applied to the right limbs may suffer extinction when they are crossed into the left hemispace (Bartolomeo, Perri, & Gainotti, 2004). When the ulnar (small finger-sided) and the radial (thumb-sided) edge of the left hand are touched simultaneously, neglect will affect the edge that happens to lie on the left side. Ulnar touch is neglected when the hand is palm down, and radial touch is neglected when the hand is palm up (Moscovitch & Behrmann, 1994; Mattingley & Bradshaw, 1994). The dependence of touch detection on the location of the limb in extrapersonal space indicates that the hand is an ambiguous object that participates in both own body and extrapersonal space.

Autoscopy and Out-of-Body Exprience

These rare but fascinating phenomena have in common that one's own body is perceived like a person in external space. In autoscopy the affected subjects see a double of themselves, whereas in out-of-body experience (OBE) they see their own body from a location other than the physical body, most frequently from above (see Devinsky et al., 1989; Brugger, Regard, & Landis, 1997; Feinberg, 2001; Blanke et al., 2004, for reviews). The two phenomena may merge when the autoscopic double captures the subject's identity, who then sees his or her own body from the perspective of the double.

Autoscopy and OBE are transient phenomena that occur mostly in states of lowered vigilance, as, for example, in epileptic seizures or in high-mountain climbing without oxygen. They are typically associated with a strong emotional experience and ideas of impending death. Whereas seeing one's double frequently evokes mortal terror or suicidal ideations, OBE may be associated with a feeling of intense happiness and of release from earthly trouble. The latter association is remarkable in that OBE may occur in situations of extreme danger and threats of death. It seems to the affected person that the soul is finally leaving the body and looking back on it from above, being elevated both spatially and spiritually (Devinsky et al., 1989).

OBE and autoscopy are frequently correlated with vestibular sensations (Critchley, 1950; Blanke et al., 2004). OBE is more likely to affect persons in a supine position and to be accompanied by sensations of flying and floating by the disembodied self. Autoscopy is more likely to affect sitting or upright persons and to be associated with illusions of rotation or shifting of one's body. At least OBE may thus be referred to as "vestibular capture," which employs visual imagery of one's own body for reconciling visual perception with an overwhelming simultaneous vestibular illusion of being lifted to the top of the room. The idea that OBE and autoscopy are fantasy attempts to integrate conflicting input from different sensory channels with the body image is endorsed by reports of illusory movements of body parts preceding or accompanying them (Devinsky et al., 1989; Blanke et al., 2002). But whereas illusions concerning the configuration and shape of one's body can affect persons with normal mental capacities, alterations of vigilance seem to be necessary for rendering the self liable to sacrifice its place within its own and only body for the sake of concordance among synchronous sensory experiences.

The Neural Substrate of the Image of One's Own Body

The examples analyzed so far demonstrate that the image of one's own body results from integration of synchronous afferences from different senses into a coherent spatial structure. If we were to make a guess as to where in the brain such integration could possibly take place, the parietal lobes would be the most plausible candidates. They receive input from the primary somatosensory and visual cortex and are the primary cortical target areas of vestibular input. They also possess close reciprocal connections with the premotor cortices, which enables fast transmission of information about motor commands. Parietal lobe areas are thus in an optimal position for integrating information from vision, somatosensory, and vestibular afferences and monitoring of motor commands into a coherent image of the body. Several lines of clinical evidence support this reasoning: The few reported cases in whom a cerebral lesion abolished a phantom limb had lesions in the parietal lobe of the opposite hemisphere (Head & Holmes, 1911; Bornstein, 1949; Appenzeller & Bicknell, 1969). Lesions causing neglect of one half of the body are, like those causing extrapersonal hemineglect, centered on the inferior parietal lobe (Bisiach et al., 1986), and both autoscopy and OBE have been observed in association with damage to the inferior parietal lobe and the adjacent parieto-temporal junction (Blanke et al., 2004; Maillard et al., 2004). In an epileptic patient who had electrodes implanted on the surface of the brain for diagnostic purposes, OBE could even be provoked by stimulation of electrodes over the inferior parietal lobe (Blanke et al., 2002).

The clinical evidence does not reveal unequivocal asymmetries in the importance of right and left parietal lesions for creating the image of one's own body.

Abolishment of phantoms after parietal lesions was observed with right-sided and left-sided phantoms and was always caused by lesions in the opposite hemisphere, and autoscopy and OBE experiences were observed with both right and left inferior parietal lesions. For neglect of one half of one's own body, however, the situation is less straightforward. Although studies that searched systematically for personal hemineglect in left and right brain damaged patients found it to be equally frequent (Cocchini, Beschin, & Jehkonen, 2001; Marcel, Tegner, & Nimmo-Smith, 2004), the most dramatic manifestations occur after right-sided lesions and affect the left upper extremity (see Chapter 8). This asymmetry is the same as for extrapersonal neglect, which is generally more severe and persistent after right- than left-sided brain lesions. Such concordance may be seen as another indication of the ambiguity of the hand belonging to both extrapersonal and personal space.

The distinction between the conscious body image and processing of body information for motor control is important for deciding whether there are regions of the brain dedicated exclusively to the body image. There certainly are cortical and subcortical brain regions occupied exclusively by representations of the body. For example, the primary motor and sensory cortex both contain neurons arranged in the form of a "homunculus" that reflects the topography of the sensory receptors or muscular effectors to which they are connected. However, these body-specific brain regions subserve sensorimotor integration, which can work independently of a conscious body image. They also provide one of several sources of input to the inferior parietal lobes for creation of the body image. The inferior parietal lobes, however, are responsible for many functions in perception and comprehension of both the external world and one's own body (Warrington & Taylor, 1973; Farah et al., 1989; Jonides et al., 1998; Kourtzi & Kanwisher, 2000). Analysis of personal hemineglect yielded only equivocal evidence for sectors of the parietal lobes devoted exclusively to creating and maintaining the body image.

Recognizing the Spatial Structure of Human Bodies

Because all human bodies are essentially equal, they have the same body parts and have them in the same spatial relationships. One person can replicate the body configuration demonstrated by another person. A third party watching them can reliably decide whether the imitation is faithful or not. This essential equality extends to pictorial or sculptural representations of the human body. One can localize, on one's own body, parts designated in pictures, or vice versa, and one can imitate a body configuration shown in a picture as if the model were a human being. However, this essential equality of human bodies is obscured by superficial differences of visual appearance. Two-dimensional pictures can look very different from three-dimensional bodies, and there is great variation of size and shape among different persons' bodies. If equality of bodies is exploited for imitation of body configurations, further differences become crucial: one sees one's own body from a different perspective than one sees another person's body, one has proprioceptive information from one's own but not from another person's body, and one has to deduce motor commands for one's own body from visual analysis of a model's body.

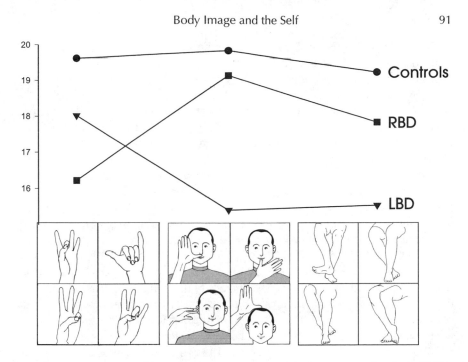

Figure 7–1. Scores of normal controls, patients with left brain damage and aphasia (LBD), and patients with right brain damage (RBD) on imitation of meaningless postures of fingers, hand, and foot. There were 10 gestures of each type, with 2 points given for correct imitation on first trial and 1 for correction after a second demonstration, yielding a maximum score of 20 for each type of gesture. Note that the sensitivity to left and right brain damage differs according to the body part. Finger postures are particularly sensitive to RBD but relatively spared by LBD. (*Source:* adapted from Goldenberg & Strauss, 2002 with permission of the publisher)

Distinguishing the common components of body structure behind their manifold appearances is facilitated by preexisting knowledge about the general structure of human bodies. Developmental data show that such knowledge is acquired during childhood: pointing to body parts reaches an adult level between 4 and 5 years of age (Poeck & Orgass, 1964) and imitation of simple body configurations like those shown in Figure 7–1 between 7 and 8 (Aouka, Goldenberg, & Nadel, 2003). It is noteworthy that at this age children have acquired not only spoken language but already the basics of writing, reading, and number processing. Clinical neuropsychology has accumulated evidence that this acquired knowledge can easily be altered or destroyed by localized brain damage and that, other than for the image of one's own body, laterality of lesions does make a crucial difference for recognition of the common structure of human bodies.

Autotopagnosia

Patients with autotopagnosia commit errors when asked to point to body parts on themselves, on another person, or on a model of the human body. They search for the body part in its vincinity, for example, for the wrist on the forearm, or they confound them with body part of similar functional properties, for example, the elbow with the knee. Both types of errors combine when they point to the nearest body part with a similar function, for example, the elbow for the wrist.

Errors occur not only when the body parts are designated by verbal command but also when they are shown on pictures or when the examiner demonstrates correct pointing and the patient tries to imitate. By contrast, the patients are able to name the same body parts when they are pointed at either on their own body or on a model, and they may be able to select a named body part when given an array of drawings of isolated body parts. Nor is there a general inability to point to the parts of their own body: they reach them accurately when asked to indicate the typical location of accessoires (e. g., a wrist watch) or the location of objects that had been temporarily fixed to a body part (Semenza, 1988; Sirigu et al., 1991; Denes et al., 2000).

Autotopagnosia thus selectively disturbs the ability to locate parts of the human body in response to an explicit request to identify them. It has been argued that the disorder is not confined to the human body but also affects pointing to single parts of other multipart objects such as bicycles (De Renzi & Scotti, 1970), but several patients with autotopagnosia could locate the parts of other multipart objects (Ogden, 1985; Semenza, 1988; Denes et al., 2000). The conclusion that the disturbance is restricted to only the human body is not straightforward. It is questionable whether the structure of bicycles involves a similar amount of subtle distinctions among easily confusable and adjacent parts as the structure of the human body. If such distinctions exist, their cognizance is reserved to experts and falls outside the scope of neuropsychological examination. By contrast, subtle distinctions among easily confusable parts of the human body are tested for diagnosing autotopagnosia and account for the majority of errors. Knowledge about the structure of the human body may be more vulnerable to brain damage because it is more fine-grained and diversified than knowledge about other multipart objects. Few persons have expert knowledge about bicycles, but all have expert knowledge about the human body.

The lesions in cases of autotopagnosia are remarkably uniform. They always affect the left inferior parietal lobe.

Finger Agnosia

Patients with finger agnosia have difficulties distinguishing their fingers when asked to move or designate only one of them. Most errors are confusions among index, middle, and ring fingers. Like autotopagnosia, finger agnosia is not restricted to verbal testing but becomes manifest also when patients are asked to show on a diagram which of their fingers had been touched or to move a finger demonstrated on a diagram (Gainotti, Cianchetti, & Tiacci, 1972; Mayer et al., 1999). Finger agnosia can occur in combination with autotopagnosia (Poncet et al., 1971; Sirigu et al., 1991) but also without it (Gerstmann, 1924; Roeltgen, Sevush, & Heilman, 1983; Mayer et al., 1999), and localization of individual fingers can be preserved in autotopagnosia (De Renzi & Scotti, 1970; Poncet et al., 1971; Assal & Butters,

1973). Autotopagnosia and finger agnosia thus must be considered independent disorders of body part localization. Another association has hitherto been examined in only a few patients and may turn out to be more reliable: These patients had similar difficulties with selection of toes as with selection of fingers (Tucha et al., 1997; Mayer et al., 1999).

Like autotopagnosia, finger agnosia can follow left inferior parietal lesions (Gerstmann, 1930; Roeltgen, Sevush, & Heilman, 1983; Mayer et al., 1999), but other than autotopagnosia it is not at all bound to this location. Group studies found finger agnosia with about equal frequency in patients with left or right brain damage (Kinsbourne & Warrington, 1962; Poeck & Orgass, 1969; Sauguet, Benton, & Hecaen, 1971; Gainotti, Cianchetti, & Tiacci, 1972).

Imitation of Meaningless Gestures

Defective imitation of meaningless gestures has traditionally been considered a symptom of apraxia. Other symptoms of apraxia are disturbed production and imitation of meaningful gestures such as waving goodbye or miming the use of a hammer and disturbed use of real objects. There are, however, patients with pure "visuo-imitative apraxia," in whom defective imitation of meaningless gestures contrasts with preservation of production and imitation of meaningful gestures and of object use (Mehler, 1987; Goldenberg & Hagmann, 1997). It thus seems justified to discuss defective imitation of meaningless gestures as a disorder on its own.

Defective imitation of meaningless gestures affects not only the translation of gestures from a model to the patient's own body but also translation to other instances of human bodies. Patients who commit errors when imitating with their own bodies commit errors also when asked to replicate the demonstrated gesture on a mannequin (Goldenberg, 1995) or to select the gesture from an array of photographs showing gestures performed by different persons and seen under different angles of view (Goldenberg, 1999).

Similar to the dissociation between autotopagnosia and finger agnosia, defective imitation of meaningless gestures can affect imitation of gestures defined by proximal body parts differently from finger postures. Patients with left brain damage have difficulties with the imitation of hand and foot postures, while imitation of finger postures is less compromised and can even be completely normal. By contrast, patients with right brain damage have severe difficulties with finger postures and some difficulties with foot postures but imitate hand postures nearly as perfectly as normal controls (Goldenberg, 1996; 1999; Goldenberg & Strauss, 2002).

Hemisphere Dominance and Body Part Coding

Autotopagnosia and finger agnosia may be combined as "body part agnosias." They differ from disturbed imitation of meaningless gestures by severity of impairment. Whereas testing for body part agnosias affords localization of only one body part, replication of meaningless gestures affords comprehension of the relationships among several body parts. The greater difficulty of imitating body configurations than of selecting single body parts explains the absence of any observation of preserved imitation of proximal gestures in autotopagnosia or of finger postures in finger agnosia. By contrast, conservation of pointing to single body parts in patients with defective imitation is frequent.

Differential sensitivity of proximal body parts and fingers to left and right brain damage is essentially the same in body part agnosias and disturbed imitation. Selection of proximal body part depends mainly on the left hemisphere and particularly the left inferior parietal lobe, whereas selection of fingers is vulnerable to lesions in both hemispheres.

It has been proposed that integrity of left parietal regions is necessary for reducing the multiple perceptual features of demonstrated body configurations to combinations of a limited number of defined body parts. Parsing body configuration into constituent body parts and their mutual relationships has been designated as "body part coding" (Goldenberg, Hermsdörfer, & Laimgruber, 2001; Goldenberg & Strauss, 2002). It requires knowledge about the defining features and boundaries of body parts. Its difficulty increases with the number of different body parts varying between configurations and with the number of features that have to be considered for identification. There are a great number of proximal body parts, and each of them has its own set of defining features (see Figure 7–1). By contrast, the fingers are a small set of uniform body parts that differ mainly in their spatial location. Knowledge about their distinctive features is reduced to knowing their positions, but because they differ only in spatial positions their perceptual distinction is difficult. This difficulty is particularly prominent for the middle three fingers, which are most vulnerable for errors in finger agnosia. Possibly, regions of the right hemisphere are involved in these fine-grained perceptual distinctions. The well-established difficulties that patients with right brain damage have with the perceptual analysis of fine-grained spatial differences supports this contention while at the same time raising doubt whether the neural substrate of distinguishing fingers is different from that subserving the analysis of extrapersonal spatial relationships.

The Nature of the Body Image

The purpose of this chapter was to explore the cognitive and neural bases of two properties of the body image that are perceived so universally and immediately as to make them plausible candidates for being based on dedicated and possibly innate neural substrates: the constancy and unity of one's own body, and the structural equality of all human bodies. I will first summarize the evidence concerning innateness and exclusivity of the neural substrate of the body image and then reconsider the likeliness of an innate and dedicated neural substrate for the body image.

The ultimate proof for an innately determined body image that manifests itself independently of experience would be the observation of a human brain born without a body and nonetheless maintaining an image of it. This is, of course, impossible. To make innateness of the body image a scientifically treatable question one must make the plausible assumption that the innately determined neural substrate supports the image of an intact body and puts constraints on distortions of that image. The existence of body part phantoms lends some support to this claim, but I have demonstrated that this support is equivocal. On the other hand, the ease of inducing distortions of the body image by experimental manipulations indicates a very weak resistance against distortions. If there are innately determined constraints, they are loose.

The dissociations between disorders of localization of proximal body parts and of fingers speak against the existence of one single region containing a coherent "master map" of the body. Discontinuous areas in both hemispheres are needed for understanding and replicating the configuration of the entire body. It remains questionable whether any of these areas is exclusively devoted to the body image or whether they are employed also for analysis of other multipart objects with similar complexity.

Conclusion

Permanence and coherence of one's own body image turns out to be a fragile outcome of fleeting integrations of synchronous afferences from vision, proprioception, and motor commands. The ability to recognize the basic commonalities between one's own and all other human bodies was shown to result from contributions of different brain areas analyzing different aspects of body structure. Nonetheless, the body image conforms quite accurately with the reality of the physical body in most circumstances of daily life and serves as an efficient template for configuration of the physical body for learning new motor skills or for miming. Fragile as it is, the body image does a good job. I think that there is no need for innately prefigured and exclusively dedicated neural representations for explaining this success. The human brain is born with a body, and there is no other part of the material world with which the human mind has as much experience as with its own body. Why should a brain capable of acquiring such complicated cultural skills as speaking, making music, and constructing and flying an airplane not be capable of creating a fairly realistic representation of its closest companion, the body? Why should the brain reserve sectors of its precious space exclusively for the body image if they can also be employed for analyzing external objects with similar properties? And why should evolution bother to provide a preconfigured image of the body if every human being has a physical body from which this image can be deduced? It seems to me that not only evidence from disorders of the body image but also considerations of biological plausibility argue against an innately prefigured body image based on exclusively dedicated areas of the brain.

References

Aglioti, S., Smania, N., Manfredi, M., & Berlucchi, G. (1996). Disownership of left hand and objects related to it in a patient with right brain damage. *NeuroReport, 8,* 293–296.

Aouka, N., Goldenberg, G., & Nadel, J. (2003). Exploring children's body knowledge via imitation of meaningless gestures. *XIth European Conference on Developmental Psychology, 17–3,* 259.

Appenzeller, O. & Bicknell, J.M. (1969). Effects of nervous system lesions on phantom experience in amputees. *Neurology, 19,* 141–146.

Assal, G. & Butters, J. (1973). Troubles du schéma corporel lors des atteintes hémisphériques gauches. *Schweizer Medizinische Rundschau, 62,* 172–179.

Bartolomeo, P., Perri, R., & Gainotti, G. (2004). The influence of limb crossing on left tactile extinction. *Journal of Neurology, Neurosurgery, and Psychiatry, 75,* 49–55.

Beschin, N. & Robertson, I.H. (1997). Personal versus extrapersonal neglect: A group study of their dissociation using a reliable clinical test. *Cortex, 33,* 379–384.

Bisiach, E., Perani, D., Vallar, G., & Berti, A. (1986). Unilateral neglect: Personal and extrapersonal. *Neuropsychologia, 24,* 759–767.

Blanke, O., Landis, T., Spinelli, L., & Seeck, M. (2004). Out-of-body experience and autoscopy of neurological origin. *Brain, 127,* 243–258.

Blanke, O., Ortigue, S., Landis, T., & Seeck, M. (2002). Stimulating illusory own-body perceptions. *Nature, 419,* 269–270.

Bornstein, B. (1949). Sur le phénomène du membre fantome. *Encéphale, 38,* 32–46.

Botvinick, M. & Cohen, J. (1998). Rubber hand "feel" touch that eyes see. *Nature, 391,* 756.

Brugger, P., Kollias, S., Müri, R.M., Crelier, G.R., Hepp-Reymond, M., & Regard, M. (2000). Beyond remembering: Phantom sensations of congenitally absent limbs. *Proceedings of the National Academy of Science of the United States of America, 97,* 6167–6172.

Brugger, P., Regard, M., & Landis, T. (1997). Illusory reduplication of one's own body: Phenomenology and classification of autoscopic phenomena. *Cognitive Neuropsychiatry, 2,* 19–38.

Cocchini, G., Beschin, N., & Jehkonen, M. (2001). The Fluff Test: A simple task to assess body representation neglect. *Neuropsychological Rehabilitation, 11,* 17–31.

Cole, J. (1995). *Pride and a Daily Marathon.* Cambridge, MA: MIT Press.

Cole, J. & Paillard, J. (1995). Living without touch and peripheral imformation about body position and movement: Studies with deafferented subjects. In: J.L. Bermudez, A. Marcel, & N. Eilan (Eds.) *The Body and the Self* (pp. 245–266). Cambridge, MA: MIT Press.

Critchley, M. (1950). The body image in neurology. *Lancet, I,* 335–341.

De Renzi, E. & Scotti, G. (1970). Autotopagnosia: Fiction or reality? *Archives of Neurology, 23,* 221–227.

Denes, G. (1990). Disorders of body awareness and body knowledge. In: F. Boller & J. Grafman (Eds.) *Handbook of Neuropsychology Volume 2* (pp. 207–228). Amsterdam: Elsevier.

Denes, G., Cappelletti, J.Y., Zilli, T., Dallaporta, F., & Gallana, A. (2000). A category-specific deficit of spatial representation: The case of autotopagnosia. *Neuropsychologia, 38,* 345–350.

Devinsky, O., Feldmann, E., Burrowes, K., & Bromfield, E. (1989). Autoscopic phenomena with seizures. *Archives of Neurology, 46,* 1080–1088.

Farah, M.J., Wong, A.B., Monheit, M.A., & Morrow, L.A. (1989). Parietal lobe mechanisms of spatial attention: Modality-specific or supramodal? *Neuropsychologia, 27,* 461–470.

Farnè, A., Pavani, F., Meneghello, F., & Ladavas, E. (2000). Left tactile extinction following visual stimulation of a rubber hand. *Brain, 123,* 2350–2360.

Feinberg, T. (2001). *Altered Egos—How the Brain Creates the Self.* Oxford: Oxford University Press.

Fink, G.R., Marshall, J.C., Halligan, P.W., Frith, C.D., Driver, J., Frackowiak, R.S.J., et al. (1999). The neural consequences of conflict between intention and the senses. *Brain, 122,* 497–512.

Frederiks, J.A.M. (1985). Phantom limb and phantom limb pain. In: J.A.M. Frederiks (Ed.) *Handbook of Neurology Vol 1 (45)* (pp. 395–404). Amsterdam: Elsevier.

Gainotti, G., Cianchetti, C., & Tiacci, C. (1972). The influence of the hemispheric side of lesion on nonverbal tasks of finger localization. *Cortex, 8,* 364–381.

Gallagher, S. (1986). Body image and body schema: A conceptual clarification. *Journal of Mind and Behavior, 7,* 541–554.

Gandevia, S.C. (1982). The perception of motor commands or effort during muscular paralysis. *Brain, 105,* 151–159.

Gerstmann, J. (1924). Fingeragnosie—eine umschriebene Störung der Orientierung am eigenen Körper. *Wiener Klinische Wochenschrift, 37,* 1010–1012.

Gerstmann, J. (1930). Zur Symptomatologie der Hirnläsionen im Übergangsgebiet der unteren Parietal- und mittleren Occipitalwindung. *Nervenarzt, 3,* 691–696.

Goldenberg, G. (1995). Imitating gestures and manipulating a mannikin—the representation of the human body in ideomotor apraxia. *Neuropsychologia, 33,* 63–72.

Goldenberg, G. (1996). Defective imitation of gestures in patients with damage in the left or right hemisphere. *Journal of Neurology, Neurosurgery, and Psychiatry, 61,* 176–180.

Goldenberg, G. (1999). Matching and imitation of hand and finger postures in patients with damage in the left or right hemisphere. *Neuropsychologia, 37,* 559–566.

Goldenberg, G. (2002). Body perception disorders. In: V.S. Ramachandran (Ed.), *Encyclopedia of the Human Brain, Vol. 1* (pp. 443–458). San Diego: Academic Press.

Goldenberg, G. (2003). Disorders of body perception and representation. In: T.E. Feinberg & M.J. Farah (Eds.) *Behavioral Neurology and Neuropsychology* (2nd ed., pp. 285–294). New York: McGraw-Hill.

Goldenberg, G. & Hagmann, S. (1997). The meaning of meaningless gestures: A study of visuo-imitative apraxia. *Neuropsychologia, 35,* 333–341.

Goldenberg, G., Hermsdörfer, J., & Laimgruber, K. (2001). Imitation of gestures by disconnected hemispheres. *Neuropsychologia, 39,* 1432–1443.

Goldenberg, G. & Strauss, S. (2002). Hemisphere asymmetries for imitation of novel gestures. *Neurology, 59,* 893–897.

Gregory, R. (1997). *Mirrors in Mind.* New York: W.H. Freeman.

Haber, W. E. (1956). Observations on phantom-limb phenomena. *Archives of Neurology and Psychiatry, 75,* 624–636.

Head, H. & Holmes, G. (1911). Sensory disturbances from cerebral lesions. *Brain, 34,* 102–254.

Jeannerod, M. (1997). *The Cognitive Neuroscience of Action.* Cambridge, MA: Blackwell Publishers.

Jonides, J., Schumacher, E.H., Smith, E.E., Koeppe, R.A., Awh, E., Reuter-Lorenz, P.A., et al. (1998). The role of parietal cortex in verbal working memory. *Journal of Neuroscience, 18,* 5026–5034.

Kinsbourne, M. & Warrington, E.K. (1962). A study of finger agnosia. *Brain, 85,* 47–66.

Kourtzi, Z. & Kanwisher, N. (2000). Imagining cognition II: An empirical review of 275 PET and fMRI studies. *Journal of Cognitive Neuroscience, 12,* 1–47.

Lackner, J.R. (1988). Some proprioceptive influences on the perceptual representation of body shape and orientation. *Brain, 111,* 281–297.

Lacroix, R., Melzack, R., Smith, D., & Mitchell, N. (1992). Multiple phantom limbs in a child. *Cortex, 28,* 503–508.

Ladavas, E., Farnè, A., Zeloni, G., & Di Pellegrino, G. (2000). Seeing or not seeing where your hands are. *Experimental Brain Research, 131,* 458–467.

Maillard, L., Vignal, J.P., Anxionnat, R., Taillander, L., & Vespignani, H. (2004). Semiologic value of ictal autoscopy. *Epilepsia, 45,* 391–394.

Marcel, A.J., Tegner, R., & Nimmo-Smith, I. (2004). Anosognosia for plegia: Specificity, extension, partiality and disunity of bodily unawareness. *Cortex, 40,* 19–40.

Mattingley, J.B. & Bradshaw, J.L. (1994). Can tactile neglect occur at an intra-limb level? Vibrotactile reaction times in patients with right hemisphere damage. *Behavioural Neurology, 7,* 67–77.

Mayer, E., Martory, M.D., Pegna, A.J., Landis, T., Delavelle, J., & Annoni, J.M. (1999). A pure case of Gerstmann syndrome with a subangular lesion. *Brain, 122,* 1107–1120.

McClelland, J.L., Rumelhart, D.E., & Hinton, G.E. (1986). The appeal of parallel distributed processing. In: D.E. Rumelhart & J.L. McClelland (Eds.) *Parallel Distributed Processing—Explorations in the Microstructure of Cognition Volume 1: Foundations* (pp. 3–44). Cambridge, MA: MIT Press.

Mehler, M.F. (1987). Visuo-imitative apraxia. *Neurology., 37, Suppl 1,* 129.

Melzack, R. (1990). Phantom limbs and the concept of a neuromatrix. *Trends in Neuroscience, 13,* 88–92.

Melzack, R., Israel, R., Lacroix, R., & Schultz, G. (1997). Phantom limbs in people with congenital limb deficiency or amputation in early childhood. *Brain, 120,* 1603–1620.

Moscovitch, M. & Behrmann, M. (1994). Coding of spatial information in the somatosensory system: Evidence from patients with neglect following parietal lobe damage. *Journal of Cognitive Neuroscience, 6,* 151–155.

Ogden, J.A. (1985). Autotopagnosia. Occurence in a patient without nominal aphasia and with an intact ability to point to parts of animals and objects. *Brain, 108,* 1009–1022.

Pavani, F., Spence, C., & Driver, J. (2000). Visual capture of touch: Out-of-the-body experiences with rubber gloves. *Psychological Science, 11,* 353–359.

Pick, A. (1915). Zur Pathologie des Bewubtseins vom eigenen Körper—Ein Beitrag aus der Kriegsmedizin. *Neurologisches Centralblatt, 34,* 257–265.

Poeck, K. (1964). Phantoms following amputation in early childhood and in congenital absence of limbs. *Cortex, 1,* 269–275.

Poeck, K. (1969). Phantome nach Amputation und bei angeborenen Gliedmabenmangel. *Deutsche medizinische Wochenschrift., 46,* 2367–2374.

Poeck, K. & Orgass, B. (1964). Die Entwicklung des Körperschemas bei Kindern im Alter von 4–10 Jahren. *Neuropsychologia, 2,* 109–130.

Poeck, K. & Orgass, B. (1969). An experimental investigation of finger agnosia. *Neurology, 19,* 801–807.

Poeck, K. & Orgass, B. (1971). The concept of the body schema: A critical review and some experimental results. *Cortex, 7,* 254–277.

Poncet, M., Pellissier, J.F., Sebahoun, M., & Nasser, C.J. (1971). A propos d'un cas d'autotopagnosie secondaire à une lésion pariéto-occipitale de l'hémisphère majeur. *Encéphale, 61,* 1–14.

Ramachandran, V.S. & Hirstein, W. (1998). The perception of phantom limbs—the D.O. Hebb lecture. *Brain, 121,* 1603–1630.

Rock, I. & Harris, C.S. (1967). Vision and touch. *Scientific American,* 96–104.

Roeltgen, D.P., Sevush, S., & Heilman, K.M. (1983). Pure Gerstmann's syndrome from a focal lesion. *Archives of Neurology, 40,* 46–47.

Saadah, E.S. M. & Melzack, R. (1994). Phantom limb experiences in congenital limb-deficient adults. *Cortex, 30,* 469–478.

Sauguet, J., Benton, A.L., & Hecaen, H. (1971). Disturbances of the body schema in relation to language impairment and hemispheric locus of lesion. *Journal of Neurology, Neurosurgery, and Psychiatry, 34,* 496–501.

Schilder, P. (1935). *The Image and Appearance of the Human Body.* London: Kegan Paul.

Semenza. (1988). Impairment of localization of body parts following brain damage. *Cortex, 24,* 443–450.

Singer, W. & Gray, C.M. (1995). Visual feature integration and the temporal correlation hypothesis. *Annual Review of Neurosciences, 18,* 555–586.

Sirigu, A., Grafman, J., Bressler, K., & Sunderland, T. (1991). Multiple representations contribute to body knowledge processing. *Brain, 114,* 629–642.

Tastevin, J. (1937). En partant de l'experience d'Aristote—les déplacements artificiels des parties du corps ne sont pas suivis par le sentiment de ces parties ni par les sensation qu'on peut y produire. *Encéphale, 33,* 57–84.

Tucha, O., Steup, O., Smely, C., & Lange, K.W. (1997). Toe agnosia in Gerstmann syndrome. *Journal of Neurology, Neurosurgery, and Psychiatry, 63,* 399–403.

Vallar, G., Rusconi, M.L., Bignamini, L., Geminiani, G., & Perani, D. (1994). Anatomical correlates of visual and tactile extinction in humans: A clinical CT scan study. *Journal of Neurology, Neurosurgery, and Psychiatry, 57,* 464–470.

van Holst, E. & Mittelstaedt, H. (1950). Das Reafferenzprinzip. Wechselwirkungen zwischen Zentralnervensystem und Peripherie. *Naturwissenschaften, 37,* 464–476.

Warrington, E.K. & Taylor, A.M. (1973). The contribution of the right parietal lobe to object recognition. *Cortex, 9,* 152–164.

Weinstein, S., Sersen, E.A., & Vetter, R.J. (1964). Phantom and somatic sensation in cases of congenital aplasia. *Cortex, 1,* 276–290.

Wolpert, D.M., Ghahramani, Z., & Jordan, M.I. (1995). An internal model for sensorimotor integration. *Science, 269,* 1880–1882.

8

Right-Hemisphere Pathology and the Self: Delusional Misidentification and Reduplication

TODD E. FEINBERG, JOHN DELUCA, JOSEPH T. GIACINO, DAVID M. ROANE AND MARK SOLMS

There are several neurological conditions that have particular relevance for our understanding of the neurobiology of the self. Patients with these disorders have neurological perturbations of the self in which brain dysfunction creates a transformation of *personal significance.* In this chapter we consider select neuropathological disorders of the self that can be grouped into two related conditions: *delusional misidentification syndromes (DMS)* and *delusional reduplication syndromes (DRS).* While these disorders may occur in the absence of gross brain pathology, the principle focus of our analysis is instances of these disorders in which gross neuropathology can be clearly demonstrated by structural imaging. We focus on the relationship between these two syndromes and the broader syndrome of *confabulation* and explore through new cases and literature review how brain pathology creates misidentification or reduplication of the body and self, other persons, and places of personal significance. We investigate *(1)* the clinical features of these syndromes, *(2)* the manner in which these specific conditions differ from other more general neuropathological disorders, *(3)* the neuroanatomical substrates of these conditions, and *(4)* possible explanations for these disorders.

Delusional Misidentification and Reduplication Syndromes

Delusional Misidentification Syndromes

Delusional misidentification syndromes (DMS) are conditions in which a patient consistently misidentifies persons, places, objects, or events. The most commonly reported form of misidentification for persons is known as Capgras syndrome. First reported by Capgras and Reboul-Lachaux (1923), the essence of the disorder lies in the delusional belief that a person or persons have been replaced by "doubles" or imposters. A related type of misidentification is the Frégoli syndrome (Courbon & Fail, 1927). This condition involves the belief that a person who is well known to the patient is really impersonating, and hence taking on the appearance of, a stranger in the patient's environment. Vié (1930) hypothesized that Capgras syndrome represents the illusion of negative doubles and Frégoli represents the illusion of positive doubles. Christodoulou (1976; 1977) suggested that Capgras syndrome is characterized by the "hypoidentification" of a person known by the patient who is felt to be an imposter, while Frégoli syndrome is the manifestation of "hyperidentification," in which a known person could be seen in the guise of others. Feinberg and Roane (Feinberg, 1997a; Feinberg, 2001; Feinberg & Roane, 1997a; 1997b; 2003a) suggested the various delusional misidentification syndromes cleave along the dimension of *personal relatedness* based on the pattern of identification between the self and other persons, objects, events, or experiences. According to this viewpoint, Capgras syndrome represents *under-personalized* and Frégoli syndrome *over-personalized* misidentification.

Delusional Reduplication Syndromes

A condition related to DMS is the delusional reduplication syndrome (DRS). Some patients with DMS reduplicate, or double, the misidentified entity(ies). For example, a patient with Capgras Syndrome may deny the identity of an actual spouse and claim that there are two spouses, the actual and the imposter. However, not every patient with DMS reduplicates the misidentified entity(ies) and the issue of reduplication, in and of itself, is unrelated to the primary condition. The patient with DRS, on the other hand, claims the existence of a fictitious person or place, often a double of an actual person or place, without the misidentification of the reduplicated entity(ies).

Delusional Misidentification and Reduplication Syndromes and Focal Neuropathology

There are a minimum of six DMS/DRS that are reported as occurring in neurological patients with focal brain pathology (Table 8–1).

Capgras Syndrome (Under-Personalization) for Persons, Places, or Body Parts

There are several reports of Capgras syndrome for persons occurring in the setting of focal brain lesions. One of the first reported and perhaps the best know is the case reported by Alexander and coworkers (1979) of a 44-year-old man who sustained a traumatic brain injury and right frontotemporal encephalomalacia. This

Table 8–1. Reported cases of delusional misidentification and reduplication after focal brain lesions

Syndrome	Age/Sex	Authors
Capgras for persons		
CP1	37/M	Hayman and Abrams (1977; case 1)
CP2	44/M	Alexander et al. (1979)
CP3	31/M	Staton et al. (1982)
CP4	67/M	Jocic and Staton (1993)
CP5	30/M	Hirstein and Ramachandran (1997)
CP6	51/M	Mattioli et al. (1999)
Capgras for environment		
CE1	71/M	Kapur et al. (1988)
CE2	81/M	Moser et al. (1998)
Capgras for arm (asomatognosia)		
CA1	79/F	Feinberg (1997)
CA2	55/F	Feinberg (2001; Shirley p.18)
CA3	62/M	Feinberg (2001; Jack p. 21)
Frégoli for persons		
FP1	60/F	Ruff & Volpe (1981; case 4)
FP2	66/F	de Pauw et al. (1987)
FP3	27/M	Burgess et al. (1996)
FP4	61/M	Feinberg et al. (1999)
FP5	27/F	Box et al. (1999)
FP6	54/F	Feinberg (2001; Fannie p. 43)
FP7	41/M	Patient L.A. (this chapter)
Frégoli for environment		
FE1	49/M	Benson et al. (1976; case 1)
FE2	72/M	Vighetto et al. (1980)
FE3	64/F	Ruff & Volpe (1981; case 1)
FE4	64/M	Ruff & Volpe (1981; case 2)
FE5	29/M	Ruff & Volpe (1981; case 3)
FE6	60/F	Ruff & Volpe (1981; case 4)
FE7	41/M	Patient L.A. (this chapter)
Delusional reduplication (without misidentification) of self or other persons		
DR1	42/M	Baddeley and Wilson (1986; RJ).
DR2	63/M	Feinberg (1997; 2001)
DR3	16/M	Bouvier-Peyrou (2000)
DR4	65/F	Feinberg (2001; Linda p. 63)

patient claimed that his first and actual wife and five children had been replaced by substitutes. Another well-known instance of this disorder was described by Staton and colleagues (1982), who described a 31-year-old man, who 8 years after a traumatic brain injury that resulted in right frontotemporal and parietal injury, claimed that his parents, siblings, and friends were not "real" but were "look-alikes" or "doubles" of the originals.

Patients have also been described who had Capgras-type misidentification for their homes. Kapur and coworkers (1988) described a patient who claimed his actual home was not his "real" home, although he recognized that the facsimile home had the same ornaments and bedside items as the original. Moser and colleagues (1998) reported an 81-year-old man who after an acute right frontal infarct believed that his real home was the "twin" of the original.

Finally, the syndrome of *asomatognosia* (Feinberg, Haber, & Leeds, 1990; Meador et al., 2000) denotes a condition in which the patient demonstrates delusional misidentification of a part of the body. The most common clinical setting in which asomatognosia occurs is in a patient with a right-hemisphere lesion and left hemiplegia who denies that the left arm belongs to him or her. It generally occurs in association with hemispatial neglect. Jacques Vié (1930; 1944a; 1944b; 1944c) was perhaps the first to note that the delusional misidentification syndromes such as Capgras syndrome were related to asomatognosia. Vié pointed out that in several neurological syndromes including asomatognosia, systematic and selective misidentifications occurred that could not be explained solely on the basis of factors such as generalized confusion. More recently, Feinberg and Roane (1997a; 1997b, 2003a) have argued that asomatognosia can be understood as a Capgras syndrome for the arm in which the personal relationship with the body part is lost. As in Capgras syndrome, in which a person is recognized but the psychological identity is denied, the patient with asomatognosia may recognize that the arm *should be* the patient's arm but disavows ownership of the limb.

The syndrome of asomatognosia is related to anosognosia, the unawareness or denial of illness. (Weinstein & Kahn, 1955; Feinberg, 2001).The patient with anosognosia for hemiplegia appears unaware or adamantly denies that the arm is paralyzed. It is more common and more severe after right-hemisphere lesions. However, anosognosia and asomatognosia are dissociable in the sense that not all anosognosic patients have asomatognosia, and not all asomatognosic patients deny illness or even hemiplegia.

The following dialogue was obtained from a patient with standard asomatognosia. This patient is a woman in her 70s with a right hemisphere stroke in the middle cerebral distribution and a left hemiplegia:

FEINBERG: *I want to ask you again now. What is this over here? Take a look at this over here. What is this?*

MIRNA: *Your fingers.*

FEINBERG: *My fingers?*

MIRNA: *Yes.*

FEINBERG: *Look at them again, take a good look. OK . . . tell me what they are.*

MIRNA: *Fingers. . . . I see fingers and a pocket.*

FEINBERG: *Take a good look. What is it? [tapping the back of her hand].*

MIRNA: *The back of your hand.*

FEINBERG: *The back of my hand?*

MIRNA: *Yes.*

FEINBERG: *Suppose I told you this was your hand?*

MIRNA: *I wouldn't believe you.*

FEINBERG: *You wouldn't believe me?*

MIRNA: *No, no.*

FEINBERG: *This is your hand.*

MIRNA: *No.*

FEINBERG: *Look, here's your right hand and here's your left hand.*

MIRNA: *OK.*

FEINBERG: *Now, What's this [holding out her left hand]?*

MIRNA: *The back of your hand!*

Some patients with asomatognosia simply attribute ownership of the limb to the doctor, claiming it's "your hand" or "the doctor's hand." These simple misidentifications can often be quickly corrected when the error is pointed out to the patient. In other patients, such as the case described above, *the misidentifications are delusional,* and patients cling to their misidentifications despite correction. Additionally, some patients produce names for their arms that can be interpreted as *personifications* (Critchley, 1955) or *metaphors* (Weinstein & Friedland, 1977; Weinstein, 1991) for the arm. Terms for the arm such as "a piece of rusty machinery," "my dead husband's hand," or "a bag of bones" indicate the patient has an altered sense of themselves in relation to the arm. Personification and metaphor are evident in the following case (Feinberg, 2001) of a woman in her 50s who had a large right-hemisphere infarct and described a feeling of alienation from her left arm:

SHIRLEY: *It took a vacation without telling me it was going. It didn't ask, it just went.*

FEINBERG: *What did?*

SHIRLEY: *My pet rock. [She lifted her lifeless left arm with her right arm to indicate what she was talking about.]*

FEINBERG: *You call that your pet rock?*

SHIRLEY: *Yeah.*

FEINBERG: *Why do you call it your pet rock?*

SHIRLEY: *Because it doesn't do anything. It just sits there.*

FEINBERG: *When did you come up with that name?*

SHIRLEY: *Right after it went plop. I thought I'd give it a nice name even though it was something terrible.*

FEINBERG: *Do you have any other names for it?*

SHIRLEY: *Her. She belongs to me so she's a her. She's mine but I don't like her very well. She let me down.*

FEINBERG: *In what way?*

SHIRLEY: *Plop plop rock rock nothing. I was on my way home out the door and then she went and did this [pointing to her left arm]. She didn't ask if she could [shaking her head back and forth]. I have to be the boss not her [pointing to her left arm].*

Frégoli Syndrome (Over-Personalization) for Persons or Places

There are many reports of patients with brain lesions who develop Frégoli syndrome for persons or places. Ruff and Volpe (1981, case 4) reported a 60-year-old woman who after removal of a right frontal subdural hematoma claimed that the patient in the bed next to her was her husband. She was actually pleased that her husband no longer snored. Feinberg and colleagues (1999) described a 61-year-old man who sustained a traumatic brain injury with right frontal and left temporoparietal contusions. He developed Frégoli misidentifications for many staff members of his rehabilitation hospital, claiming they were actually sons, daughters-in-law, coworkers, and town officials, and he even claimed an ice skater on TV was himself.

Frégoli syndrome for place refers to patients who misidentify their current and unfamiliar environments, such as a hospital room or rehabilitation hospital, for places of greater personal significance, such as their homes or job sites. The syndrome has also been termed *reduplicative paramnesia,* since some patients maintain they are in *both* a correct and incorrect location, and the disorder was often seen in association with memory impairment. However, because many of these patients misidentify their environments without reduplicating them, the term *Frégoli syndrome for environment* is a better descriptor of the syndrome. Further, the term *Frégoli syndrome for environment* brings this condition into relationship to the other delusional misidentification syndromes.

Some patients demonstrate Frégoli syndrome for *both* persons and their environments. This was the case with patient L.A. (Table 8–1, case FP7 and FE7), a 41-year-old man with a right frontal intracranial hemorrhage and subarachnoid hemorrhage secondary to an arteriovenous malformation. The patient had confabulation, claimed he was at work, and misidentified multiple staff workers as people from his workplace. The examination was performed in a rehabilitation facility in New Jersey:

EXAMINER: *What are you doing here?*

PATIENT: *I'm working.*

EXAMINER: *OK. And what are you working at?*

PATIENT: *I'm trying to learn from them.*

EXAMINER: *OK. Is this part of your job?*

PATIENT: *Yes.*

EXAMINER: *And what's your job?*

PATIENT: *I'm a computer person.*

EXAMINER: *So that's what you're doing here? Computers? . . . And you're at work here?*

PATIENT: *Yes.*

EXAMINER: *Do you get paid your regular salary?*

PATIENT: *Yes.*

EXAMINER: *Where are we right now?*

PATIENT: *We're at [name of his company] in New York . . . My office is right around the corner [pointing]. If they have problems with their computers I solve them.*

EXAMINER: *[Pointing to a therapist of the facility that the patient had previously claimed he knew] And you know her from . . . ?*

PATIENT: *Yes. [names his company]*

EXAMINER: *Co-worker? What's her job?*

PATIENT: *Her job is to do research on certain items and then bring them to [his company] . . . She works with somebody else . . . She comes to me for the type of information I need to connect for her . . . that's the time we have connection. Otherwise there isn't any connection . . . when she has problems with her computer she comes to me.*

Delusional Reduplication (Without Misidentification) of Self or Other Persons

There is another and final group of delusional confabulatory patients who reduplicate persons or places but who do not misidentify the reduplicated entities. For example, Weinstein, Kahn, and Morris (1956) described patients with brain injuries who expressed the delusion that they were the parent of a fictitious child, a condition they termed the *phantom child syndrome*. They observed that a unique feature of the delusion was that the "patients often ascribed to the 'phantom child' the same illness or disability that they themselves had." For example, a woman with a pituitary tumor and blindness claimed she had a child who was "sick and blind," and a 21-year-old soldier with a head injury and bilateral leg weakness claimed he had a 3-year-old "daughter" who had paralysis of both legs from polio. In some patients the "phantom child" embodied personal concerns other than illness. For instance, a woman who felt abused by the nursing staff claimed she had a "baby" that the nurses had "harmed and even killed."

The following case (Feinberg, 1997a; 2001; Table 8–1, case DR2) illustrates this condition. A 63-year-old man sustained a ruptured anterior cerebral artery aneurysm and bilateral frontal infarctions. Neuropsychological testing showed impairments in attention, memory, and executive functioning. He displayed anosognosia for his cognitive impairments and denied his hospitalization, stating he was "a guest" with the "Optimists club" to "help out."

The patient was the biological father of three children but never adopted any children. Although estranged from his wife since his injury, he claimed the existence of a child that he was planning to adopt. He denied his own impairments but asserted the adopted child "has problems" and complained about the way the doctor's were treating "the child":

SAM: *I feel like I've got a little more ability than they give me credit for.*

EXAMINER: *So one last question: Has this aneurysm or the consequences of this aneurysm changed your life in any way at all?*

SAM: *No.*

EXAMINER: *So basically your life is the way it was before?*

SAM: *Yeah, like the way it was before. We have another baby . . . we've just adopted, and I have three children of my own. I've got my own house.*

EXAMINER: *When did you adopt a baby?*

SAM: *We haven't gotten the final result, but about a month ago.*

EXAMINER: *They said you could have the baby?*

SAM: *But the baby has problems now. They're trying to sort out the problems before, you know, somebody really adopts it . . . the baby. They want to make sure it's the right direction.*

EXAMINER: *Who's actually adopting the baby?*

SAM: *Me and my wife.*

EXAMINER: *Have you seen the baby at all?*

SAM: *Well, we've seen pictures. And I've seen the baby in person, too.*

EXAMINER: *And where does the baby live now?*

SAM: *The baby lives with the mother, and I think it's the mother of the boy that was dumped . . . and the mother would like to have the baby. I guess she lost her sons he might as well have the baby. That's a little problem there.*

EXAMINER: *You said before the baby has some problems.*

SAM: *That's what the psychologists are telling the guy who is in charge of the hospital. You know it's like they say certain things I go along with and certain things I don't go along with. I think there's too much pressure on the kid to really give an honest answer. I don't think a kid who is 6 or 7 years old is capable of giving you the right answer.*

EXAMINER: *What kind of problems does this child have?*

SAM: *I don't know . . . to tell you the honest truth, I don't know. I know this kid has been in the hospital off and on for a couple of years, and they kind of rate them as far as progress goes or things like that. [The patient was being rated during the interview.]*

EXAMINER: *How do they rate them?*

SAM: *I guess they must rate them when they don't hear the things they want to hear . . . like the kid is not accomplishing anything, which I think is very unfair to basically analyze a kid that way.*

Review of Previously Reported Cases

In order to better understand the features of delusional misidentification and reduplication after focal brain lesions and elucidate the underlying neuropathology of these disorders, we analyzed a series of previously published cases of these conditions. We also included the unreported case described above, L.A., in the analysis.

The criteria for inclusion in our series were patients who displayed stable misidentification(s) or reduplication(s) of the Capgras or Frégoli type in the pres-

ence of focal brain pathology. Case descriptions also had to provide sufficient clinical detail to determine the nature and stability of the misidentification and adequate neuroanatomical detail to determine the anatomical focus of the brain lesion.

Cases were categorized according to the predominant type of misidentification into six classes: *(1)* Capgras syndrome for person(s), *(2)* Capgras for environment, *(3)* Capgras for the arm (asomatognosia), *(4)* Frégoli syndrome for per-
son(s), *(5)* Frégoli for environment, and *(6)* delusional reduplication (without
misidentification) for the self or other persons. There were a total of 27 cases reviewed. Two cases who had prominent misidentification for both persons and the
environment appeared in both categories (Table 8–1).

The nature of the misidentification or reduplication is shown in Table 8–2. It
is apparent that there are consistent patterns within categories. In all patients with
Capgras misidentification for persons (group 1), the misidentified individuals were
persons close to them, and all persons with Capgras for environment (group 2)
misidentified their homes. In contrast, all patients with Frégoli misidentification
for persons (group 3) mistook relative strangers for persons who were either relatives or well known to them and all patients with delusional reduplicative paramnesia (Frégoli for environment) misidentified their current environment for their
homes or hometowns. Patients with Capgras syndrome for the arm (delusional asomatognosia) tended to misidentify their arms as belonging to relatives, and patients
with delusional reduplication without misidentification replicated either their-
selves or relatives. In other words, all delusional misidentifications overwhelmingly
involved either the self or significant others, especially relatives.

Table 8–3 enumerates the anatomical findings. For the purposes of comparison,
we used the basic anatomical format of Burgess and coworkers (1996). A 2 × 4
(hemisphere × brain region) chi-square test revealed no significant interaction
($X^2(3) = 4.17$, p > .05). This indicated that DMS did not vary across brain region in
terms of hemisphere. However, a likelihood ratio test revealed that the occurrence
of right frontal damage (28 of 29 cases) was significantly above chance (p < .001).
We then examined the main effects for hemisphere and brain region. In terms of
hemisphere, all 29 patients (100%) suffered some degree of right-hemisphere damage, while only 15 (51.72%) suffered some degree of left-hemisphere damage. This
difference was found to be significant employing a chi-square test ($X^2(1) = 4.45$,
p < .03), indicating that the greater distribution of right-hemisphere cases was
likely not due to chance. In terms of exclusive damage, there were 14 (48.28%)
cases with right-hemisphere damage only. There were no (0%) cases with left-
hemisphere damage only. Using a binomial test, this difference was found to be
significant (p < .001). These data indicate an overwhelming bias toward right-
hemisphere damage in terms of DMS.

In terms of lesion location, 10 (34.48%) of the cases had frontal damage only.
There were no cases of any other brain region exclusively leading to DMS (i.e.,
there were no parietal-only cases, etc.). This difference was found to be significant
(p < .002), indicating that exclusive frontal damage is overrepresented in DMS.

Neuropsychological findings are summarized in Table 8–4. In accordance
with the predominance of right-hemisphere pathology, almost all patients in
whom the neuropsychological data were reported demonstrated a combination of

Table 8–2. Clinical features of cases with delusional misidentification and reduplication after focal brain lesions

Syndrome	Age/Sex	Misidentified individual(s)	Selective and consistent	Refactory to correction
Capgras for persons				
CP1	37/M	parents, ex-wife, siblings, physicians	NA	NA
CP2	44/M	wife and children	+	+
CP3	31/M	parents and siblings, cousin, pet cat, himself	+	NA
CP4	67/M	wife	+	+
CP5	30/M	father, mother, self, grandfather	+	+
CP6	51/M	wife, daughters, relatives	+	+
Capgras for environment				
CE1	71/M	home	+/−	NA
CE2	81/M	home	+	+
Capgras syndrome for arm (asomatognosia)				
CA1	79/F	husband's arm	+	+
CA2	55/F	little Suzy's arm	+	+
CA3	62/M	mother-in-law's arm	+	+
Frégoli for persons				
FP1	60/F	stranger for husband	+	+
FP2	66/F	strangers for married cousin and lady friend	+	NA
FP3	27/M	fellow patient for prior nurse who was having an affair with patient's wife	+	+
FP4	61/M	relative strangers and fellow patients for sons, daughter-in-law, coworkers, friends, boss, town mayor, himself	+	+
FP5	27/F	fellow patient for mother	+	+
FP6	54/F	fellow patient for coworker	+	+
FP7	41/M	therapist for coworker	+	+
Frégoli for environment				
FE1	49/M	hospital in home town	+	+
FE2	72/M	while in hospital claimed he was in home town	+	+
FE3	64/F	hospital in home town	+	+
FE4	64/M	hospital annex in home town	+	+
FE5	29/M	branch of hospital in home town	+	NA
FE6	60/F	hospital in home town	+	NA
FE7	41/M	hospital for workplace	+	+
Delusional reduplication (without misidentification) of self or other persons				
DR1	42/M	reduplicated brother with similar injury to patient's	+	+
DR2	63/M	reduplicated child with simlar history to patient's	+	+
DR3	16/M	reuplicated self that (unlike patient) was healthy	+	+
DR4	65/F	reduplicated cousins with same illness as patient	+	+

NA, not assessed.

Table 8–3. Neuroanatomical findings in delusional misidentification and reduplication after focal brain lesions

Syndrome	Age/sex	Right hemisphere lesion(s)					Left hemisphere lesion(s)					Etiology
		Front	Temp	Pariet	Occip	Other	Front	Temp	Pariet	Occip	Other	
Capgras for persons												
CP1	37/M	+		+		BG						AVM
CP2	44/M	+	+				+					TBI
CP3	31/M	+	+	+	+		+					TBI
CP4	67/M	+	+	+		BG						CVA
CP5	30/M	+					+					TBI
CP6	51/M	+	+				+	+				TBI
Capgras for environment												
CE1	71/M	+										AVM
CE2	81/M	+					+			+		CVA contusions
Capgras for arm (asomatognosia)												
CA1	79/F	+	+	+								CVA
CA2	55/F	+	+	+								CVA
CA3	62/M	+	+	+	+							CVA

Frégoli for persons

	Age/Sex									Etiology
FP1	60/F	+								TBI
FP2	66/F	+	+							CVA
FP3	27/M	+	+							TBI
FP4	61/M	+		+				+		TBI
FP5	27/F	+		+						TBI
FP6	54/F	+				+				cerebral metateses
FP7	41/M	+								AVM

Frégoli for environment

	Age/Sex									Etiology
FE1	49/M	+	+							TBI
FE2	72/M	+		+						CVA
FE3	64/F	+								cerebral tumor
FE4	64/M	+		+						AVM
FE5	29/M	+		+						ICH
FE6	60/F	+								TBI
FE7	41/M	+				+				AVM

Delusional reduplication (without misidentification) of self or other persons

	Age/Sex									Etiology
DR1	42/M	+				+				TBI
DR2	63/M	+				+				ACoA
DR3	16/M	+				+	+			TBI
DR4	65/F	+				+				ACoA
Total	**29**	**28**	**9**	**13**	**3**	**14**	**2**	**1**	**1**	

Table 8–4. Neuropsychological and neuropsychiatric findings in cases of delusional misidentification and reduplication after focal Brain lesions

Syndrome	Age/Sex	Memory impairments	Perceptual impairments	Executive impairments	Other confabulations	Other delusions or psychiatric features
Capgras for persons						
CP1	37/M	not noted	constructional	NA	—	delusions, hallucinations
CP2	44/M	mild nonverbal	visuospatial	+	—	prior paranoia
CP3	31/M	non-verbal	isuospatial	+	—	suspicious, "victimized," derealization
CP4	67/M	verbal, nonverbal	visuospatial	NA	+	depression, anosognosia/denial
CP5	30/M	NA	mild visuoperpceptual	NA	—	—
CP6	51/M	verbal, nonverbal, autobiographical	visuospatial	+	+	delusions
Capgras for environment						
CE1	71/M	nonverbal	visuospatial	+	—	—
CE2	81/M	verbal, nonverbal	not noted	+	—	—
Capgras for arm (asomatognosia)						
CA1	79/F	nonverbal, verbal	left hemineglect	NA	+	—
CA2	55/F	nonverbal	left hemineglect	NA	—	—
CA3	62/M	nonverbal, verbal	left hemineglect	NA	+	anosognosia

Frégoli for persons

FP1	60/F	nonverbal, verbal	visuospatial	+	—	paranoia	—
FP2	66/F	nonverbal	NA	NA	—	paranoia	—
FP3	27/M	nonverbal, verbal	visuospatial, visuoperceptual, prospognosia	+	—	paranoia	—
FP4	61/M	nonverbal, verbal	visuoperceptual	+	+		—
FP5	27/F	nonverbal, verbal	visuospatial, visuoperceptual	+	+	Cotard delusion	—
FP6	54/F	nonverbal, verbal	NA	NA	—	anosognosia/denial, misidentified person had patient's illness	
FP7	41/M	non-verbal and verbal	visuospatial	+	+		—

Frégoli for environment

FE1	49/M	intact verbal during DMS	NA	NA	—		h/o alcoholism
FE2	72/M	nonverbal	visuospatial	NA	—	paranoia	—
FE3	64/F	nonverbal	visuospatial	+	—		—
FE4	23/F	nonverbal	visuospatial	NA	—		—
FE5	29/M	nonverbal	visuospatial	+	—		—
FE6	60/F	nonverbal, verbal	visuospatial	+	—		—
FE7	41/M	nonverbal, verbal	visuospatial	+	+		—

Delusional reduplication (without misidentification) of self or other persons

DR1	42/M	autobiographical	constructional	+	+	anosognosia/denial	
DR2	63/M	nonverbal, verbal	NA	+	+	"psychological breakdown," anogonosia/denial	
DR3	16/M	retrograde amnesia and verbal	intact	NA	+	the "other self" was healthy	
DR4	65/F	anterograde and retrograde	visuospatial	NA	+	anosognosia	

NA, not assessed.

memory (primarily nonverbal), perceptual, and executive impairments. Interestingly, most patients did not demonstrate other confabulations or delusional impairments, indicating that the misidentifications and reduplications in these patients were specific.

Common Features Among the Syndromes

This analysis suggests that neurological cases of delusional misidentification and reduplication share a number of features, and further that these features distinguish these conditions from simple unawareness and confabulation in general:

1. *The misidentifications in these syndromes reflect alterations in personal significance.* Table 8–2 clearly indicates that one of the salient features of this particular variety of confabulation is that the misidentifications and reduplications that these patients display are almost wholly with reference to persons, places, and events of personal significance, such as the body, family, current location, job situation, and other emotionally charged topics. This feature is of particular interest since most of the traditional ways of subtyping confabulation do not address the issue of personal significance. However, Feinberg (1997a, 1997b) and Feinberg and Roane (1997a, 1997b) have emphasized that patients who display personal confabulation tend to do so within domains of personal significance. This feature was highlighted by Weinstein and coworkers with confabulation and denial of illness (Weinstein & Kahn, 1955), however we did not find anosognosia a universal feature in our review.

2. *The misidentifications are generally selective and consistent.* The same aspects of the self and environment are repeatedly misidentified. This suggests that whatever the mechanisms of these conditions, they cannot be explained by a generalized memory or perceptual impairment.

3. *Some patients with DMS and DRS appear to be unaware of or to minimize their neurological, neuropsychological, or personal problems in general.* Although not a universal feature of all cases, many cases, particularly those with delusional reduplication without misidentification, displayed frank denial or anosognosia. In patients with Frégoli like delusional confabulatory misidentifications, the misbeliefs generally put patients in a better position than they were in reality. These patients tended to locate themselves in comfortable, familiar surroundings and claimed they were at home or at work while they actually were located in a hospital or rehab facility. If they were aware that they were in a hospital, they tended to mislocate the hospital closer to their home or to a location significantly related to their past. For these reasons, Ruff and Volpe (1981) argued that there might be some wish-fulfilling aspects to these delusions.

4. *The misidentifications and confabulations are refractory to correction.* The misidentifications were delusional. In spite of the apparent illogical nature of the delusions, and in spite of repeated correction by examiners and family members, patients held to their delusional misidentifications

or reduplications. This suggests that there is an impediment or resistance to the truth. Indeed, these patients may have explicit or implicit knowledge regarding their true locations, illnesses, and other issues that they seem unaware of and confabulate about (Feinberg 1997b; Feinberg & Roane, 1997a; 2003a; Weinstein, 1991; Weinstein, Friedland, & Wagner, 1994). These features help distinguish this class of behavior from other forms of confabulation (e.g., amnesiac confabulation) or unawareness in general. If we are to understand the mechanisms of these conditions, their delusional nature must be explained.

5. *Right-hemisphere dysfunction is especially implicated in these disorders.* Right frontal dysfunction was a nearly universal feature of all cases regardless of type of delusional misidentification or reduplication.

Explaining Delusional Misidentification and Reduplication

There have been many attempts to explain delusional misidentification that account for some of the features of these disorders. The proposed mechanisms can be divided between "negative" theories that emphasize the deficits (in a Jacksonian sense; Taylor, 1958) seen in patients with these disorders versus the "positive" theories that emphasize the features of these conditions not explained by the deficits alone (Table 8–5).

"Negative" Theories

Spatial Disorientation
Spatial disorientation is often cited as a factor in the origin of reduplicative paramnesia (see, for example, Benson, Gardner, and Meadows, 1976; Ruff & Volpe, 1981) and is likely to be a prerequisite for delusional misidentification for place. Indeed,

Table 8–5. Negative and positive features of delusional misidentification and reduplication after focal brain lesions

Negative features	Positive features
Spatial disorientation	Paranoia
Visuoperceptual disturbance	Delusional nature
Hemispatial neglect	Wish-fulfillment
Executive dysfunction	Defensive operations: projection and denial
Retrograde and anterograde amnesia	
Autobiographical memory loss	
Temporal context confusion	
Reality monitoring failure	
Anatomical disconnection	
Disturbance of self-representation/ego functions	

visuospatial disorders including hemispatial neglect were noted in nearly all cases in this series (Table 8–4). This finding was common even in cases of Capgras or Frégoli for persons. Visuospatial disorientation, however, does not explain why patients are always disoriented to a place closer to home or why the disorientation is delusional and refractory to correction,

Anatomical Disconnection

Some theories have attributed DMS, especially Capgras syndrome for persons, to anatomical disconnection. Alexander, Stuss, and Benson (1979) argued that a deep right frontal lesion could functionally disconnect temporal and limbic regions from the damaged frontal lobe. This disconnection could result in a disturbance in familiarity of people and places, and the presence of frontal pathology could lead to an inability to resolve the cognitive conflict. Staton, Brumback, and Wilson (1982) proposed that disconnection of the hippocampus from other parts of the brain important for memory storage could result in an inability to associate new information with previous memories, leading to reduplication.

Some investigators have suggested that Capgras syndrome is caused by visuo-anatomical disconnection. Ellis and Young (1990), among others, based on the finding that some patients with prosopognosia have covert (emotional) but not overt recognition of faces (Bauer, 1984; 1986), suggested that patients with Capgras syndrome have overt but not covert recognition of faces. This covert recognition is subserved by a "dorsal route" that runs between the visual cortex and the limbic system via the inferior parietal lobule. A lesion in the dorsal system would allow explicit but not implicit (emotional) recognition, and they suggest this accounts for the occurance of Capgras syndrome. Similarly, Hirstein and Ramachandran (1997) and Ramachandran (1998) suggested that a disconnection between the infero-temporal cortex and the amygdala could allow the patient to correctly identify faces but not experience the appropriate emotion connected to familiar faces and that this discrepancy leads to delusional misidentification.

In our series of reviewed cases in Table 8–3, within the left hemisphere the temporal and parietal lobes were overwhelmingly spared in cases of Capgras syndrome for persons and environment. Therefore, if there is an anatomical disconnection, it would have to be in the nondominant hemisphere. Within the right hemisphere, two of five cases of Capgras syndrome for persons and both cases of Capgras syndrome for place had temporal-sparing lesions, and three of five cases of Capgras for environment and both cases of Capgras syndrome for place had parietal-sparing lesions. On the other hand, all eight cases of Capgras syndrome for persons or places had nondominant frontal lesions. Therefore, if anatomical disconnection is important, it appears that a disconnection of nondominant frontal structures, as suggested by Alexander, Stuss, and Benson (1979), is most likely to play a role in the etiology of Capgras syndrome.

It should also be noted that theories such as that of Ellis and Young (1990) and Hirstein and Ramachandran (1997) that emphasize visuoanatomical disconnection cannot account for most cases of Capgras syndrome since this is a multimodal disorder not confined to the visual modality. Furthermore, when we consider the

DMS and DRS syndromes as a whole, formulations that emphasize anatomical disconnection seem most suitably applicable only to the Capgras syndrome in which there is a failure to match a current experience with premorbid memories, resulting in the underidentification of particular entities. As noted above, Capgras syndrome is a disorder of *underpersonalization* in which there may be confabulation of *imaginary differences* between the misidentified entity and the original, but Frégoli syndrome is a disorder of *overpersonalization* in which there is the confabulation of *imaginary resemblances* between the misidentified entity and the original. It remains to be explained how a disconnection of current experience from premorbid memory could explain overrelatedness to one's environment.

Some partial answers to this latter question may come from Rapcsak and colleagues (1996, case 21), who described a patient without prosopagnosia who displayed false recognition (overidentification) of faces. This pattern developed after the patient underwent the surgical removal of a right prefrontal lesion. They attributed the patient's pattern of impairment to an intact reflexive face recognition system but an impaired reflective or strategic face processing system, leading this patient to mistake an unknown face for one in memory. While the authors do not state whether the patient had delusional misidentification, this type of disturbance could help explain some instances of visual overidentification of faces, but this account does not explain selectivity, refractoriness, delusional nature, or multimodality.

Memory and Executive Impairments and the Possible Role of Confabulation
In contrast to the lack of significant perceptual impairments in this series, memory and executive impairments were found in nearly all cases of DMS and DRS in which these functions were assessed. Since many of the current cognitive and neuropsychological theories of the origin of confabulation implicate some combination of memory impairment and executive dysfunction (Stuss et al., 1978; DeLuca, 1993; 2000), this finding raises the question of the relationship between DMS/DRS and confabulation. Furthermore, since patients with DMS of the Frégoli (overpersonalized) variety claim that they are familiar with relatively unfamiliar persons or places, and patients with confabulation may mistake past for current environmental stimuli (Levin, 1945), it is relevant to consider whether theories of the origin of confabulation can help explain some aspects of the origin of the DMS and DRS syndromes.

Confabulation has been broadly defined as an erroneous statement that is made without a conscious effort to deceive (Berlyne, 1972) or "statements or actions that involve unintentional but obvious distortions" (Moskovitch & Melo, 1997). Korsakoff (1889; Victor & Yakovlev, 1955) first observed the tendency of patients with what is now known as Wernicke-Korsakoff syndrome to display both amnesia and confabulation ("pseudoreminiscences"), and many authors subsequently confirmed confabulation in Korsakoff syndrome (Bonhoeffer, 1901,1904; Van der Horst, 1932; Williams & Rupp, 1938; Talland,1961; 1965).

Korsakoff (1892; Victor & Yakovlev, 1955) observed that during confabulation "patients confused old recollections with the present impressions. Thus, they may believe themselves to be in the setting (or circumstances) in which they were 30 years ago, and mistake persons who are around them now for people who were around them at that time" (Victor, Adams, & Collins, 1989). Other authors have also noted that mistaking current for past experience may contribute to confabulation. Thus, Kraepelin (1904; 1907; 1919) distinguished two subtypes of confabulation, one of which he called *simple confabulation,* caused in part by errors in the temporal ordering of real memories. The other variety he called *fantastic confabulations,* which was bizarre and patently impossible statements not rooted in true memory. Berlyne (1972) found this distinction useful and suggested that momentary confabulation had to be provoked by questions from the examiner and that the content of such confabulation consisted of true memories that were temporally displaced. Van der Horst (1932) and Williams and Rupp (1938) also noted that many confabulations were rooted in true memory and derived from preserved past memories. As an example of this phenomenon, Talland (1961) commented that amnesiac confabulators tended to misidentify their doctors as old acquaintances.

These observations fit with one current and popular theory of confabulation that posits that confabulation results from *temporal context confusion* due to frontal-executive dysfunction. According to this account confabulation results from inaccurate identification of the temporal order in which information is stored (Schnider, Von Danilsen, & Gutbrod, 1996; Schnider et al., 1996; Schnider & Ptak, 1999; Schnider et al., 2000; Schnider, 2003) and suggests that spontaneous confabulation occurs because these patients cannot establish the appropriate contrast between current or ongoing experience and memories of past events due to an inability to suppress activated but irrelevant memory traces.

Other theories posit that deficient strategic retrieval is the primary deficit in confabulation. This explanation of confabulation (Moscovitch, 1989, 1995; Moscovitch & Melo, 1997) proposes that there are two components involved in memory retrieval. Associative retrieval is considered to be relatively automatic and does not require frontal or executive intervention. A second retrieval process, strategic retrieval, may be necessary to guide continuation of the search. Strategic retrieval is conscious, effortful, and self-directed and requires frontal functions. Confabulation is presumed to be the result of a breakdown in strategic retrieval processes involved in memory search, temporal ordering, and output monitoring. The predisposition to confabulation increases when a particular cognitive subsystem (e.g., memory) is damaged and produces faulty output (e.g., failure to remember) in addition to impaired output monitoring (e.g., unawareness of response discrepancies).

Cognitively based theories of confabulation could help explain some of the *negative* features of DMS and DRS. Temporal context confusion or retrieval defects could cause old memories to be confused with recent memories, explaining in part why patients with DMS and DRS believe they are located in previously known locations or are performing well-known social roles. However, these explanations are incomplete when attempting to address the *positive* features reported in DMS and DRS such as why only certain entities are misidentified (selectivity) and why persons or places of personal significance are typically the subject of the DMS and DRS. General theories of confabulation also fail to explain why most confabulators, following anterior communicating artery (AcoA) aneurysms, do not display a "delusional" fabric to their confabulations (DeLuca, 2000), but patients with DMS and DRS cling to their misidentifications in spite of correction (delusional aspects). For instance, Patterson and Zangwill (1944) noted that their patients with reduplicative paramnesia who misidentified their current location to a geographical location closer to their actual home were *refractory to correction, and this could not be solely explained on the basis of memory loss.* Their patients might accept the correct orientation in an "abstract geographical" sense, such as knowing the correct locale "according to the map," but still maintain they "felt" they were located closer to home. Patterson and Zangwill observed that while amnesia was initially present, the "retention deficit cleared rapidly" and

> there was failure to adjust the drive to the true nature of the environment even when cognitive recovery had proceeded far enough to permit and sustain proper orientation. The very fact that the patient remained disoriented for so long suggests that a strong desire was actively inhibiting the cognitive mechanisms which normally subserve orientation.

Subsequent authors also emphasized the delusional quality of the statements of some patients with misidentification. Thus, Weinstein (1996), with specific reference to patients who adamantly maintain an incorrect orientation in spite of correction, referred to this variety of disorientation as "symbolic or delusional environmental disorientation." Burgess and coworkers (1996) in a broader context referred to a variety of delusional confabulation as "delusional paramnesic misidentification" or "delusion with paramnesia" to emphasize the link to memory disorders. These considerations suggest that the delusional aspects are an important distinguishing feature between DMS/DRS and confabulation in general.

Additional observations support the notion that delusional misidentification can be partially dissociated from confabulation in general. Box, Laing, and Kopelman (1999) described a 27-year-old woman who developed Frégoli misidentifications after a traumatic brain injury. Initially the patient had inconsistent and short-lived confabulations that resolved, but this patient later went on to demonstrate more stable Frégoli misidentification. There is evidence as well that DMS of the Capgras variety can be dissociated from confabulation. Mattioli, Miozzo, and Vignolo (1999) reported a 51-year-old man with right frontopolar, right temporal, and bilateral frontobasal hypodensities after traumatic brain injury who developed confabulation in personal recollections and on long-term verbal memory testing and Capgraslike misidentifications for his wife, daughters, and house. During a year follow-up period, the patient's confabulations improved to the point at which deficits were restricted to verbal memory tasks. However, the patients "delusional misidentification of his wife and home remained stable in time, independent of the degree of memory loss, and impervious to correction and to all attempts at reality testing." Taken together, these considerations suggest that there is evidence that DMS and DRS can be considered a delusional disorder apart from more generalized forms of confabulation.

Finally, there is an additional line of evidence that suggests that patients with DMS and DRS differ from the broader class of confabulatory patients. Numerous studies have demonstrated that ventromedial frontal damage is critical for the occurrence of spontaneous confabulation (Alexander & Freedman, 1984; Vikki, 1985; Fischer et al., 1995; Moskovitch & Mello, 1997; Ptak & Schnider, 1999; Stuss et al., 1978; Schnider & Ptak, 1999; Feinberg & Giacino, 2003; for reviews see DeLuca, 2000; Johnson et al., 2000). DeLuca and coworkers (1991; 1993; 2000) provided additional support for the role of combined basal forebrain and frontal damage in producing confabulation in ACoA patients.

However, there do not appear to be strongly lateralized effects when a broad range of confabulatory patients is considered. Indeed, in the largest literature review of confabulatory patients ever performed, Johnson and coworkers (2000) did an extensive analysis of the anatomical features of confabulatory patients. These authors *specifically eliminated* cases with confabulation manifesting as Capgras syndrome, reduplicative paramnesia, and Anton's syndrome. They also excluded confabulation associated with anosognosia for hemiplegia. In the ACoA group, the patient population for which the largest number of cases had anatomical data reported, there were approximately equal numbers of left- (14) and right- (15) hemisphere cases and marginally more unilateral (29) than bilateral (22) cases. Therefore, there is no evidence to suggest laterality effects in confabulatory patients when considered as a group.

In contrast, in the present series there was a highly significant laterality effect favoring right frontal dysfunction. This finding is consistent with prior studies that found that right hemisphere dysfunction is particularly common in delusional misidentification of places and persons (Alexander, Stuss, & Benson, 1979; Feinberg & Shapiro, 1989). Feinberg and Shapiro found that in reported cases of misidentification–reduplication in which cerebral dysfunction was unilateral, there was a highly significant right-hemispheric predominance in reduplication. This finding has been subsequently confirmed by others (Förstl et al., 1991; Fleminger & Burns, 1993; Burgess et al., 1996). Therefore, the finding of strong right frontal hemisphere predominance in the present series indicates that delusional misidentification and reduplication can be distinguished both clinically and neuroanatomically from confabulation.

"Reality Monitoring" Defect

Finally, Johnson and coworkers (1991; 2000) suggest a reality monitoring framework or a source monitoring framework to explain some aspects of confabulation (for review, see Johnson et al., 2002). According to the reality monitoring framework (Johnson, 1991), confabulations result from a failure to discriminate between memories and internally derived thoughts. According to the source monitoring framework, disturbances in the "encoding, retrieval, and evaluation" of perceptions and memories lead to a failure to distinguish veridical memory from self-generated confabulations. Confabulation in this view results from a failure of judgment processes that determine whether the perceptual information in a memory represents a true memory or imagination and additional judgments upon how this information conforms to previously acquired knowledge (Johnson et al., 2000).

A failure of reality monitoring could help explain why some confabulations appear to be "wish-fulfilling," but it does not explain why confabulations may become delusional in some patients and not others, and why patients with DMS or DRS, in contrast to patients with confabulation in general, have right frontal lesions. It also does not explain why the misidentifications in these cases are so selective or why patients do not have a generalized impairment in reality testing. As noted in Table 8–4, most of these cases do not show generalized confabulations or delusions in other domains.

"Positive" Theories

The *negative* neurological features listed in Table 8–5 are the result of a loss of neurological functions, and the majority of patients with significant right-hemisphere pathology will display these features. On the other hand, the question remains why the vast majority of patients with right-hemisphere lesions, including many with right frontal lesions, do not demonstrate delusional misidentification or reduplication. In order to answer this question, one must consider the *positive* neurological features in these cases that are the result of the functions of the remaining brain (Taylor, 1958).

In some instances it is not entirely clear whether a characteristic is a negative or positive feature of a disorder. For example, is the delusional nature of these disorders a positive or negative feature of these conditions? Delusions in general have been reported to occur with increased frequency in the presence of right-hemisphere pathology (Levine & Grek, 1984). Malloy and Richardson (1994), in a literature review of a wide variety of content-specific delusions, including delusional misidentification, sexual delusions, and somatic delusions, found a high incidence of lesions of the frontal lobes and right hemisphere, and Kumral and Özturk (2004) found delusional ideation in 15 of 360 stroke patients that was associated with right posterior temporoparietal lesions.

Alexander, Stuss, and Benson (1979) attributed the delusional ideation of a patient with Capgras syndrome to the presence of bilateral frontal deficits leading to a failure to resolve conflicting or competing information. However, one of the striking features of Table 8–4 is that five of six cases of Capgras misidentification involving persons had either prior or current paranoia, suspiciousness, or depression. Indeed, in the Alexander, Stuss, and Benson (1979) case the patient suffered from "grandiose and paranoid delusions, and had auditory hallucinations" prior to the brain injury that led to his Capgras delusions. This raises the possibility that in some cases premorbid personality features or psychopathology, especially *paranoia,* perhaps subserved by brain areas left undamaged by the cortical lesions, played a positive role in the production of these symptoms. Three of seven cases with Frégoli syndrome for persons had paranoia or other delusions, so the same association with psychopathology was present in this group, but not to the extent seen in patients who displayed Capgras for persons.

An entirely different picture emerges in the cases with Frégoli for place. In this group no patients were reported to be paranoid or demonstrate other evidence of psychopathology. However, in every instance the patients' conviction that they were close to or actually in their homes could not be corrected. Patterson and

Zangwill (1944) hypothesized that their patients' failure to accept evidence that conflicted with their delusional disorientation was related to their patients' desire to return home (see also Turnbull, Berry, & Evans, 2004; and Fotopoulou, Solms, & Turnbull, 2004, for a discussion of these issues). They argued that "a strong desire was actively inhibiting the cognitive mechanisms which normally subserve orientation" and that these patients were oblivious to the conflict presented by their dual orientation and would confabulate explanations when confronted with the disparity. The authors interpreted the delusional disorientation on the basis of both the *negative features*—in a Jacksonian sense (Taylor, 1958)—of anterograde and retrograde amnesia, restriction of perception, and a defect in judgment in which there is a failure to correct incompatible interpretations, as well as the positive features of motivation.

Ruff and Volpe (1981) also suggested that motivation might play a role in the maintenance of delusional disorientation. These authors described four patients who misidentified the location of their hospital rooms and claimed the hospital was located within their homes or that the hospital was moved into their houses. These authors suggested that a multiplicity of neurological and psychological factors created the delusional beliefs, and among these were motivational factors:

> all our patients insisted that they were at home. When they recovered each claimed that their confabulated stories resulted from a desire to be at home. Though it is difficult to know how the desire may have contributed to the formation of environmental reduplication in our patients, others have suggested that motivation may be essential in the formation and pattern of reduplication. . . . In summary, environmental reduplication in each of our patients was associated with a right parietal or frontal cerebral lesion, impaired spatial perception and visual memory, confusion or apathy early in the hospital course, and a strong desire to be at home.

Therefore, within the Frégoli group there is evidence that *motivation,* or *wishfulfillment,* is important in the creation and maintenance of the delusion.

Finally, there may be a role for a disturbance in *ego functions* in the creation of delusional misidentification and reduplication. For instance, in the delusional asomatognosia cases, the arm is not simply misidentified, it is projected onto another person close to the patient. Further, in the cases with delusional reduplication without misidentification, the patients' own disabilities are often projected onto external fictitious or reduplicated persons (Table 8–4). Thus, these cases demonstrate the potential role of psychological *projection* in the adaptation to the impairments. This is also the group in which anosognosia is most apparent.

Delusional Misidentification and Reduplication and the Self

In order to account for the five distinguishing features of delusional misidentification and reduplication enumerated above and at the same time account for the positive features noted in Table 8–5, we propose the following account for the etiology of these disorders. In addition to the perceptual, memory, and executive impairments enumerated in Table 8–5, patients with delusional misidentification and reduplication suffer from disorders of *ego boundaries* and *ego functions*. These findings indicate that the right hemisphere may be dominant for the self and self-related functions, and an important negative feature of right-hemisphere damage in this series appears to be a disturbance *of self* and *self-related functions*. This could account for why the misidentifications were almost universally and *selectively* about aspects of the self or others of personal significance and why the delusional misidentifications were *consistently* within this domain.

This hypothesis is consistent with the suggestion that delusional misidentification including its confabulatory aspects should be viewed as disorders of personal relatedness and the self (Feinberg, 1997a; 1997b; 2001); Feinberg & Roane, 1997a; 1997b) and account for disorders in which there is underrelatedness, overrelatedness, or both between the self and the environment. It also could explain why in this series there is the nearly universal presence of right frontal damage, as there is increasing evidence that the right hemisphere plays a dominant role in self-representation (for review, see Keenan et al., 2000; Keenan, Gallup, & Falk, 2003). For example, in an fMRI study of self-face presentation, Kircher and co-workers (2001) found that self-faces activated almost twice as much area in the right hemisphere compared to unfamiliar faces and 1.3 times greater when compared to familiar faces. In another study subjects were anesthetized during a presurgical WADA test and subsequently presented with a morphed face made up of a composite of their own face and that of a famous person. Subjects more readily identified the morphed face as their own when the right hemisphere was active (left hemisphere inactivated). Conversely, they identified the face as a famous person when the right hemisphere was inactive (Keenan et al., 2001). Other studies have shown right-hemisphere dominance for self-face recognition (Keenan et al., 2001; Keenan, Gallup, & Falk, 2003; Platek et al., 2004; Sugiura et al., 2000) as well as other self-related abilities including autobiographical memories (Calabrese et al., 1996; Fink et al., 1996; Markowitsch et al., 2000; Nakamura et al., 2001; see Decety & Sommerville, 2003, for review).

According to the proposed account, right frontal hemisphere damage creates a disturbance in ego functions that mediate the relationship between the self and the world both for personally significant incoming afferent information as well as for self-generated affects and drives. Thus, there is a *two-way disturbance* between the self and the environment specifically with regard to personal relatedness that could lead to disorders of *both* under- and overrelatedness to the environment. Without the mediation of right frontal regions that subserve certain self-related functions, patterns of personally significant incoming information may be disconnected from a feeling of familiarity (Alexander, Stuss, & Benson, 1979; Feinberg, 1987) or personal relatedness (Feinberg, 1997; 2001). On the other hand, in the presence of internally derived motives, such as the desire to be home, without the appropriate mediation of the ego functions of the right frontal regions, the wish may appear in the patient's mind as an externalized reality. In a similar fashion, in delusional asomatognosia, when the right frontal regions fail to establish the appropriate ego boundaries, the feelings of alienation from the arm result in the unmediated projection of the arm directly into the environment. Finally, in the case of delusional reduplication without misidentification, as occurs, for example, in the "phantom child syndrome," personal affects and feelings are projected onto fictitious others in the environment.

A potential factor linking right-hemisphere pathology to disturbed ego boundaries emphasizes the special role for the right hemisphere in spatial cognition. An accurate representation of the self–nonself boundary requires intact spatial cognition, since this boundary depends fundamentally on a concrete spatial distinction (perhaps the most basic of all such distinctions). Right-hemisphere damage that impairs spatial cognition therefore predisposes these patients to disturbances of ego boundaries. These disturbances consist not only of *deficits* of veridical self–nonself space representation, but also of the *release* of more primitive (affectively driven) representations of ego boundary, whereby the self represents space according to wishes rather than the unwelcome current reality (Kaplan-Solms & Solms, 2000).

Conclusions and Implications

According to Freud:

> Pathology has made us acquainted with a great number of states in which the boundary lines between the ego and the external world become uncertain or in which they are actually drawn incorrectly. There are cases in which parts of a person's own body, even portions of his mental life—his perceptions, thoughts and feelings—appear alien to him and as not belonging to his ego; there are other cases in which he ascribes to the external world things that clearly originate in his own ego and that ought to be acknowledged by it. Thus even the feeling of our own ego is subject to disturbances and the boundaries of the ego are not constant. (Freud, 1930, p. 66)

This statement could easily have been written to apply to the disorders enumerated in this chapter. It appears that the negative features of delusional misidentification and reduplication may be attributed to deficits produced by right frontal damage resulting in the disturbances of ego boundaries and ego functions. On the other hand, it follows that the positive features of the syndrome noted in Table 8–5—the verbally expressed defensive and motivated features of delusional misidentification—might be the product of the relatively intact left hemisphere or axial motivational system. Further, as Freud (1925) postulated a developmental progression from "pleasure-ego" to "reality-ego," our proposed mechanism may be described as a regression from a reality-ego to pleasure-ego construal of the self–nonself boundary (Kaplan-Solms & Solms, 2000).

Without the mediation of the right frontal lobe, the patient may display the negative features of an inappropriate alienation from items of personal relevance or, conversely, the positive features of inappropriate externalization of internal states, affects, and motivation. It is within the domain of these positive features that individual differences in motivation, personality, and adaptation may come into play that help explain why only a minority of patients with right frontal injury develop these disorders. Premorbid trends in personality type may not necessarily result in overt pathology and may not be apparent even to persons close to the patient. Under conditions of ambiguity (as in projective psychometric measures such as the Rorschach test), specific themes may emerge. Personal themes concerning work, family, and other emotionally salient material may be identified in those individuals that develop these delusional conditions, thus differentiating them from others with more random forms of confabulation.

References

Alexander, M.R. & Freedman, M. (1984). Amnesia after anterior communication artery aneurysm rupture. *Neurology, 34,* 752–757.

Alexander, M.P., Stuss, D.T., & Benson, D.F. (1979). Capgras syndrome: A reduplicative phenomenon. *Neurology, 29,* 334–339.

Baddeley, A.D. & Wilson, B. (1986). Amnesia autobiographical memory and confabulation. In: D.C. Rubin (Ed.) *Autobiographical Memory.* Cambridge: Cambridge University Press.

Baddeley, A.D. & Wilson, B. (1963). Frontal amnesia and the dysexecutive syndrome. *Brain and Cognition, 7,* 212–230.

Barbizet, J. (1963). Defect of memorizing of hippocampal-mammillary origin: A review. *Journal of Neurology, Neurosurgery and Psychiatry, 26,* 127–135.

Bauer, R.M. (1984). Autonomic recognition of names and faces: A neuropsychological application of the Guilty Knowledge Test. *Neuropsychologia, 22,* 457–469.

Bauer, R.M. (1986). The cognitive psychophysiology of prosopagnosia. In: H. Ellis, M. Jeeves, F. Newcombe, & A. Young (Eds.) *Aspects of Face Processing* (pp. 253–267). Dordrecht: Martinus Nijhoff.

Benson, D.F., Djenderedjian, A., Miller, B.L., et al. (1996). Neural basis of confabulation. *Neurology, 46,* 1239–1243.

Benson, D.F., Gardner, H., & Meadows, J.C. (1976). Reduplicative paramnesia. *Neurology, 26,* 147–151.

Berlyne, N. (1972). Confabulation. *British Journal of Psychiatry, 120,* 31–39.

Bonhoeffer, K. (1901). *Die akuten Geisteskrankheiten der Gewohnheitstrinker.* Jena: Gustav Fischer.

Bonhoeffer, K. (1904). Der Korsakowsche Symptomenkomplex in seinen Beziehungen zu den verschiedenen Krankheitsformen. *Allg Z Psychiatry, 61,* 744–752.

Bouvier-Perrou, M., Landis, T., & Annoni, Jean-Marie. (2000). Self-duplication shifted in time: A particular form of delusional misidentification syndrome. *Neurocase, 6,* 57–63.

Box, O., Laing, H., & Kopelman, M. (1999). The evolution of spontaneous confabulation, delusional misidentification and a related delusion in a case of severe head injury. *Neurocase, 5,* 251–262.

Burgess, P.W., Baxter, D., Martyn, R., & Alderman, N. (1996). Delusional paramnesic misidentification. In: P.W. Halligan & J.C. Marshall (Eds.) *Method in Madness: Case Studies in Cognitive Neuropsychiatry* (pp. 51–78). East Sussex, UK: Psychology Press.

Calabrese, P., Markowitsch, H.J., Durwen, H.F., Widlitzek, H., Haupts, M., Holinka, B., & Gehlen, W. (1996). Right temporofrontal cortex as critical locus for the ecphory of old episodic memories. *Journal of Neurology, Neurosurgery, and Psychiatry, 61,* 304–310.

Capgras, J. & Reboul-Lachaux, J. (1923). L'illusion des "sosies" dans un delire systematise. *Bulletin de Société Clinique de Médicine Mentale, 11,* 6–16.

Christodoulou, G.N. (1976). Delusional hyper-identifications of the Fregoli type. *Acta Psychiatrica Scandinavica, 54,* 305–314.

Christodoulou, G.N. (1977). The syndrome of Capgras. *British Journal of Psychiatry, 130,* 556–564.

Christodoulou, G.N. (1991). The delusional misidentification syndromes. *British Journal of Psychiatry, 14,* 65–69.

Christodoulou, G.N. (1986). Role of depersonalization-derealization phenomena in the delusional misidentification syndromes. *Bibliotecha Psychiatrica, 164,* 99–104.

Conway, M.A. & Tacchi, P.C. (1996). Motivated confabulation. *Neurocase, 2,* 325–339.

Courbon, P. & Fail, G. (1927). Syndrome d'ilusion de Frégoli et schizophrénie. *Bulletin de Société Clinique de Médicine Mentale, 15,* 121–24.

Critchley, M. (1955). Personification of paralyzed limbs in hemiplegics. *British Medical Journal, 30,* 284–287.

Dalla Barba, G. (1993). Confabulation: Knowledge and recollective experience. *Cognitive Neuropsychology, 10(1),* 1–20.

Decety, J. & Sommerville, J.A. (2003). Shared representations between self and other: A social cognitive neuroscience view. *Trends in Cognitive Science, 12,* 527–533.

DeLuca, J. & Cicerone, K.D. (1991). Confabulation following aneurysm of the anterior communicating artery. *Cortex, 27,* 417–424.

DeLuca, J. (1993). Predicting neurobehavioral patterns following anterior communicating artery aneurysm. *Cortex, 29,* 639–647.

DeLuca, J. A. (2000). Cognitive neuroscience perspective on confabulation. *Neuro-Psychoanalysis, 2,* 119–132.

de Pauw, K.W. (1994). Delusional misidentification: A plea for an agreed terminology and classification. *Psychopathology, 27,* 123–129.

de Pauw, K.W., Szulecka, T.K., & Poltock, T.R. (1987). Frégoli syndrome after cerebral infarction. *Journal of Nervous and Mental Diseases, 175,* 433–438.

Dohn, H.H. & Crews, E.L. (1968). Capgras syndrome: A literature review and case series. *Hillside Journal of Clinical Psychiatry, 8,* 56–74.

Ellis, H.D. & Young, A.W. (1990). Accounting for delusional misidentification. *British Journal of Psychiatry, 157,* 239–248.

Feinberg, T.E. (1997a). Some interesting perturbations of the self in neurology. *Seminars in Neurology, 17,* 129–135.

Feinberg, T.E. (1997b). Anosognosia and confabulation. In: T.E. Feinberg & M.J. Farah (Eds.) *Behavioral Neurology and Neuropsychology.* (pp. 369–390). New York: McGraw-Hill.

Feinberg, T.E. (2001). *Altered Egos: How the Brain Creates the Self.* New York: Oxford University Press.

Feinberg, T.E., Eaton, L.A., Roane, D.M., & Giacino, J.T. (1999). Multiple Fregoli delusions after traumatic brain injury. *Cortex, 35,* 373–387.

Feinberg, T.E. & Giacino, J.T. (2003). Confabulation. In: T.E. Feinberg & M.J. Farah (Eds.) *Behavioral Neurology and Neuropsychology, 2nd Edition.* (pp. 363–372). New York: McGraw-Hill.

Feinberg, T.E., Haber, L.D., & Leeds, N.E. (1990). Verbal asomatognosia. *Neurology, 40,* 1391–1394.

Feinberg, T.E. & Roane, D.M. (1997a). Anosognosia, completion and confabulation: The neutral-personal dichotomy. *Neurocase, 3,* 73–85.

Feinberg, T.E., & Roane, D. (1997b). Misidentification syndromes. In: T.E. Feinberg & M.J. Farah (Eds.) *Behavioral Neurology and Neuropsychology* (pp. 391–397). New York: McGraw-Hill.

Feinberg, T.E., & Roane, D. (2003a). Misidentification syndromes. In: T.E. Feinberg & M.J. Farah (Eds.) *Behavioral Neurology and Neuropsychology* (pp. 373–381). New York: McGraw-Hill.

Feinberg, T.E. & Roane, D.M. (2003b). Anosognosia. In: T.E. Feinberg & M.J. Farah (Eds.) *Behavioral Neurology and Neuropsychology*. New York: McGraw-Hill.

Feinberg, T.E., Roane, D.M., & Ali, J. (2000). Illusory limb movements in anosognosia for hemiplegia. *Journal of Neurology, Neurosurgery, and Psychiatry, 68,* 511–513.

Feinberg, T.E. & Shapiro, R.M. (1989). Misidentification-reduplication and the right hemisphere. *Neuropsychiatry, Neuropsychology, and Behavioral Neurology, 2,* 39-48.

Fink, G.R., Markowitsch, H.J., Reinkemeier, M., Bruckbauer, T., Kessler, J., & Heiss, W.D. (1996). Cerebral representation of one's own past: Neural networks involved in autobiographical memory. *Journal of Neuroscience, 16,* 4275–4282.

Fischer, R.S., Alexander, M.P., D'Esposito, M., & Otto, R. (1995). Neuropsychological and neuroanatomical correlates of confabulation. *Clinical and Experimental Neuropsychology, 17,* 20–28.

Fleminger, S. & Burns, A. (1993). The delusional misidentification syndromes in patients with and without evidence of organic cerebral disorder: A structured review of case reports. *Biological Psychiatry, 33,* 22–32.

Förstl, H., Almeida, O.P., Owen, A., et al. (1991). Psychiatric, neurological and medical aspects of misidentification syndromes: A review of 260 cases. *Psychological Medicine, 21,* 905–950.

Fotopoulou, A., Solms, M., & Turnbull, O.H. (2004). Wishful reality distortions in confabulation: A case report. *Neuropsychologia, 42,* 727–744.

Freud, S. (1925). *Negation.* Standard Edition, 19. (p. 233–239). London: Hogarth Press, 1961.

Freud, S. (1930). *Civilization and Its Discontents, Standard Edition,* 21 (p. 66). London: Hogarth Press, 1961.

Hakim, H., Verma, N.P., & Greiffenstein, M.F. (1988). Pathogenesis of reduplicative paramnesia. *Journal of Neurology, Neurosurgery, and Psychiatry, 51,* 839–841.

Hayman, M.A. & Abrams, R. (1977). Capgras' syndrome and cerebral dysfunction. *British Journal of Psychitary, 130,* 68–71.

Hirstein, W., & Ramachandran, V.S. (1997). Capgras syndrome: A novel probe for understanding the neural representation of the identity and familiarity of persons. *Proceedings of the Royal Society of London B, 264,* 437–444.

Johnson, M.K. (1991). Reality monitoring: Evidence from confabulation in organic brain disease patients. In: G.P. Prigatano & G.L. Schacter (Eds.) *Awareness of Deficit after Brain Injury: Clinical and Theoretical Issues* (pp. 176–197). New York: Oxford University Press.

Johnson, M.K., Hayes, S.M., D'Esposito, M., & Raye, C.L. (2000). Confabulation. In: J. Grafman & F. Boller (Eds.) *Handbook of Neuropsychology, 2nd Ed.* (pp. 383–407). Amsterdam: Elsevier Science.

Joseph, A.B. (1968). Focal central nervous system abnormalities in patients with misidentification syndromes. In: G.N. Christodoulou (Ed.) *The Delusional Misidentification Syndromes* (p. 68). Basel: Karger.

Kaplan-Solms, K. & Solms, M. (2000). *Clinical Studies in Neuro-Psychoanalysis.* London: Karnac Books.

Kapur, N. & Couglan, A.K. (1980). Confabulation and frontal lobe dysfunction. *Neurology, Neurosurgery, and Psychiatry, 43,* 461–463.

Kapur, N., Turner, A., & King, C. (1988). Reduplicative paramnesia: Possible anatomical and neuropsychological mechanisms. *Neurology, Neurosurgery, and Psychiatry, 51,* 579–581.

Keenan, J.P., Wheeler, M.A., Gallup, G.G., & Pascual-Leone, A. (2000). Self-recognition and the right prefrontal cortex. *Trends in Cognitive Science, 4,* 338–334.

Keenan, J.P., Nelson, A., O'Connor, M., & Pascual-Leone, A. (2001). Self-recognition and the right hemisphere. *Nature, 409 (6818),* 305.

Keenan, J.P., Gallup, G.G., & Falk, D. (2003). *The Face in the Mirror: The Search for the Origins of Consciousness.* New York: Harper Collins/Ecco.

Kircher, T.T., Senior, C., Phillips, M.L., Rabe-Hesketh, S., Benson, P.J., Bullmore, E.T., Brammer, M., Simmons, A., Bartels, M., & David, A.S. (2001). Recognizing one's own face. *Cognition, 78,* B1–B15.

Korsakoff, S.S. (1889). *Psychic Disorder in Conjunction with Peripheral Neuritis.* Translated and republished by M. Victor & P.I. Yakovlev. (1955). *Neurology, 5,* 394–406.

Kraepelin, E. (1904). *Lectures on Clinical Psychiatry.* Translated by T. Johnstone. London: Bailliere, Tindall, & Cox.

Kraepelin, E. (1907). *Clinical Psychiatry: A Textbook for Students and Physicians.* Translated by A.R. Diefendorf. New York: MacMillan.

Kraepelin, E. (1919). *Dementia Praecox and Paraphrenia.* Translated by R.M. Barclay. Edinburgh, UK: E. & S. Livingstone.

Kumral, E. & Özturk, Ö. (2004). Delusional state following acute stroke. *Neurology, 62,* 110–113.

Levin, M. (1945). Delirious disorientation: The law of the unfamiliar mistaken for the familiar. *Journal of Mental Science, 91,* 447–53.

Levine, D.N. & Grek, A. (1984). The anatomic basis for delusions after right cerebral infarction. *Neurology, 34,* 577–582.

Malloy, P.F. & Richardson, E.D. (1994). The frontal lobes and content-specific delusions. *Journal of Neuropsychiatry and Clinical Neurosciences, 6,* 455–466.

Markowitsch, H.J., Thiel, A., Reinkemeier, M., Kessler, J., Koyuncu, A., & Heiss, W.D. (2000). Right amygdalar and temporofrontal activation during autobiographic, but not during fictitious memory retrieval. *Behavioral Neurology, 12,* 181–190.

Mattioli, F., Miozzo, A., & Vignolo. (1999). Confabualtion and delusional misidentification: A four year follow-up study. *Cortex, 35,* 413–422.

Meador, K.J., Loring, D.W., Feinberg, T.E., Lee, G.P., & Nichols, M.E. (2000). Anosognosia and asomatognosia during intracarotid amobarbital inactivation. *Neurology, 55,* 816–820.

Moscovitch, M. (1989). Confabulation and the frontal systems: Strategic vs. associative retrieval in neuropsychological theories of memory. In: H.L. Roediger & F.M. Craik (Eds.) *Varieties of Memory and Consciousness: Essays in Honour of Endel Tulving* (pp. 133–160). Hillsdale, NJ: Lawrence Erlbaum.

Moscovitch, M. (1995). Confabulation. In: D.L. Schacter (Ed.) *Memory Distortion: How Minds, Brains and Societies Reconstruct the Past* (pp. 226–251). Cambridge, MA: Harvard University Press.

Moscovitch, M. & Melo, B. (1997). Strategic retrieval and the frontal lobes: Evidence from confabulation and amnesia. *Neuropsychologia, 35,* 1017–1034.

Moser, D.J., Cohen, R.A., Malloy, P.F., Stone, W.M., & Rogg, J.M. (1998). Reduplicative paramnesia: Longitudinal neurobehavioral and neuroimaging analysis. *Journal of Geriatric Psychiatry and Neurology, 11,* 174–80.

Nakamura, K., Kawashima, R., Sugiura, M., Kato, T., Nakamura, A., Hatano, K.,

Nagumo, S., Kubota, K., Fukuda, H., Ito, K., & Kojima, S. (2001). Neural substrates for recognition of familiar voices: A PET study. *Neuropsychologia, 39,* 1047–1054.

Patterson, A. & Zangwill, O.L. (1944). Recovery of spatial orientation in the post-traumatic confusional state. *Brain, 67,* 54–68.

Pick, A. (1903). On reduplication paramnesia. *Brain, 26,* 260–267.

Platek, S., Keenan, J.P., Gallup, G.G., & Mohamed, F. (2004). Where am I? The neurological correlates of self and other. *Cognitive Brain Research, 19,* 114–122.

Price, B.H. & Mesulam, M. (1985). Psychiatric manifestations of right hemisphere infarctions. *Journal of Nervous and Mental Diseases, 173,* 610–614.

Ptak, R. & Schnider, A. (1999). Spontaneous confabulations after orbitofrontal damage: The role of temporal context confusion and self-monitoring. *Neurocase, 5,* 243–250.

Ramachandran, V.S. (1998). Consciousness and body image: Lessons from phantom limbs, Capgras syndrome and pain asymbolia. *Philosophical Transactions of the Royal Society of London B, 353,* 1851–1859.

Rapcsak, S.Z., Polster, M.R., Glisky, M.L., & Comer, J.F. (1996). False recognition of unfamiliar faces following right hemisphere damage: Neuropsychological and anatomical observations. *Cortex, 32,* 593–611.

Ruff, R.L. & Volpe, B.T. (1981). Environmental reduplicaton associated with right frontal and parietal lobe injury. *Journal of Neurology, Neurosurgery and Psychiatry, 44,* 382–86.

Schnider, A. (2003). Spontaneous confabulation and the adaptation of thought to ongoing reality. *Nature Reviews Neuroscience, 4,* 662–671.

Schnider, A, von Daniken, C., & Gutbrod, K. (1996). Disorientation in amnesia. A confusion of memory traces. *Brain, 119,* 1627–1632.

Schnider, A., Gutbrod, K., Hess, C.W., et al. (1996). Memory without context: Amnesia with confabulations after infarction of the right capsular genu. *Journal of Neurology Neurosurgery, and Psychiary, 61,* 186–193.

Schnider, A. & Ptak, R. (1999). Spontaneous confabulators fail to suppress currently irrelevant memory traces. *Nature Neuroscience, 2,* 677–681.

Schnider, A., Ptak, R., von Daniken, C., et al. (2000). Recovery from spontaneous confabulations parallels recovery of temporal confusion in memory. *Neurology, 55,* 74–83.

Staton, R.D., Brumback, R.A., & Wilson, H. (1982). Reduplicative paramnesia: A disconnection syndrome of memory. *Cortex, 18,* 23–36.

Stuss, D.T., Alexander, M.P., Lieberman, A., & Levine, H. (1978). An extraordinary form of confabulation. *Neurology, 28,* 116–172.

Stuss, D.T. (1991). Disturbance of self-awareness after frontal system damage. In: G.P. Prigatano & D.L. Schacter (Eds.) *Awareness of Deficit After Brain Injury: Clinical and Theoretical Issues* (pp. 63–83). New York: Oxford University Press.

Sugiura, M., Kawashima, R., Nakamura, K., Okada, K., Kato, T., Nakamura, A., Hatano, K., Itoh, K., Kojima, S., & Fukada, H. (2000). Passive and active recognition of one's own face. *Neuroimage, 11,* 36–48.

Talland, G.A. (1961). Confabulation in the Wernicke-Korsakoff syndrome. *Journal of Nervous and Mental Diseases, 132,* 361–381.

Talland, G.A. (1965). *Deranged Memory.* New York: Academic Press.

Taylor, J. (1958). *Selected Writings of John Hughlings Jackson.* New York: Basic Books.

Turnbull, O.H., Berry, H., & Evans, C.E. (2004). A positive emotional bias in confabulatory false beliefs about place. *Brain and Cognition, 55,* 490–494.

Ullman, M. (1960). Motivational and structural factors in denial of hemiplegia. *Archives of Neurology, 3,* 306–318.

Van Der Horst, L. (1932). Uber die Psychologie des Korsakowsyndroms. *Monatschr Psychiatry and Neurology, 83,* 65–84.

Victor, M., Adams, R.D., & Collins, G.H. (1989). *The Wernicke-Korsakoff Syndrome and Related Neurological Disorders due to Alcoholism and Malnutrition,* 2nd ed. Philadelphia: Davis.

Victor, M., & Yakovlev, P.I. (1955). SS Korsakoff's psychic disorder in conjunction with peripheral neuritis: A translation of Korsakoff's original article with brief comments on the author and his contribution to clinical medicine. *Neurology, 5,* 394–406.

Vié, J. (1930). Un trouble de l'identification des personnes: L'illusion des sosies. *Annales Médico- Psychologiques (Paris), 88,* 214–237.

Vié, J. (1944a). Les meconnaissances systematiques. *Annales Médico- Psychologiques (Paris), 102,* 410–455.

Vié, J. (1944b). Le substratum morbide et les stades evolutifs des meconnaissances systematiques. *Annales Médico-Psychologiques (Paris), 102,* 410–455.

Vié, J. (1944c). Etude psychopathologique des meconnaissances systematiques. *Annales Médico-Psychologiques (Paris), 102,* 1–15.

Vighetto, A., Aimard, G., Confavreux, C., & Devic, M. (1980). Une observation anatomo-clinique de fabulation (ou délire) topografique. *Cortex, 16,* 501–507.

Vilkki, J. (1985). Amnesic syndromes after surgery of anterior communicating artery aneurysms. *Cortex, 21,* 431–444.

Weinstein, E.A. (1996). Symbolic aspects of confabulation following brain injury: Influence of premorbid personality. *Bulletin of the Menninger Clinic, 60,* 331–350.

Weinstein, E.A. & Kahn, R.L. (1952). Non-aphasic misnaming (paraphasia) in organic brain disease. *Archives of Neurology and Psychiatry, 67,* 72–79.

Weinstein, E.A, & Kahn, R.L. (1955). *Denial of Illness.* Springfield, IL: Charles C. Thomas.

Weinstein, E.A., Kahn, R.L., & Morris, G.O. (1956). Delusions about children following brain injury. *Journal of Hillside Hospital, 5,* 290–298.

Weinstein, E.A. & Friedland, R.P. (1977). Behavioral disorders associated with hemi-inattention. In: E.A. Weinstein & R.P. Friedland (Eds.) *Advances in Neurology.* (pp. 51–62). New York: Raven Press.

Weinstein, E.A. & Kahn, R.L. (1950). The syndrome of anosognosia. *Archives of Neurology and Psychiatry, 64,* 772–791.

Weinstein, E.A. & Kahn, R.L. (1955). *Denial of Illness.* Springfield, IL: Charles C. Thomas.

Weinstein, E.A. & Cole, M. (1964a). Concepts of anosognosia. In: L.E. Halpern (Ed.) *Dynamic Neurology.* (pp. 254–273). Jerusalem: Jerusalem Post Press.

Weinstein, E.A., Cole, M., Mitchell, M.S., & Lyerly, O. (1964b). Anosognosia and aphasia. *Archives of Neurology and Psychiatry, 10,* 376–386.

Weinstein, E.A. (1991). Anosognosia and denial of illness. In: G.P. Prigatano & D.L. Schacter (Eds.) *Awareness of Deficit after Brain Injury: Clinical and Theoretical Issues* (pp. 240–257). New York: Oxford University Press.

Weinstein, E.A., Friedland, R.P., & Wagner, E.E. (1994). Denial/unawareness of impairment and symbolic behavior in Alzheimer's disease. *Neuropsychiatry, Neuropsychology, and Behavioral Neurology, 7,* 176–184.

Weinstein, E.A. & Friedland, R.P. (1977). Behavioral disorders associated with hemi-inattention. In: E.A. Weinstein & R.P. Friedland (Eds.) *Advances in Neurology* (pp. 51–62). New York: Raven Press.

Williams, H.W. & Rupp, C. (1938). Observations on confabulation. *American Journal of Psychiatry, 95,* 395–405.

9

The Mirror Sign Delusional
Misidentification Symptom

KAREN SPANGENBERG POSTAL

> . . . the mirror of the mind is the face, its index the eyes.
> *Cicero*

Beginning in toddlerhood, the act of looking into a mirror is associated metaphorically with self-reflection. What more devastating blow to the self, then, is the loss of the capacity to recognize oneself in the mirror? Delusional misidentification symptoms (DMS) have been hailed as excellent examples of the interaction between neuropathological and psychological processes (Flemminger, 1994). The mirror sign, a bizarre DMS involving the misidentification of oneself in the mirror, presents investigators with just such a unique opportunity to track the pathophysiology of a delusional phenomenon. In this chapter the mirror sign is described from phenomenological, neuropathological, and neuropsychological perspectives. The chapter begins with a case description of an elderly woman who saw the image of herself as a little girl when she looked in the mirror (Spangenberg, Wagner, & Bachman, 1998).

CASE EXAMPLE

MH appeared to be a perfectly normal elderly southern lady, meticulously polite with a soft-spoken manner. Two of MH's seven children accompanied her to the office visit. They reported that she was in her normal "right mind" until the previous year when she underwent cataract surgery followed by a hypotensive crisis. At that point there was an abrupt change in her mental status. She "went crazy" hallucinating that a little girl was living in her house. It soon became clear to them that she "saw" the girl only when looking in the mirrors of her home, particularly the bathroom. Seven months later, MH was admitted to the hospital with a urinary tract infection. Her symptom appeared to worsen at that point. She would see the "little girl" in all types of reflective surfaces, not just mirrors. When she walked down the street to go shopping, she would see the girl in the reflections of store windows. MH began to conclude at that point that the "girl" was following her around town. She also began to make other types of visual errors, mistaking a coat hanging across the room for a person and feeling that large crowds of people were watching her from across the street. A personality change accompanied the worsening of MH's symptoms. Her children described her as "sweet and retiring" before and increasingly irritable and paranoid after the symptoms worsened.

Remarkably, given her highly unusual chief complaint, during the several-hour neurological and neuropsychological portions of the examination, MH displayed no peculiar behavior. Even when administered the Geriatric Mood Inventory (Yesavage et al., 1983) and given ample opportunity to discuss emotional issues, no mention was made of the "little girl" by the patient. Had family members not brought up the symptom, no portion of the patient interview or standard neuropsychological evaluation would have surfaced it.

To investigate MH's reaction to the mirror, she was presented with a small hand-held mirror. For the first time in the examination, she became animated, stating "That girl! What is she doing here? I thought she was only back home!" Agitated, she began a lengthy tirade implicating "the girl" in a scheme to move into her home and drain her resources. "I just can't afford to feed two people!" Interestingly, when asked to describe the girl in the mirror, she stated that the girl "favored her [resembled her]" but was much younger than herself. She looked like MH did when MH was a young girl.

When confronted with the fact that she was looking at a reflection of herself in the mirror, MH adamantly denied it, stating "It's that girl!" To clarify whether there was a dissociation between her ability to recognize others and herself in the mirror, an examiner then tilted the mirror at an angle so that the patient saw the examiner rather than herself. MH was easily able to recognize the examiner but unable to recognize herself. Even after extensive coaching about the mirror and its reflection, she maintained the misperception that her reflection was that of the little girl.

A CT scan of MH's head demonstrated significant periventricular white matter change in the bilateral parieto-occipital watershed regions, particularly involving the right posterior parietal region. White matter changes were also apparent bifrontally. An MRI scan of the head demonstrated lacunar infarcts in the right basal ganglia region and both thalami and mild generalized atrophy. Results of the diagnostic examinations, including neuropsychological testing described below, indicated acute mild onset vascular dementia with disproportional right hemispheric symptoms.

Epidemiology

Mirror Sign as a Delusional Misidentification Symptom

Fascinating symptoms involving the misidentification of self, others, place, time, and objects have all been reported in the psychiatric and neurological literatures and eventually classified under a broader category of delusional misidentification symptoms (DMS) by Christodoulou (1986; see also chapter 8 this volume). The mirror sign is largely considered a DMS characterized by an inability to recognize one's own image in the mirror, usually in the presence of an intact ability to recognize others in the mirror (Foley & Breslau, 1982).

There is some disagreement in the categorization of specific subtypes of DMS, with several different classification systems and inconsistent agreement on inclusion and exclusion criteria (see Markova & Berrios, 1994, for a review). Weinstein

(1994) categorized the various DMS as all "doubling" place, person, time, body parts, or self. This is consistent with case reports describing the mirror sign as a "Capgrass syndrome for the mirror image," (Gluckman, 1968; Feinberg & Shapiro, 1989) Others treat the mirror sign as a distinct DMS subcategory (Mendez et al., 1992). Less often, the mirror sign has been excluded altogether from the larger DMS category, based on its emergence in the context of prominent global cognitive deterioration (Cummings, 1985; Forstl et al., 1991b).

Whether the inability to recognize oneself in the mirror in the context of global profound neurocognitive deficits represents true mirror sign is a salient question. Cummings (1985) suggests that the mental confusion and diffuse cerebral pathology associated with dementia in general is likely to result in simple, transient delusions and does not categorize these simple delusions with other DMS. The mirror sign is noted as an example of such delusions. Likewise, Forstl and colleagues (1991b) suggest that distinctions between types of DMS (including mirror sign) may not be necessary in cases with prominent global cognitive impairment, as is typical in Alzheimer dementia (AD). In this vein, Grewel (1994) demonstrated that the inability to recognize oneself in the mirror was strongly associated with severe dementia, while patients who were only moderately demented usually retained this ability. Similarly, Biringer, Anderson, and Strubel (1988) found that none of their profoundly demented patients could self-recognize, while 50% of their severely and 100% of their moderately demented patients could recognize themselves in a mirror. Given the prominent association between the inability to recognize oneself in the mirror and increasing dementia severity, neuropsychological data establishing the fixed, focal nature of the symptom, independent of a global dementia, would appear necessary to distinguish a legitimate mirror sign delusional misidentification symptom from general cognitive disorganization. Such data have been described in case examples (Feinberg & Shapiro, 1989; Spangenberg, 1998; Breen et al., 2001), lending support for the mirror sign's inclusion in the broader DMS category as a distinct entity.

Prevalence of the Mirror Sign
Forstl and coworkers (1994a) appropriately point out that delusional misidentification symptoms "are neither syndromes or diseases" and can occur in a variety of diseases affecting different systems of the brain. Although DMS as a whole have been noted in an array of diseases in psychiatric and neurological populations, specific mention of the mirror sign is rarely included. The exception to this is the Alzheimer disease literature, in which several epidemiologic studies of DMS include the mirror sign. The prevalence of the mirror sign within these studies varies considerably, between 2% and 22%. For example, Mendez and coworkers (1992) reported that out of a sample of 217 patients diagnosed with dementia of the Alzheimer type, 5 (2.3%) exhibited the mirror sign. Forstl and coworkers (1991b) examined 128 Alzheimer patients, 5.5% of whom exhibited mirror sign. In another series of studies, Forstl and colleagues (1994a) reported prevalences of 4% and 22% in a consecutive series of 56 and 50 patients, respectively. Although the mirror sign has been primarily reported in the context of AD, individual cases of mir-

ror sign have been reported in the context of vascular dementia (Spangenberg, Wagner, & Bachman, 1998; Breen, Caine, & Coltheart, 2001) and schizophrenia (Gluckman, 1968).

Screening Procedures in the Clinical Evaluation of the Mirror Sign
One of the problems with estimating the prevalence of the mirror sign is that it may be overlooked in the course of a typical neurological or neuropsychological workup. One approach to determining whether patients exhibit the mirror sign is to ask the patients' family members. Unfortunately, few rating scales specifically address the mirror sign. For example, a current mainstay of neuropsychiatric research in demented populations is the BEHAV-AD (Reisberg et al., 1987). Although specific questions address the Capgras delusion, no question asks about mirror sign. Even scales designed specifically to address delusions (e.g., Dementia Psychosis Scale, Migliorelli et al., 1995) may not include the mirror sign, although some do (e.g., Coulmbia University Scale for Psychopathology in Alzheimer's Disease; Devanand et al., 1992).

Another approach to determining whether the mirror sign is present is to perform bedside testing. Spangenberg, Wagner, and Bachman (1998) use a mirror sign clinical protocol in which patients are presented with a hand-held mirror and allowed to respond spontaneously. They are next asked to identify the person in the mirror. A dissociation is then tested for between their ability to recognize themselves and others in the mirror by tilting the mirror and asking them to identify the examiner who is in view. Others have described more elaborate procedures to test for the presence of the mirror sign. Biringer, Anderson, and Strabel (1988) borrowed a strategy from the developmental psychology literature designed to determine toddlers' ability to recognize themselves in the mirror. This involves surreptitiously placing a mark on the patients' faces and then turning them toward a mirror. If a patient reacts to the mark verbally or tries to manually interact with the mark (e.g., touch it on their own face), then mirror self-recognition can be inferred. To clarify that general inattention or lack of concern is not the cause of patients' failure to respond to the facial mark, a second procedure is used, furtively placing a mark on the patients' hands and recording the reaction. Although clearly superior for research purposes, using the furtive marking method as part of a screening procedure for mirror sign in a clinical setting would very likely alienate higher-functioning patients!

Other DMS Accompanying the Mirror Sign:
The Case of the Phantom Boarder

Delusional misidentification symptoms are often found to coexist (Joseph, 1986). However, Breen, Caine, and Coltheart (2001) point out that the phantom boarder delusional misidentification symptom (PBS), the delusional belief that another person is living in one's home, may actually be a result of patients misidentifying their mirror image (and doctors and family members misidentifying the delusion). The association between PBS and the mirror sign was addressed by Hwang, Yang, and Tsai (2003), who studied PBS in 240 demented patients. Of these, 21% of the subset who believed that a phantom boarder was in their home also misidentified their mirror images. In contrast, only 3% of the sample who did not have PBS misidentified their mirror images. This study suggests that there is indeed a connection between the mirror sign and PBS. Given this data, when PBS is reported, further investigation of the possibility that the mirror sign is also present is warranted.

Phenomenology

Overt vs. Covert Self-Recognition in Mirrors

An interesting phenomenon has been reported in cases of mirror sign in which patients cannot recognize themselves yet use the mirror as if they did. Bologna and Camp (1997) tested mirror recognition in 15 severely demented Alzheimer patients, 3 of whom met criteria for mirror sign. All three demonstrated primping behavior when given a comb, even though they could not identify themselves as the person in the mirror. The dissociation was startlingly underscored when each participant both primped and had a conversation with "the other" in the mirror during the same 5-minute rating interval.

Because Bologna and Camp's patients were all globally demented, as were a series of patients studied in a similar manner by Biringer, Anderson, and Strubel (1988), it is not clear whether the dissociation would be present in patients in whom the mirror sign was a focal symptom. In other words, in a less-demented individual, would the automatic and procedural reaction to the mirror (primping) cue a realization that they were therefore looking at themselves in the mirror? The answer is apparently "no." Breen, Caine, and Coltheart (2001) reported a nonglobally demented patient, FE, who continued to shave in front of a mirror despite demonstrating the mirror sign. Additionally, when asked if the "stranger" in the mirror was bald, FE tilted his head in the mirror to look, clearly demonstrating a dissociation in inplict and explicit self-recognition behavior.

Intact Recognition of Self in Photographs in Mirror Sign Patients
Another interesting phenomenon reported in published mirror sign cases is the intact ability of patients to recognize themselves in photographs despite an inability to recognize themselves in mirrors. For example, Phillips, Howard, and David (1996) reported that an 80-year-old woman, EF, was able to recognize herself in photographs but could not recognize herself in the mirror. Breen and coworkers (2000) reported a similar phenomenon with their patient, FE, noting that he was able to recognize a past representation of himself (the photo) but was not able to recognize a concurrent representation (the mirror). Phillips and colleagues pointed out that this was consistent with models of visual processing that hold that an expected image is compared with the actual image before recognition takes place. If the patient's expected image is erroneous (e.g., an earlier memory of what one looks like in the mirror) then a "match" does not occur, and recognition does not take place.

In this vein Mendez and coworkers (1992) noted that damage to the temporal and limbic areas that commonly occurs in AD may cause poor integration of visual perception and memory, "decoupling" patients' perceptions from appropriate memory. Defective formation of new visual memories may also underlie patients' outdated expectations for how they should appear in the mirror (Silva et al., 2001). Our patient MH's insistence that her mirror reflection was that of a little girl who looked like her when she was a little girl supports this hypothesis.

Paranoia and Aggression Accompanying the Mirror Sign
In a description of seven patients who exhibited mirror sign, Foley and Breslau (1982) noted that paranoia often accompanied the symptom. The "stranger" in the mirror was typically regarded as an undesirable character or someone intending harm. Mendez and coworkers (1992) reported that four out of five of their subjects who demonstrated the mirror sign had angry and paranoid reactions to their mirror images. In the case of MH, paranoid ideation developed about the "little girl" in the mirror, particularly when she began to see the little girl in all reflected surfaces, not just mirrors. The finding that paranoia often accompanies the mirror sign, and in the case of MH, increased as the symptom generalized to any reflective surface, is consistent with Flemminger's (1992) model of DMS, which predicts that paranoia will escalate as a result of a cycle of distorted visual hypotheses that are confirmed in the context of poor basic visual perception.

The tendency of the misidentified persons to be the objects of anger and suspicion has been established for delusional misidentification symptoms as a whole (Silva et al., 1997). Cummings (1985) noted that aggressively acting on delusional beliefs was common in his series of patients with organic delusions. In Forstl and coworkers' (1991a) series of 260 DMS cases, physical aggression was reported in 18%. The issue of why some patients with delusional misidentification symptoms display an angry reaction, however, has not been well addressed. Silva and colleagues (1997) hypothesized that the temporal and limbic structures involved in faulty facial perception may also be involved in aggression in these patients.

Mirror Agnosia

Do patients with the mirror sign understand what a mirror is and use it appropriately? Ramachandran, Altschuler, and Hillyer (1997) described four patients who displayed "mirror agnosia" following right-hemisphere stroke with left hemispatial neglect. When a mirror was placed on their right side, reflecting objects on their neglected left side, the patients tried to reach into the mirror to grasp the objects. Remarkably, this occurred even when the patients could verbally state that they were looking into a mirror. None of the patients were reportedly demented and were otherwise noted to be logical in their thought processes. Interestingly, when a mirror was placed in front of them, reflecting objects just beyond their right visual field, patients appropriately reached for the objects behind their shoulders. Binkofski and colleagues' (1999) study of 13 patients with mirror agnosia concluded that hemispatial neglect was not a necessary condition for the symptom. MRI studies demonstrated that lesions of overlap occurred in the posterior angular gyrus and superior temporal gyrus on either the right or the left. Unfortunately, whether the patients exhibited the mirror sign was not addressed in either study.

Breen, Caine, and Coltheart (2001) described a patient with mirror sign, TH, who also demonstrated striking mirror agnosia. Neuroradiological studies revealed subcortical ischemic changes, a small cortical infarct in the posterior right frontal lobe, and bilateral profusion deficits in the posterior parietal cortices. TH demonstrated accurate semantic knowledge of mirrors. There was no hemispatial neglect. When an experiment similar to Ramachandran's was carried out, TH was unable to accurately reach for objects behind both his right and left shoulders, instead scratching the mirror or attempting to reach behind it.

Although Breen and colleagues (2001) reported two cases of mirror sign, the mirror agnosia experiment was performed on only one. As no other published cases of mirror sign specifically tested for the presence of mirror agnosia, the prevalence of this interesting phenomenon in cases of mirror sign is not yet known.

Disordered Body Schema

In studies that addressed the pathogenesis of the mirror sign there has been a focus on the potential breakdown of the visuoperceptual system. Potential breakdown of the body schema or internal representation of body image has not been well addressed, although Feinberg (1997) has pointed out the similarity in the disorders of Capgras, mirror sign, and asomatognosia, considering asomatognosia to be a form of DMS, with loss of relatedness to the self as the common denominator.

In a review of the neural bases of body image awareness, Berlucchi and Aglioti (1997) describe the body schema as a mental construct that is the final result of systematic and mutually reinforcing interactions between somatosensory and visual input. Right hemispheric brain lesions have been shown to induce profound changes in the body schema, termed asomatognosia. For example, a patient might deny that a hemipelegic left limb is his or her own (Gerstmann, 1942). Asomatognosia has also been demonstrated during intercaratoid amobarbital inactivation (Wada test) of the non-language-dominant hemisphere (Meador et al., 2000).

Interestingly, asomatognosia has been reported to be induced in patients by asking them to look in a mirror. Paysant et al. (2004) reported the presence of mirror-induced asomatognosia in 12 of 16 right side stroke patients. Even though many of their subjects had experienced asomatognosia in the acute phases following their strokes, none demonstrated the symptom at the time of the study. The symptom was reactivated in the context of looking in a conventional or inverted mirror. Patients again began to experience their limbs as strange, changed in form, or belonging to someone else. Mirrors have been shown to affect body schemas in individuals without brain lesions as well, such as amputees, in whom use of a mirror can generate phantoms (Ramachandran, Rogers-Ramachandran, & Cobb, 1995). It is possible, then, that the mirror sign represents for some patients a mirror-induced disruption in their facial body schema associated with right-hemisphere lesions. This would answer the conundrum of patients with mirror sign correctly identifying others in a mirror.

Personal Relatedness and Affective Response to the Stranger in the Mirror
What role does a patient's affective response play in the formation of the mirror
sign and other DMS? To answer this question, Ellis and Young (1990) applied
Bauer's (1984) two route facial processing theory to Capgras syndrome. Bauer had
discovered that some prosopagnosics demonstrated increased skin conductance
response (SCR) to familiar faces, despite having lost the ability to consciously recognize faces. Two distinct and simultaneous routes to facial processing were proposed to account for this dissociation, with affective and covert recognition following a "dorsal visual-limbic pathway," and conscious recognition following a
"ventral visual-limbic pathway." While prosopagnosia was shown to involve disordered conscious visuospatial recognition in the context of somewhat preserved
(but unconscious) emotional response, Ellis and Young proposed that Capgras represented the inverse: a disorder of reasonably intact conscious visuospatial recognition and disordered emotional response. Studies of SCR of patients with Capgras syndrome indeed demonstrate reduced emotional response to familiar faces
(Ellis et al., 1997). Ellis and Young felt that this diminished emotional response was
often pervasive, effecting personal belongings and sense of place as well as identification of people. Applying this theory to the mirror sign, Breen et al. (2000)
tested their patient, FE, to determine whether he displayed a reduced sense of familiarity for his personal possessions. Consistent with the theory, he made several
errors when presented with objects that his wife felt should have had strong personal significance. He also made errors of hyperfamiliarity to unknown faces.
Breen and coworkers thought either diminished or excessive affective responses
could represent substrates of the mirror sign, although no SCR results have been
reported in their or other mirror sign patients.

Facial Processing

Facial processing deficits have been demonstrated in DMS (Young et al., 1990).
Neuropsychological evaluation of facial processing in patients with mirror sign
has been carried out by two investigators. Phillips, Howard, and David (1996) attempted formal facial processing testing with their patient EF. This was hampered,
however, by EF's difficulty understanding directions and poor concentration in the
context of moderate Alzheimer dementia. Breen, Caine, and Coltheart (2001) carried out extensive formal testing of their patients' facial processing abilities. These
evaluations are more enlightening, as focal facial processing deficits could be differentiated in these patients from low scores on tests resulting from global cognitive decline. Interestingly, although both patients demonstrated the mirror sign,
only one, FE, was found to have significant facial processing deficits on formal
testing. FE was impaired on simple face matching tasks and severely impaired on
the Benton Facial Recognition Test (Benton et al., 1983). He was mildly impaired
on a task that required him to judge facial gender. He was unable to name any of
the famous faces on the Albert Famous Faces Task and felt that many of the famous faces were personally familiar to him. He was able to recognize and correctly name photos of relatives. He also rated most photos of strangers as familiar.
Breen and colleagues felt that this testing indicated that EF demonstrated poor

structural encoding of faces. The striking differences in the performances on facial processing tasks for their two patients supports Flemminger's (1994) notion that delusional misidentification symptoms likely represent the final common pathway of a variety of possible cognitive deficits.

Neuroradiographical Findings

In cases of delusional misidentification symptoms that have an established cerebral pathology, right hemispheric dysfunction, occasionally in the presence of bifrontal pathology, has been identified on neuroradiographic studies (Benson, Gardner, & Meadows, 1976; Cutting, 1991; Forstl et al., 1991b, 1994a; Flemminger, 1992). Feinberg and Shapiro (1989) noted, however, that bilateral cerebral dysfunction was also a common substrate, concluding that right dysfunction alone or in concert with left dysfunction was associated with DMS. Weinstein (1994) similarly noted that right-side lesions associated with DMS typically had widespread effects (e.g., hemorrhages) suggesting widely spaced networks of dysfunction and interaction of the hemispheres were likely contributors to the clinical symptoms. Likewise, Cummings (1985) noted the contribution of disordered limbic and cortical connections in the development of delusions, pointing out that regardless of the location of the cortical lesion, inputs from cortical regions to the limbic system will be necessarily disrupted.

Similar to other DMS, a review of mirror sign case studies that report neuroradiographic data reveals primarily diffuse, mild bilateral changes such as atrophy and periventricular white matter changes. However, when focal lesions were present, they were located in the right hemisphere (see Table 9–1). In a rare prospective study of neuroanatomical correlates of DMS that addressed mirror sign as a distinct category, Forstl et al. (1991b) reported that no significant anatomical differences emerged between Alzheimer patients without DMS and Alzheimer patients with mirror sign, although there was a trend for a larger left anterior brain area and right lateral ventricle, suggestive of right frontal atrophy.

Neuropsychological Findings

While available neuroradiographic evidence suggests both diffuse and right hemispheric dysfunction, reports of mirror sign that include neuropsychological evaluations (for those patients who are not moderately to severely demented) typically note striking deficits in right-hemisphere-mediated cognition. That is, the neuropsychological data seem to underscore the importance of the right neuroradiographical involvement (see Table 9–1). The neuropsychological findings of the patient MH are illustrative of cognitive findings in other cases with mirror sign and are described below. Visual perception deficits emerged at the visual associative level, a substantial Wechsler Adult Intelligence Scale Verbal IQ/Performance IQ split was in evidence, and weak visual memory and poor orientation were discovered. These findings are similar to other reported cases of DMS implicating promi-

Table 9–1. Case descriptions of patients with mirror sign reported in the English language literature

Authors	Name	Neuropsychological findings	Neuroradiographic findings	Diagnosis
Gluckman, 1968	None given	Bedside only	Air encephalogram: atrophy	Paranoid schizophrenia
Cummings, 1985	Case 1	MMSE = 9; Bedside testing only	CT: atrophy	AD
Feinberg and Shapiro, 1989	SM	Focal right hemisphere impairment and mild diffuse cerebral dysfunction	MRI: mild atrophy and R temporal parietal atrophy	None provided
Molchan et al., 1990	HT	13 mmse; 59 wms; draw clock poor- no detailed neuropsych	None reported	AD
	LB	12 mmse; clock, calculation, block design poor; no detailed neuropsych	None reported	AD
Forstl et al., 1991b	Ms. A	Bedside cognitive testing only; global cognitive deficts aparent	CT: mild atrophy	AD
Mendez, 1992	Case 2	None reported; "intact facial recognition"	None reported	AD
Phillips et al., 1996	EF	MMSE = 10; "moderately severe global dementia"; facial processing deficits	CT: normal	AD
Spangenberg et al., 1998	MH	RH findings	CT: Watershed infarction, particularly R posterior parietal; MRI: R basal ganglion infarcts, bilateral thalami	VD
Breen et al., 2001	TH	Profound right hemisphere dysfunction; mirror agnosia	CT normal; MRI: diffuse cerebral atrophy, ischemic white matter changes, small cortical infarct posterior R frontal lobe	Atypical dementia-AD vs. Lewy Body
	FE	Profound right hemisphere findings; Facial processing deficits	Multiple periventricular white matter infarcts; chronic small vessel white matter ischemia; MRI: atrophy and age-associated white matter high signal intensity	VD

nent right hemispheric involvement, memory dysfunction, and poor orientation (Patterson & Mack, 1985; Forstl et al., 1991b, 1994b).

MH's Mayo-corrected (Ivnik, Malec, & Smith, 1992) scores on the Wechsler Adult Intelligence Scale, Revised (Wechsler, 1981) revealed a 25-point VIQ/PIQ discrepancy demonstrating diminished visual perceptual abilities (VIQ = 86; PIQ = 61; FSIQ = 75). Visual perceptual examination was suggestive of deficits at the visual associative level. Visual tracking, visual fields, shape recognition and matching, and identification or recognition of line drawings were grossly intact. That said, MH made a few perceptual errors on the Modified Boston Naming Test (Consortium to Establish Registry for Alzheimer's Disease [CERAD] battery, Morris et al., 1989), such as mistaking card 3, "whistle," for a key. MH was also able to identify objects around the room, a performance inconsistent with visual agnosia. There was no evidence of prosopagnosia, as MH was able to identify family members during the examination and pictures of relatives and examiners. Her response to the Boston Diagnostic Aphasia Exam's cookie thief picture (Goodglass & Kaplan, 1983) suggested the presence of some elements of simultanagnosia. A constructional apraxia surfaced on the CERAD neuropsychological battery's Constructional Praxis Task (1 of 11 correct).

Conversely, MH's performance on language tests indicated grossly intact receptive and expressive language abilities. On the Boston Diagnostic Aphasia Exam, she was able correctly to identify and name 18 of 18 items on card 2 (shapes, objects, and numbers). The patient was able accurately to read 10 of 10 words on Card 5.

MH demonstrated a lateralized pattern of impairment on memory testing. Her attentional abilities were grossly intact, with repetition of digits forward to 7 (82nd percentile) and backward to 4 (48th percentile). Acquisition, retention, and retrieval of verbal information was grossly within normal limits (Weschler Memory Scale, Revised Logical Memory I 17th percentile, Logical Memory II 26th percentile), while visual memory performance was remarkably impaired (Visual Reproduction I 1st percentile, Visual Reproduction II 4th percentile).

MH was not administered extensive tests of frontal-executive network functioning. In the other reported cases of mirror sign with available neuropsychological data, testing of complex problem solving revealed essentially normal findings in two of three cases. For example, Feinberg and Shapiro's (1989) patient demonstrated normal abstract reasoning on the Raven's progressive matrices (47th percentile; Raven, 1965). One of Breen, Caine, and Coltheart's (2001) patients, TH, likewise demonstrated normal reasoning skills on the Similarities subtest of the Weschler Intelligence Scale (50th percentile).

Implications for the Etiology of Mirror Sign: A Final Common Pathway

Neuroradiographic and neuropsychological studies of mirror sign have demonstrated that right-hemisphere dysfunction in the context of relative preservation of left hemispheric abilities are common substrates for the mirror sign. Investigators have clarified some specific aspects of right hemispheric dysfunction that may contribute to the manifestation of mirror sign, including change in affective function, impairment of facial processing, and mirror agnosia. Preservation of other right hemispheric-mediated functions including intact ability to recognize others in the mirror, intact ability to recognize themselves and others in photographs, and procedural use of the mirror suggest that global right hemispheric dysfunction per se is not the primary etiological factor. Breen and colleagues' cases demonstrate clearly that mirror sign can develop with or without a significant face processing deficit. Similarly, while other aspects of right-hemisphere function have been identified as playing a role in the manifestation of mirror sign, these clearly occur in patients who do not display the symptom and cannot account alone for its development.

Feinberg and Shapiro (1989) and others have suggested that bifrontal pathology contributes to patients' impairment in evaluating the incongruity of the perception created by faults in the visuoperceptual system. That is, although visuoperceptual mistakes arising from some aspect of right hemispheric dysfunction produce a faulty mirror image, the frontal pathology impairs patients' ability to consider explanations other than "there is a stranger in the mirror." Macrae and Trolle's (1956) case report of a prosopagnosic patient illustrates this point well. In the early phase of recovery from traumatic brain injury he questioned whether his mirror reflection was himself, "even though he knew it could be none other, on several occasions grimaced or stuck out his tongue 'just to make sure.' By carefully studying his face in the mirror he slowly began to recognize it . . . he relied on the hair . . . and on two small moles on his left cheek" (pp. 95–96). Rather than accept the initial impression that his mirror reflection was not his own, this patient reasoned that it had to be his own face and used feedback cues such as sticking out his tongue and nonfacial cues such as hair to counteract the effect of the initial misperception. Presumably the frontal–executive network functions of self-monitoring and flexible reasoning were preserved enough in this man to counteract the initial faulty percept caused by the profound facial processing deficits associated with his prosopagnosia. Interestingly, he was reportedly impaired on the similarities subtest of the Weschler-Bellevue intelligence test, suggesting "concretistic thinking" to the authors. This raises the question of what type and how much frontal dysfunction would be necessary to produce the reasoning deficit associated with mirror sign.

Ramachandran, Altschuler, and Hillyer (1997) refer to a "domain specific tolerance for absurdities" in their series of patients with mirror agnosia. The patients' intellectual reasoning capacity was felt to have become "selectively distorted" to accommodate the mirror agnosia. The patients were noted to reason well in other domains. Although this intact reasoning was not demonstrated via formal testing, the magnitude of a reasoning deficit that could explain a patient's lack of concern with the proposition of reaching into a mirror to grasp an object would presumably be obvious without formal testing. This also would appear to hold true for mirror sign. Although frontal dysfunction is commonly mentioned as a contributing etiological factor, the magnitude of reasoning deficit needed to accept the proposition that a stranger is staring back when one looks in the mirror has not been convincingly reported in existing case reports (e.g., Breen, Caine, & Coltheart's, 2001, patient TH scored in the average range on a test of novel abstract reasoning).

Interestingly, Fink and coworkers (1999) reported that the ventrolateral right prefrontal cortex was activated in their PET studies when normal patients were faced with conflicting or incongruent visual feedback. The area was considered to be responsible for monitoring and bringing to consciousness awareness of such conflict. If mirror sign evolves in the context of conflict between an internal representation of the mirror self-image and disordered visual perception, impairment in this cortical area could contribute to a specific lapse of reasoning necessary to create the symptom.

While many authors conclude that frontal dysfunction in addition to specific visuoperceptual deficits is necessary to develop a delusional misidentification symptom, some (Flemminger, 1994; Feinberg, 1997) go further in suggesting that a psychological response to the organic impairment is important for the development of mirror sign and similar symptoms. Flemminger (1994) has produced an elegant theory of the development of DMS that could explain the importance of the role of a patient's psychological response to perceptual deficits in developing mirror sign.

Flemminger's model uses the notion of top-down visual processing, which holds that prior to "seeing," individuals use initial sense data to generate a hypothesis about what they are looking at. The hypothesis is then matched to the actual visual image. At this stage deficits at any of the visuoperceptual processing levels described above, including mirror agnosia, facial processing deficits, and impaired affective response, could interfere with a sound match. A judgment is then made about the validity of the percept. Once the percept is accepted, it drives future hypotheses about what one is likely to see, thus perpetuating a vicious cycle.

Applying this model to mirror sign, an individual might look in the mirror with a reasonable hypothesis of seeing her own image. A new onset deficit interfering with visuoperception, such as poor facial processing or mirror agnosia, would result in no "match" between the hypothesis and what is seen. Then, shaky reasoning might result in the temporary conclusion that she is not seeing herself in the mirror. The next time she looks into a mirror, a new hypothesis about what she might see is now waiting to be used, that of a stranger in the mirror. An individual who feels disconnected and alienated from herself in some way (perhaps due to the ego dystonic nature of new onset faulty perception following a stroke), may be less likely to evaluate the faulty hypothesis as unreasonable. Thus, some aspect of poor visual perception and/or elements of self-alienation may interact in a vicious top-down perceptual processing cycle to create the mirror sign as the final common outcome.

Acknowledgment
I am grateful to William Postal, M.D., for insightful comments on the manuscript.

References

Bauer, R. (1984). Autonomic recognition of names and faces: A neuropsychological application of the guilty knowledge test. *Neuropsychologia, 22,* 457–469.

Benson, D.F., Gardner, H., & Meadows, J. (1976). Reduplicative paramnesia. *Neurology, 26,* 147–51.

Benton, A., Hamsher, K., Varney, N., & Spreen, O. (1983). *Facial Recognition: Stimulus and Multiple Choice Pictures.* New York: Oxford University Press.

Berlucchi, G., & Aglioti, S. (1997) The body in the brain: Neural bases of corporeal awareness. *Trends in Neurosciences, 20(1),* 560–564.

Binkofski, F., Buccino, G., Dohle, C., Seitz, R., & Freund, H. (1999). Mirror agnosia and mirror ataxia constitute different parietal lobe disorders. *Annals of Neurology, 46(1),* 51–61.

Biringer, F., Anderson, J., & Strubel, D.S. (1988). Self-recognition in senile dementia. *Experimental Aging Research, 14(4),* 177–180.

Bologna, S., & Camp, C. (1997). Covert versus overt self-recognition in late stage Alzheimer's disease. *Journal of the International Neurological Society, 3,* 195–198.

Breen, N., Caine, D., Coltheart, M., Hendy, J., & Roberts, C. (2000). Towards an understanding of delusions of misidentification: Four case studies. *Mind and Language, 15(1),* 74–110.

Breen, N., Caine, D., & Coltheart, M. (2001). Mirrored-self misidentification: Two cases of focal onset dementia. *Neurocase, 7,* 239–254.

Burns A., Jacoby, R., & Levy, R. (1990). Psychiatric phenomena in Alzheimer's disease II: Disorders of perception. *British Journal of Psychiatry, 157,* 76–81.

Christodoulou, G.N. (1986). Role of depersonalization-derealization phenomena in the delusional misidentification syndromes. *Bibliotheca Psychiatrica, 164,* 99–104.

Cummings, J. (1985). Organic delusions: Phenomenology, anatomical correlations, and review. *British Journal of Psychiatry, 146,* 184–97.

Cutting, J. (1991). Delusional misidentification and the role of the right hemisphere in the appreciation of identity. *British Journal of Psychiatry Supplement, 14,* 70–75.

Devanand, M., Miller, L., Richards, M., Marder, K., Bell, K., Mayeux, R., & Stern, Y. (1992). The Columbia University scale for psychopathology in Alzheimer's disease. *Archives of Neurology, 49,* 371–376.

Ellis, H., Young, A. (1990). Accounting for delusional misidentification. *Brittish Journal of Psychiatry, 157,* 239–248.

Ellis, H., Young, A., Quayle, A., & DePauw, K. (1997). Reduced autonomic responses to faces in Capgras delusion. *Proceedings of the Royal Society, London (B), 264,* 1085–1092.

Feinberg, T., & Shapiro, R. (1989). Misidentification-reduplication and the right hemisphere. *Neuropsychiatry, Neuropsychology, and Behavioral Neurology, 1,* 39–48.

Feinberg, T. (1997). Some interesting perturbations of the self in neurology. *Seminars in Neurology, 17(2),* 129–135.

Fink, G., Marshall, J., Halligan, P., Frith, C., Driver, J., Frackowiak, R., & Dolan, R. (1999). The neural consequences of conflict between intention and the senses. *Brain, 122,* 497–512.

Flemminger, S. (1992). Seeing is believing: The role of "preconscious" perceptual processing in delusional misidentification. *British Journal of Psychiatry, 160,* 293–303.

Flemminger, S. (1994). Delusional misidentification: An exemplary symptom illustrating an interaction between organic brain disease and psychological process. *Psychopathology, 27,* 161–167.

Foley, J., & Breslau, L. (1982). A new syndrome of delusional misidentification. *Annals of Neurology, 12,* 76.

Forstl, H., Osvaldo, P., Owen, A., Burns, A., & Howard, R. (1991a). Psychiatric, neurologic, and medical aspects of misidentification syndromes: A review of 260 cases. *Psychological Medicine, 21,* 905–910.

Forstl, H., Burns, A., Jacoby, R., & Levy, R. (1991b). Neuroanatomical correlates of clinical misidentification and misperception in senile dementia of the Alzheimer's type. *Journal of Clinical Psychiatry, 52,* 268–271.

Forstl, H., Burns, A., Levy, R., & Cairns, N. (1994a). Neuropathological correlates of psychotic phenomena in confirmed Alzheimer's disease. *British Journal of Psychiatry, 165,* 53–59.

Forstl, H., Besthron, C., Burns, A., Geiger-Kabisch, C., Levy, R., & Sattel, A. (1994b). Delusional misidentification in Alzheimer's disease: A summary of clinical and biological aspects. *Psychopathology, 27,* 194–199.

Gerstmann, J. (1942). Problem of imperception of disease and of impaired body territories with organic lesions. *Archives of Neurology and Psychiatry, 48,* 890–913.

Gluckman, L. (1968). A case of Capgras syndrome. *Australian New Zealand Journal of Psychiatry, 2,* 39–43.

Goodglass, H., & Kaplan, E. (1983). *The Assessment of Aphasia and Related Disorders.* Philadelphia: Lea & Feiger.

Grewel, R. (1994). Self-recognition in dementia of the Alzheimer type. *Perceptual and Motor Skills, 79(2),* 1009–1010.

Hwang, J., Yang, C., Tsai, S. (2003). Phantom boarder symptom in dementia. *International Journal of Geriatric Psychiatry, 18,* 417–420.

Ivnik, R., Malec, J., & Smith, G. (1992). Mayo's older Americans normative studies: WAIS-R norms for ages 56 to 97. *Clinical Neuropsychologist—Supplement, 6,* 1–30.

Joseph, A.B. (1994). Observations on the epidemiology of the delusional misidentification syndromes in the Boston metropolitan area: April 1983–June 1984. *Psychopathology, 27,* 150–153.

Joseph, A.B. (1986). Focal central nervous system abnormalities in patients with misidentificationn syndromes. *Bibliotheca Psychiatrica, 164,* 68–79.

Kirov, G., Jones, P., & Lewis, S.W. (1994). Prevalence of delusional misidentification syndromes. *Psychopathology, 27(3–5),* 148–149.

Macrae, D., & Trolle, E. (1956). The defect of function in visual agnosia. *Brain, 79(1),* 94–110.

Markova, I., & Berrios, G. (1994). Delusional misidentification: Facts and fancies. *Psychopathology, 27,* 136–143.

Meador, K., Loring, D., Feinberg, T., Lee, G., & Nichols, M. (2000). Anosognosia and asomatognosia during intracarotid amobarbital inactivation. *Neurology, 55,* 816–820.

Mendez, M., Martin, R., Smyth, K., & Whilehouse, P. (1992). Disturbances of person identification in Alzheimer's disease. *Journal of Nervous Mental Disease, 180,* 94–96.

Mendez, M.F. (1992). Delusional misidentification of persons in dementia. *British Journal of Psychaitry, 160,* 414–416.

Migliorelli, R., Petracca, G., Teson, A., Sabe, L., Leiguarda, R., & Starkstein, S. (1995). Neuropsychiatric and neuropsychological correlates of delusions in Alzheimer's disease. *Psychological Medicine, 25(3),* 505–514.

Molchan, S., Martinez, R., Lawlor, B., Grafman, J., & Sunderland, T. (1990). Reflections of the self: Atypical misidentification and delusional syndromes in two patients with Alzheimer's disease. *British Journal of Psychiatry, 157,* 605–608.

Morris, J., Heyman, A., Mohs, R., Hughes, M., van Belle, G., Fillenbaum, G., Mellitis, E., & Clark, C. (1989). The consortium to establish a registry for Alzheimer's disease (CERAD). Part I. Clinical and neuropsychological assessment of Alzheimer's disease. *Neurology, 39,* 1159–1165.

Paysant, J., Beis, J., Chapelain, L., & Andre, J. (2004). Mirror asomatognosia in right lesions stroke victims. *Neuropsychologia, 42,* 920–925.

Patterson, M., & Mack, J. (1985). Neuropsychological analysis of a case of reduplicative paramnesia. *Journal of Clinical and Experimental Neuropsychology, 7,* 111–121.

Phillips, M., Howard, R., & David, A. (1996). "Mirror, mirror on the wall, who." Towards a model of visual self-recognition. *Cognitive Neuropsychiatry, 1(2),* 153–164.

Ramachandran, V., Rogers-Ramachandran, D., & Cobb, S. (1995). Touching the phantom limb. *Nature, 377,* 489–490.

Ramachandran, V., Altschuler, E., & Hillyer, S. (1997). Mirror agnosia. *Proceedings of the Royal Society of London Biological Science, 264(1382),* 645–647.

Raven, J. (1965). *Guide to the Standard Progressive Matrices.* London: H.K. Lewis.

Reisberg, M., Borenstein, M., Salob, S., Ferris, S., Franssen, M., & Georgotas, A. (1987). Behavioral symptoms in Alzheimer's disease: Phenomenology and treatment. *Journal of Clinical Psychiatry, 48(5, suppl),* 9–15.

Silva, J., Leong, G., Rhodes, L., & Weinstock, R. (1997). A new variant of "subjective" delusional misidentification associated with aggression. *Journal of Forensic Science, 42(3),* 406–410.

Silva, J., Leong, G., Weinstock, R., & Ruiz-Sweeney, M. (2001). Delusional misidentification and aggression in Alzheimer's disease. *Journal of Forensic Science, 46(3),* 581–585.

Spangenberg, K., Wagner, M., & Bachman, D. (1998). Neuropsychological analysis of a case of abrupt onset mirror sign following a hypotensive crisis in a patient with vascular dementia. *Neurocase, 4,* 149–154.

Weinstein, E. (1994). The classification of delusional misidentification symptoms. *Psychopathology, 27,* 130–135.

Wechsler, D. (1981). *Manual for the Wechsler Adult Intelligence Scale—Revised.* New York: Psychological Corporation.

Wechsler, D. (1987). *Manual for the Wechsler Memory Scale—Revised.* New York: Psychological Corporation.

Yesavage, J., Brink, T., Rose, T., Lum, O., Huang, V., Ady, M., & Leirer, V. (1983). Development and validation of a geriatric depression screening scale: A preliminary report. *Journal of Psychiatric Research, 17,* 37–49.

Young, A., Ellis, H., Szulecka, T., & de Pauw, K. (1990). Face processing impairments and delusional misidentification. *Behavioral Neurology, 3(3),* 153–168.

10

Disorders of the Self in Dementia

WILLIAM W. SEELEY AND BRUCE L. MILLER

We experience the self as a unified whole, yet self-representation by the brain requires an interconnected hierarchy of parts that can be selectively dismantled by neurological disease. This idea is readily illustrated with the dementias, in which progressive regional degeneration can alter one aspect of the self while sparing others. In this chapter we summarize the evolution of self-representational capacities, outline the acquisition of the self during human development, and offer associations between the self's functional subcomponents and the brain structures that support them. From that perspective we discuss how the self can be unmade in patients with dementia.

Evolutionary Pressures and the Phylogeny of Self

Nervous systems that dynamically represent the state of the body confer a greater survival advantage than those that do not. Self-representation, in its simplest forms, evolved in vertebrate species remote from humans to allow reflexive integration of complex behavior with homeostatic needs and the environment (Churchland, 2002). Conscious awareness of the body state is improbable in reptiles, questionable in birds, but likely supported to some degree by the neocortex of even primitive mammals (Eccles, 1992). More abstract self-awareness may be unique to humans and great apes (Gallup, 1987; Parker, 1997), suggesting that it evolved within the past 10 to 15 million years. Selective pressures that forged this competence are much debated, but hypotheses include reliance upon arboreal locomotion (Povinelli & Cant, 1995), apprenticeship demands of tool-based fruit extraction (Parker, 1997), spatial and temporal variability in ripe fruit resources (Potts, 2004), and increasing size, complexity, and fluidity of social groupings (Joffe & Dunbar, 1997). These ecological challenges favor a brain's use of abstract mental representations of stimuli that can be re-created and manipulated after removal of those stimuli and, still more evolved, recognition of the self as a permanent object, "me," that can act with agency upon the environment. Thus, an orangutan unable to mentally model her weight (with or without a clinging infant) against the stability of the next tree branch stood to pass few of her genes on to posterity. Chimpanzees best at harvesting dispersed fruit ranges would have been those able to imitate tool use modeled by others, track when last a territory was foraged, and predict when it would reripen. Fission–fusion social groupings favored apes that could maintain mental representations of themselves in relation to conspecifics well enough to reassure allies and deceive rivals. These cognitive achievements served as the foundations upon which human self- and other-awareness would build (Table 10–1).

In the common chimpanzee (Pan troglodytes), self-recognition in mirrors begins in early adolescence and seems to decline with advancing age (de Veer et al. 2003). To date orangutans, gorillas, and chimpanzees have all been shown to display mirror self-recognition behaviors not present in monkeys (Gallup, 1970; Patterson, 1984). The status of cetaceans remains uncertain (Hart & Whitlow, 1995; Marten & Psarakos, 1995). In primates the evolution toward increasing self-awareness has been paralleled by brain characteristics that distinguish hominoids, including progressive encephalization with disproportionate expansion of the frontal lobes, hemispheric lateralization, and maturational delay.

Recently, two further specializations of great apes have been recognized. First, the Lamina I homeostatic afferent pathway runs directly from the spinal cord to the posterior ventromedial nucleus of the thalamus (VMpo), a structure that is discernible only in primates and is considerably more prominent in the human brain (Craig, 2002). In addition, although most neuronal types have been conserved across primate species, humans and great apes share a new class of spindle-shaped projection neurons, clustered in layer 5b of the anterior cingulate (ACC) and agranular frontoinsular cortices (Von Economo, 1926; Nimchinsky et al., 1995; Nimchinsky et al., 1999). The concentration of these cells is greater in humans than in chimpanzees, which, in turn, have more than gorillas, which have more than orangutans. The functions and projection targets of these neurons remain unknown, but their circumscribed distribution and species selectivity suggest a link to functions that distinguish great apes and humans from other primates (Allman et al., 2001).

Ontogeny of Self: A Recapitulation and Beyond

The earliest representations of self in humans are present at birth, as the newborn's developing nervous system surveys the body's needs and—as any parent will attest—promotes behaviors to ensure that those needs are met. Primitive awareness of the self as distinct from the environment surfaces by 3 months of life, as experimentalist infants detect the link between their actions and the kinesthetic–proprioceptive, vestibular, tactile, auditory, and visual coherencies they produce (Rochat, 1998). A calibrated body schema emerges, followed by the ability to construct an ego-centered extrapersonal space and move through it with a sense of personal agency. From 7 to 12 months of age, infants improve steadily at object permanence tasks (Diamond & Goldman-Rakic, 1989), and by 15 to 24 months they show convincing signs of mirror self-recognition, such as attempts to remove

Table 10–1. Phylogeny, Ontogeny, Anatomy, and Degenerations of the Self

Level of self-representation	Minimal Self							Longitudinal Self			
	Unconscious body state	Semiconscious body state	Egocentric extrapersonal space	Sense of motor agency	Mirror self-recognition	Self-conscious feeling states, embarrassment	Self-evaluative emotions	SITS	Cued event memory	Autonoetic consciousness	Abstract self-knowledge
Phylogeny	Vertebrates	Birds Mammals	Birds? Mammals	Monkeys	Great apes Dolphins?	Humans Great apes	Humans	Humans	Great apes	Humans	Humans
Ontogeny	In utero	Birth	3 months	3–4 months	15–24 months	22–30 months	3–4 years	??	2–4 years	4–5 years	14–18 years
Neuroanatomy*	Brainstem Hypothalamus	SI, SII, DPI	R > L Fronto-parietal network	SMC, AI, dACC	R VLPFC R temp pole	VMpo, DPI R > L AI, VMPFC	DMPFC, AI, temp poles	DMPFC	Medial temporal, occipital	DMPFC, precuneus, R VLPFC	Lateral temporal
Relevant Dementias	—	—	PCA: AD, CBD, DLB, CJD	AHP: CBD, AD, CJD	AD, DLB	fvFTD, tvFTD	fvFTD tvFTD	fvFTD	AD	fvFTD, AD	tvFTD

*In humans. ACC, anterior cingulate cortex; AD, Alzheimer disease; AHP, alien hand phenomena; AI, anterior insulae; CBD, corticobasal degeneration; CJD, Creutzfeldt-Jacob disease; DLB, dementia with Lewy bodies; DMPFC, dorsomedial prefrontal cortex; DPI, dorsal posterior insula; fvFTD, frontal variant frontotemporal dementia; PCA, posterior cortical atrophy; SMC, supplementary motor cortex; VLPFC, ventrolateral prefrontal cortex; VMPFC, ventromedial prefrontal cortex; VMpo, ventromedial nucleus of thalamus, posterior part; SITS, stimulus-independent thoughts; tvFTD, temporal variant frontotemporal dementia.

covertly placed rouge marks from their noses (Lewis & Brooks-Gunn, 1979; Anderson, 1984). Signs of embarrassment follow late in the second year and are typically preceded by mirror self-recognition (Lewis, 1997). Appreciation of standards and self-descriptive utterances surface midway through the second year (Kagan, 1982), around when toddlers begin to collect knowledge of prior events, though they remain unable to reexperience those events in the absence of cues (Levine, 2004).

As children enter their third year, human-specific self-representational capacities emerge. The combination of self-consciousness and social standards leads to self-evaluative emotions, such as shame, guilt, and pride. Self-recognition in videotapes improves, even when tested after a delay (Povinelli & Simon, 1998), suggesting that a more longitudinal sense of self has taken hold. Children begin to assemble their past into a story line of remembered episodes to which they can mentally transport themselves in time and space (Snow, 1990; Levine, 2004). Construction of the self marches forward throughout childhood, but it is not until adolescence that a more abstract and reflective conception of past, present, and future selves is seen (Parker, 1997). By early adulthood priorities and allegiances are formed, self-statements about personal characteristics, or "self-schemata," are structured (Markus, 1977), and—barring acquired cerebral disease—the self's framework remains stable throughout the life cycle (Finn, 1986; Costa & McCrae, 1988).

Neuroanatomy of the Self

The growing literature on the self suggests that late-evolving and late-maturing brain regions support the most complex self-representational achievements of human development. To discuss the neuroanatomy of the self, however, requires definition of its phenomenological makeup. Some authors separate the self into a *minimal* self, the immediate experience of one's person, unextended in time, and a more longitudinal, or *narrative*, self, having a personal past and future (see Gallagher, 2000, for a review). The minimal self represents both the body state and the contents of consciousness. Damasio (1999) further divides the minimal self into a "protoself" (body state, unconscious) and "core self" (conscious thought). The more longitudinal, self, also referred to as the "extended self" (Neisser, 1988) or "autobiographical self" (Damasio, 1999), is comprised of elements that persist about an individual outside a given moment in time. We prefer the term *longitudinal self* because it highlights the essence of the construct, time and continuity, and leaves room for personal knowledge, attitudes, tendencies, beliefs, affiliations, the stories we weave about them, and the memories that frame and secure them.

The minimal self provides a platform for the longitudinal self, but each system influences the workings of the other. The minimal self can bring elements of the longitudinal self into consciousness, but the longitudinal self renders an impression of the self over time. Its readout is iteratively modified and updated by the perceptions of the minimal self, which, in turn, are filtered through the longitudinal self's working model.

The Minimal Self: "This Is How I Am Right
Now (whether I know it or not)"

Phylogenetically ancient systems, rooted in the brainstem and hypothalamus, are the homeostatic bedrock of the minimal self. These networks represent the physical self and support its most basic needs, largely beneath the surface of awareness. The conscious components of the minimal self are of more direct relevance to disorders of self in dementia. These layered self-representations, perceived together, provide the streaming subjective experience that defines human mental life.

The minimal self has a wondrous capacity to take inventory of the body, surveying from above to ensure that its parts are conditioned to operate. An experience familiar to many comes after a serious fall or blow; an evaluative process shifts the mental set toward physical self-examination. If I want to check the integrity of my right fifth toe, I need only to direct my attention toward it, and my brain provides an answer. Anatomic and functional imaging studies suggest that homeostasis-related afferent information from the entire body first reaches the cortex in the dorsal posterior insulae, whether it pertains to temperature, pain, itch, muscle fatigue, thirst, or hunger (Peyron, Laurent, & Garcia-Larrea, 2000; Craig, 2002).

In humans incoming body state data undergo further processing by the ipsilateral anterior insula before being re-represented by the anterior insula of the non-dominant hemisphere, providing a substrate for *evaluative* interoception (Craig, 2002; Critchley et al., 2004). Insular connections to limbic and paralimbic structures, such as the amygdala, ACC, and orbitofrontal cortex, allow motivation of behavior toward escape from ongoing bodily harm, risk, or deficiency. Empathy for another's visceral state, such as a spouse's experience of pain, recruits the same anterior insular regions and the ACC but not discriminative pain processors such as the dorsal posterior insula and parietal operculum (Singer et al., 2004). The insulae also transmit efferent signals to the viscera, helping to coordinate autonomic responses (Augustine, 1996; Kuniecki et al., 2003). Access of body signals to consciousness is under top-down regulatory control, as evidenced by our ability to disregard most of the information that the insulae receive. Right dorsolateral prefrontal activity, in particular, diminishes the correlation between insular activity and pain intensity–unpleasantness, perhaps by actively shifting attention away from the body (Lorenz, Minoshima, & Casey, 2003).

Once the body state is represented, its movement requires construction of a body-centered world map. Positions of the head, trunk, and limbs are charted, facilitating gaze and reaching toward visual and auditory targets. These processes are embedded in a bilateral fronto-cingulo-parietal spatial attentional matrix that draws heavily upon the right hemisphere (Mesulam, 1981; Corbetta, 1998; Astafiev et al., 2003).

Coupling of actions to a sense of agency may also involve the anterior insulae, which register multimodal feedback about self-generated actions (Farrer & Frith, 2002; Farrer et al., 2003). In keeping with the right hemisphere's dominance for representing the body state, recognizing distorted images of one's face appears to involve several regions of the right prefrontal cortex (Keenan et al., 2000; Platek et al., 2004).

Just as the machinations of the bowel and flutters of the heart are cortically represented, the brain's intrinsic spontaneous activities — thoughts — are broadcast on the screen of consciousness. Spontaneous thoughts are a core feature of the minimal self and have characteristics of both action and perception. Like actions, thoughts are generated using a range of volition (sometimes none at all), are marked with a sense of ownership and agency, and are subject to feedback control by the sensory consequences of their execution. Like perceptions, spontaneous thoughts have modality-specific features; they are the imagery and inner dialogue that compose reflection, detached from the external environment but cast in its likeness.

Evidence for the neural basis of "stimulus-independent thoughts" (SITS) has linked this key element of the self to the medial prefrontal cortex (McGuire et al., 1996). In functional imaging paradigms subjects scanned during "rest" conditions show a pattern of brain activations, referred to by Raichle and colleagues as the default mode network (Raichle et al., 2001; Greicius et al., 2003), which includes the dorsomedial (Brodmann areas [BA] 8, 9, and 10 and the paracingulate sulcus, 32) and ventromedial (BA 32, 25) prefrontal cortex, posterior cingulate/precuneus, and bilateral posterior parietal cortex. Cognitively demanding, externally driven tasks activate, in proportion to degree of difficulty, the rostral ACC (BA 24, 32) but deactivate the default mode network (Gusnard & Raichle, 2001). The exception occurs during judgments about the current mental state of the self or another, in which case the default mode network, especially the dorsomedial frontal cortex, is activated compared to tasks that concern the outside world (Gusnard et al., 2001; Gusnard & Raichle, 2001) or do not require mental state judgments (Vogeley et al., 2001). Thus, two adjacent regions, rostral ACC and medial superior frontal cortex, maintain a dynamic interplay while competing for the attentional resources of the minimal self. When situations demand outward focus and muted self-examination, the ACC takes control. Turning attention inward calls upon slightly more rostral medial frontal cortex.

The Longitudinal Self: "This Is How I Am, Was, and Will Be"

Patients with global amnesia demonstrate that the minimal self can persist, stranded in the moment, without the privilege of mental time travel that episodic memory affords (Scoville & Milner, 1957). An integrated longitudinal self, however, requires alignment of one's current mental state with enduring semantic knowledge of personal traits, goals, beliefs, and values. To do so requires autonoetic consciousness, the seamless access to episodic memories of past, present, and future selves (Wheeler, Stuss, & Tulving, 1997) that grounds semantic self-knowledge and infuses it with emotional meaning. When an overworked single mother must reconcile her exhaustion with the needs of her ailing 4-year-old, she may call upon both semantic self-statements ("I am a good mother") and projections of herself into prior situations (the way she felt after successfully managing her child's first major illness) or imaginable futures (her feelings should the child be harmed by her neglect). Self-schemata carved by decades of emotionally intense experiences ("I am an American," "I am a brother," "I am a doctor") are particularly resistant to change, but an adaptive longitudinal self can remodel itself in the face of changing life circumstances. It is flexible but not flimsy.

The capacity to reflect upon the minimal and longitudinal selves calls upon overlapping neural systems. Functional imaging studies in which subjects judge the self-descriptiveness of adjectives (Craik et al., 1999; Kelley et al., 2002; Fossati et al., 2003; Schmitz, Kawahara-Baccus, & Johnson, 2004), self-statements, such as "I am a good friend" (Johnson et al., 2002), or opinions, such as "George Bush is a good president" (Zysset et al., 2002) all demonstrate medial prefrontal activation. Therefore, to assess one's *traits* employs some of the same neural machinery used to assess one's *state*. This finding seems straightforward: to judge the "goodness of fit" between a descriptor and semantic self-knowledge (trait judgment) requires access to the self's immediate disposition toward the descriptor (state judgment). In addition, to evaluate the longitudinal self requires episodic and emotional memory retrieval. Recruitment of medial parietal regions (posterior cingulate and precuneus) appears in self-referential tasks with a longitudinal component (Vogeley et al., 2001; Johnson et al., 2002; Kelley et al., 2002; Zysset et al., 2002; Seger, Stone, & Keenan, 2004), can be less prominent in those without one (Gusnard et al., 2001), and may reflect the use of recalled perceptual imagery. Furthermore, self-judgments impose temporal indexing and monitoring demands upon episodic retrieval (Tulving et al., 1994) that may relate to participation of right lateral prefrontal cortex in assessments of the self as opposed (Craik et al., 1999) or in relation (Vogeley et al., 2001) to others. The clinical implications of this network's organization are important. Superior medial prefrontal lesions should impede self-examination, disconnecting cognition from an emotional sense of one's goals and constraining the adaptive deployment of episodic memory. In contrast, more posterior lesions of the medial cinguloparietal transition zone should dilute the richness of the episodic memories themselves but spare the drive toward self-reflection. In either case, right lateral prefrontal injury should hinder supervision of episodic retrieval and yield a disorderly sense of one's self in time.

Dementia, Regional Vulnerability, and the Fracturing of Self Through De-development

Tragically, the distributed self-representational networks so carefully assembled during development are not immune to neurological disease. With degenerative dementias, patients suffer progressive regional degeneration that erodes the architecture of the self. Family members remark that their loved one is "no longer himself" or "not the person she used to be." Their statements reflect the bias that the self is unitary, and on one level, it is. Losing any core aspect of one's cognitive or emotional makeup yields a categorically different person. Nonetheless, patients with dementia remind us that the self is multifaceted, its parts selectively vulnerable to neurodegenerative injury.

The dementias can be described by their clinicoanatomic features, such as "posterior cortical atrophy syndrome" or "corticobasal syndrome," or by underlying histopathologic entities, such as Alzheimer disease (AD) or corticobasal degeneration (CBD). Correspondence between these levels of description is not always straightforward. In the remaining sections, we use both anatomic and histopathologic terminology but highlight anatomy, under the presumption that changes in self are more the result of the brain regions affected than the molecular pathophysiology. We propose that some disorders of self arise due to loss of self-representation, while others result from excessive attention to self-relevant data.

Disorders of the Minimal Self

Fragmentation of Ego-Centered Extrapersonal Space:
The Posterior Cortical Atrophy Syndrome
When patients present with a slowly progressive disturbance of visual and spatial processing, they are described clinically as having the posterior cortical atrophy syndrome. Most often AD is found at autopsy (Ross et al., 1996; Hof et al., 1997). When the disease affects the occipital regions, a primary visual disorder occurs featuring distortion of form, altered colors, and eventually cortical blindness (Victoroff et al., 1994; Chan, Crutch, & Warrington, 2001). More dorsal parieto-occipital involvement, however, yields patients who cannot center themselves in space. Visual search and reaching are haphazard and ineffective. Objects cannot be perceived in relation to one another. An egocentric perspective no longer grounds the extrapersonal space, yet patients may show great insight, referring to their new selves who are unable to interpret the visual world. Thus, the longitudinal self accommodates the change in the minimal self. Family members note that the patient is still emotionally accessible, still the person they have always known.

Feedback Dyscontrol of Self-initiated Movement: Alien
Limb Phenomena in Corticobasal Degeneration
Just as the brain can endow our movements with a sense of agency and ownership, disease can strip these features away. In corticobasal degeneration (CBD) there is progressive atrophy of frontal, parietal, insular, and basal ganglia structures, often with marked asymmetry. Patients develop progressive limb rigidity, slowness, and apraxia, often with cortical motor signs such as myoclonus, dystonia, and postural tremor. Alien limb phenomena (ALP), a group of related motor abnormalities, are seen in up to 42% of CBD patients (Kompoliti et al., 1998) and in other settings such as anterior callosotomy (Akelaitis, 1944) and anterior communicating artery aneurysm rupture (Fisher, 1963), as well as in other dementias (Boeve et al., 1999). ALP can take various simple forms including undetected drifting off or levitation of one limb, bizarre posturing, or movements of one hand that mirror those of the other. At times patients describe their limb by saying "It just does not do what I want it to do" (Rinne et al., 1994), suggesting that their sense of motor agency for the limb is altered. Movements proceed in an involuntary, frustrating, and often debilitating fashion. In some cases these unbidden movements involve elaborated reflexes seen in infants, such as a fixed or tonic grasp, but more complex forms of conflict and interference between the hands have been described (Fisher, 2000). For example, a patient may button her blouse with the right hand, only to unbutton

it with the left. Fisher (2000) noted that these seemingly competitive movements, though tagged as unwilled by their owners, often occur in the nondominant hand during execution of voluntary, skilled, and routinely bimanual acts that have specific roles for each hand (e.g., dominant hand leads shirt buttoning, nondominant leads unbuttoning), leading him to suggest that nondominant hand participation was appropriate but temporally estranged from the intended act. In extreme cases CBD patients may rate their limb as foreign to them, saying "It does not belong to me" (Rinne et al., 1994). The precise injuries that render limb movements unbidden or disowned in ALP remain to be clarified. Even when an entire half of the body is disowned, however, patients safeguard a sense of who they are and what it means to possess the intact side. The longitudinal self is updated to resolve the discrepancy between its image of the body and the flood of dissonant input that the minimal self provides.

Imposters in the Mirror: Self-Misidentification Phenomena
in Alzheimer's Disease and Dementia with Lewy Bodies
When dementia disrupts mirror self-recognition, it is usually in the context of a posterior temporoparietal illness that is worse in the right hemisphere (Breen, Caine, & Coltheart, 2001). The diagnosis is typically AD (Forstl et al., 1994) or dementia with Lewy bodies. Because Chapter 9 reviews the mirror misidentification syndrome in detail, it will not be discussed further here.

Disruptions of Body State Monitoring: Hypochondriasis and Interoceptive
Agnosia in Frontotemporal Lobar Degeneration
Frontotemporal lobar degeneration (FTLD) refers to a group of disorders that cause progressive degeneration within the frontal, insular, anterior temporal, and striatal regions (Rosen et al., 2002; Broe et al., 2003), as shown in Figure 10–1. Clinically recognizable subtypes exist (Neary et al., 1998), including a frontal variant (fvFTD), in which social and behavioral symptoms predominate (Miller et al., 1991); a temporal variant (tvFTD, also known as semantic dementia), which causes loss of semantic knowledge when it affects the dominant hemisphere (Hodges et al., 1992) but emotional disturbance with nondominant temporal disease (Edwards-Lee et al., 1997; Thompson, Patterson, & Hodges, 2003, Seeley et al., in press); and progressive nonfluent aphasia, which results from degeneration of anterior perisylvian language areas (Mesulam, 1982). In tvFTD and fvFTD, contrasting symptoms illuminate how the healthy brain keeps track of the body.

    In tvFTD there is striking, often asymmetric, anterior temporal atrophy, but symptoms suggest that both sides are typically involved by 3 years into the illness (Seeley et al., 2004). Independent of the more affected hemisphere, patients come to interact with their environment in a rigid and compulsive manner (Rosso et al., 2001). Resulting behaviors are driven toward stimuli least devalued by the illness, such that left-predominant tvFTD patients often gravitate toward visual–nonverbal stimuli (sticks, coins, insects, soda cans), while right tvFTD patients are preoccupied with words and symbols (extensive note writing, card games, Scrabble®) (Seeley et al., 2004). Heightened visual attention, especially in left tvFTD, can lead to one

Posterior insula   **Subgenual & rostral ACC/SFG**

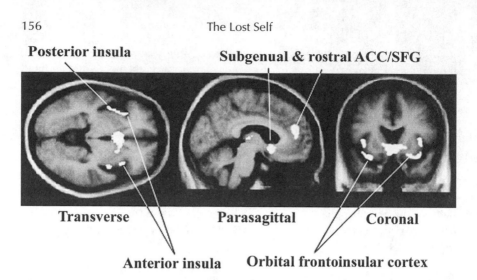

Transverse   **Parasagittal**   **Coronal**

Anterior insula   **Orbital frontoinsular cortex**

Figure 10–1. Schematic view of overlapping neurodegeneration in the frontal and temporal variants of frontotempemporal dementia. White stippling is superimposed on regions atrophic in both disorders when compared to healthy controls. The anatomy of FTLD is the anatomy of higher-order self-representation (see Table 10–1). ACC = anterior cingulate cortex, SFG = superior frontal gyrus

of the best-known consequences of the disorder, the birth of artistic creativity (Miller et al., 1996; Miller et al., 2000). As the bitemporal disease unfolds, however, both word and object landscapes lose meaning.

In some tvFTD patients the focus turns inward, and the body becomes the object of fixation. Somatic concerns result, and patients complain of new headaches, joint and muscle pains, gastrointestinal upset, itchiness, and other afflictions for which no cause can be found (Edwards-Lee et al., 1997; Gregory, 1999). Patients make compulsive trips to the bathroom, sensing their bladders full despite recent evacuation. Others believe that they have acquired life-threatening illnesses, such as AIDS or cancer (Box 10–1, Figure 10–2).

Symptomatically, exaggerated responses to pain and temperature are reported by caregivers for roughly half of tvFTD patients (Snowden et al., 2001). We suggest that normal interoceptive signals, represented in the posterior insulae and evaluated by the right anterior insula/ACC, can take on undue biological significance, overvalued by a self with little else left to regard. In short, it is pain without injury. The anatomic substrates of hypochondriasis in tvFTD, once determined, could help to demystify other body state representation disorders.

While tvFTD can result in hypervigilance toward body state information, the situation is reversed in fvFTD. Two fvFTD subtypes are recognized, an apathetic form (FTD-A) with more dorsomedial frontal/ACC involvement, and a disinhibited version (FTD-D) with predominant orbital frontal disease, especially on the right. As FTD-A progresses spontaneous thought and action diminish, and patients enact little more than prepotent responses to the environment, even when homeostasis is threatened. A 58-year-old FTD-A patient of ours had no perceptible verbal

Box 10–1. Somatic preoccupation in tvFTD

Patient JG was a 55-year-old former dentist with a remote history of left breast cancer treated with radical mastectomy. She was seen after an 8-year history of progressive semantic loss. At 3 years into symptoms, she made untimely and insensitive remarks to family members. As her knowledge of words failed, she became visually compulsive and began to gather dead insects and place them in plastic containers to show to her husband. She washed all dishes by hand before placing them in the dishwasher, refusing to use detergent because of concerns about residue. During the 2 weeks prior to her hospital stay, she had become preoccupied with the status of her right breast, continuously signaling to her husband for its removal. The topic became the primary focus of the couple's interaction. On examination, she was alert, attentive, and spoke fluently with 10 to 15 words, all nonspecific pronouns or high-frequency verbs. She used *house* to refer to her own body. She continuously scanned her surroundings and picked small pieces of lint from her bed sheets, gesturing toward the wastebasket. She lowered her blouse on several occasions and presented her right breast to the examiner saying, "What do we do for this?" During a 24-hour admission, she stole away from the ward and was found exploring the operative suite (eight floors down), seeking a surgeon to perform a second mastectomy. Her Mini-Mental State Exam (MMSE) score was 1/30 (one point for the copy of intersecting pentagons). Her regional atrophy pattern is shown in Figure 10–2.

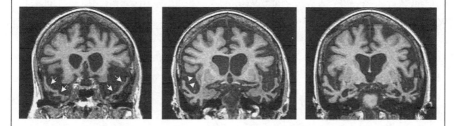

Figure 10–2. JG's T1-weighted coronal MRI shows striking atrophy of anterior temporal (white arrows), orbital frontal, and subgenual anterior cingulate cortex (ACC) regions, left worse than right. Milder atrophy of the amygdalae and relative sparing of dorsomedial frontal cortex and the right insula (white arrowheads) are seen. Did the areas of relative preservation enable her visual and somatic compulsions, brought forth by the orbital frontal and subgenual ACC pathology?

or motor reaction as she underwent radial artery puncture for blood gas sampling. When asked if the needle was painful, she responded 20 seconds later, stating simply "No pain." When asked if she felt the needle, she replied (after another 20 seconds), "I feel it." Incredulous, we asked her again if the needle hurt, and (after another 20 seconds) she reiterated, "No Pain!" In FTD-D, patients have exaggerated pain responses less often than in tvFTD (33% versus 50%) but significantly more than in FTD-a (33% versus 0%) (Snowden et al., 2001). Thus, while in tvFTD we witnessed pain without injury, in fvFTD there is injury without pain. Whether loss of subjective pain in FTD-A is driven by anterior cingulate, paracingulate, insular, or ventral striatal disease is unknown, but the deficit, perhaps a form of "interoceptive agnosia," (Nauta, 1971) simulates the loss of emotional self-awareness so characteristic of the disorder.

Loss of Stimulus-Independent Thought: The Abulia/Apathy
Syndrome in Frontal Variant Frontotemporal Dementia
Relatively early in their course, patients with FTD-A enter a state reminiscent of akinetic mutism yet continue to react to the environment through stimulus-bound behaviors, such as echolalia (repetition of another's speech), pallilalia (repetition of one's own speech), imitation, and utilization (compulsory handling of tools with use mimicry). Response initiation is delayed, and accurate responses to questions may arrive after as long as 10 minutes (personal observations). The apathetic–abulic state is in part a result of medial superior frontal/ACC pathology, including rostral BA 24 and 32 (Devinsky, Morrell, & Vogt, 1995). Patients recovering from strokes involving the ACC often report that during their acute illness not only were they not *saying* anything, they were not *thinking* anything, either (Damasio & Van Hoesen, 1983)! A similar internal milieu is suspected in FTD-A, though it is difficult to assess directly since patients do not later return to a higher level of communication. It is unclear whether the abulic state results from a failure of thought and action schemata to reach activation threshold or merely sufficient psychomotor slowing to render interpersonal communication impractical. In either case the online stream of stimulus-independent thought, perhaps a uniquely human component of the minimal self, is brought to a standstill by neurodegenerative disease.

Disorders of the Longitudinal Self

Clinging to Personal Semantics: Self-Evaluative Emotion and Shades
of Dogmatism in Temporal Variant Frontotemporal Dementia
Just as was seen for the minimal self's assessment of the body state, tvFTD and fvFTD diverge in their effects on the longitudinal self. Despite progressive deficits in emotional processing and general semantic knowledge, tvFTD patients typically retain their semantic concepts of self, along with long-held beliefs and allegiances. In some patients self-statements become the primary form of verbal communication, either for deprecation or bravado. One left tvFTD patient ruminated over his anomia and referred to himself (melodically) as "Mr. Dumb-da-dumb-dumb-dumb-dumb." A patient with right-predominant tvFTD, in contrast, often asserted "You know, I really am a tremendous golfer . . . and I come from a family of outstanding card players" and "There is absolutely nothing wrong with my intelligence . . . I assure you my intelligence is still quite exceptional." His prowess was verified; in fact, he had recently been earning master's points in tournament duplicate bridge. Thus, at least two self-evaluative emotions, shame and pride, can escalate in tvFTD, perhaps as the longitudinal self attempts its updating process in the face of skewed emotional signals.

In other tvFTD patients premorbid religious, political, or philosophical ideas are amplified (Edwards-Lee et al., 1997). These entrenched systems of under-standing the world (in relation to the self), laid down through decades of emotional experience, may be more resilient than other forms of knowledge, perhaps because they are more bilaterally represented, stored outside the temporal poles, or remain linked to surviving emotionally rich episodic memories. As knowledge about the world slips away, these personal semantic "rules" provide a sense of meaning, and behavior rushes out to greet it. As with the hypochondriasis of tvFTD, misprocessed visceral signals coming forward from the posterior insulae may also endow commonplace events and objects with a feeling of emotional significance, leading to increased piety, activism, or ideological fervor.

Identities at Risk: Autonoetic Unconsciousness and Instability of Self in Right Frontal Variant Frontotemporal Dementia
When fvFTD affects the orbital prefrontal networks out of proportion to other frontal and temporal regions, the result is often a socially disruptive phenotype. From early in their disease, patients with FTD-D become tactless, jocular, and childish yet often rigid and demanding. Social boundaries are violated, and discourse may regress to the level of the elementary school playground. Guidance of the self toward acts of personal, familial, and social responsibility is lost. Patients become imprudent with financial resources and may enter sweepstakes, donate to solicitors, or, as we recently heard from a caregiver, throw cash out of the car windows while driving down Main Street! Depth of insight into these behaviors is lacking, even among patients who have acquired the semantic knowledge that they misbehave and carry a diagnosis of FTD. When we asked one patient how his illness had affected his family, he replied, "Well, some of my behaviors are really hard on my wife and daughter." His comment, made with no outward show of emotion, came 2 weeks after he had been moved to a nursing home to protect his 9-year-old daughter from his bawdy hypersexual pranks and displays. Cognitive testing, including frontal–executive functions, was normal.

A subgroup of patients with nondominant FTD-D shows not only deteriorations of the self but lateral shifts in core aspects of the longitudinal self. A pathological flexibility develops, and the longitudinal self can evolve from one self into another (Miller et al., 2001). In our cohort this process brought unheralded changes in political orientation, religion, career, and social identity (including one man who took to dressing himself as a sailor). In another patient, RP, the sense of self was so adrift that she took on an alternate personality to anchor it. She referred to a second persona, "Jenny," in the third person and used her as a receptacle for ongoing rude behaviors that were at odds with her previously refined conduct. Despite her dysregulated approach, RP's efforts at self-reconciliation exceeded those of most, who readily incorporated the new selves as their former identities were displaced. Importantly, these patients did not lose all knowledge of who they used to be. Many of them could dispassionately report on their changed traits and affiliations. Nonetheless, when it came time to act in the world, they lacked the unity of personhood that normally binds the longitudinal self together. Republicans became Democrats; Protestants turned to Catholicism.

The cognitive neuroscience of the self has evolved considerably since our report and sheds new light on our patients' behaviors. We suggested previously that changes of self in nondominant fvFTD might reflect a loss of autonoetic consciousness, the ability to travel mentally through time. The frontal lobes contribute to this capacity, particularly to its temporal indexing and organizational demands (Wheeler, Stuss, & Tulving, 1997), and right frontotemporal circuits may be particularly important (Levine et al., 1998; Craik et al.,1999). Two recent studies provide additional support for our hypothesis by demonstrating that episodic memories are deficient in FTD regardless of the life epoch from which they are retrieved (Piolino et al., 2003; Levine, 2004). Yet, not all patients with episodic memory problems develop shifts in self. On the contrary, AD patients typically maintain a firm sense of their social identity until advanced stages of disease. This discrepancy has two possible explanations. First, in AD the amnesia exhibits a temporal gradient, such that older memories are retained better than more recent ones (Piolino et al., 2003). Thus, personal semantics tied to the reminiscence of young adulthood may buttress an AD patient's sense of identity. Second, shifts in the longitudinal self may require loss of both orderly long-term autonoetic retrieval (ventrolateral prefrontal pathology) *and* the inward-focused attention (medial frontal pathology) required to benefit from prior experiences and compare new action plans to one's visceral disposition toward them.

Summary

Human self-awareness is built upon layered and distributed but separable neural systems. These self-representations are rooted in the right hemisphere and are designed to address all human needs, from mundane to sublime. The past decade has brought the first real attempts to address the cognitive subcomponents of the self in parallel with their anatomic foundations. The task ahead is to carve out even more precise definitions that can be studied directly and applied to human disease. Though once relegated to philosophers and mystics, the structure of the self may soon become mandatory reading for neurology, psychiatry, and neuroscience trainees. For the dementia specialist the need for this evolution is transparent, as shattered selves — of one form or another — remain a daily part of clinical practice.

References

Akelaitis, A.J. (1944). Studies on the corpus callosum IV. Diagonistic dyspraxia in epileptics following partial and complete section of the corpus callosum. *American Journal of Psychiatry, 101,* 594–599.

Allman, J.M., Hakeem, A., Erwin, J.M., Nimchinsky, E. & Hof, P. (2001). The anterior cingulate cortex. The evolution of an interface between emotion and cognition. *Annals of the New York Academy Science, 935,* 107–117.

Anderson, J.R. (1984). The development of self-recognition: a review. *Developmental Psychobiology, 17(1),* 35–49.

Astafiev, S.V., Shulman, G.L., Stanley, C.M., Snyder, A.Z., Van Essen, D.C. & Corbetta, M. (2003). Functional organization of human intraparietal and frontal cortex for attending, looking, and pointing. *Journal of Neuroscience, 23(11),* 4689–4699.

Augustine, J.R. (1996). Circuitry and functional aspects of the insular lobe in primates including humans. *Brain Research Brain Research Reviews, 22(3),* 229–244.

Boeve, B.F., Maraganore, D.M., Parisi, J.E., Ahlskog, J.E., Graff-Radford, N., Caselli, R.J., Dickson, D.W., Kokmen, E. & Petersen, R.C. (1999). Pathologic heterogeneity in clinically diagnosed corticobasal degeneration. *Neurology, 53(4),* 795–800.

Breen, N., Caine, D. & Coltheart, M. (2001). Mirrored-self misidentification: Two cases of focal onset dementia. *Neurocase, 7(3),* 239–254.

Broe, M., Hodges, J.R., Schofield, E., Shepherd, C.E., Kril, J.J. & Halliday, G.M. (2003). Staging disease severity in pathologically confirmed cases of frontotemporal dementia. *Neurology, 60(6),* 1005–1011.

Chan, D., Crutch, S.J. & Warrington, E.K. (2001). A disorder of colour perception associated with abnormal colour after-images: a defect of the primary visual cortex. *Journal of Neurology, Neurosurgery, and Psychiatry, 71(4),* 515–517.

Churchland, P.S. (2002). Self-representation in nervous systems. *Science, 296(5566),* 308–310.

Corbetta, M. (1998). Frontoparietal cortical networks for directing attention and the eye to visual locations: Identical, independent, or overlapping neural systems? *Proceedings of the National Academy of Sciences, 95(3),* 831–838.

Costa, P.T., Jr., & McCrae, R.R. (1988). Personality in adulthood: a six-year longitudinal study of self-reports and spouse ratings on the NEO Personality Inventory. *Journal of Personality and Social Psychology, 54(5),* 853–863.

Craig, A.D. (2002). How do you feel? Interoception: The sense of the physiological condition of the body. *Nature Reviews Neuroscience, 3(8),* 655–666.

Craik, F.I.M., Moroz, T.M., Moscovitch M., Stuss, D.T., Winocur, G., Tulving, E., & Kapur, S. (1999). In search of the self: A positron emission tomography study. *Psychological Science, 10(1),* 26–34.

Critchley, H.D., Wiens, S., Rotshtein, P., Ohman, A. & Dolan, R.J. (2004). Neural systems supporting interoceptive awareness. *Nature Neuroscience, 7(2),* 189–195.

Damasio, A.R., & Van Hoesen, G.W. (1983). Focal lesions of the limbic frontal lobe. In: K.M.S. Heilman (Ed.) *Neuropsychology of Human Emotion* (pp. 85–110). New York: Guilford Press.

Damasio, A.R. (1999). *The Feeling of What Happens: Body and Emotion in the Making of Consciousness.* Orlando, FL: Harcourt.

de Veer, M.W., Gallup, G.G., Jr., Theall, L.A., van den Bos, R. & Povinelli, D.J. (2003). An 8-year longitudinal study of mirror self-recognition in chimpanzees (Pan troglodytes). *Neuropsychologia, 41(2),* 229–234.

Devinsky, O., Morrell, M.J. & Vogt, B.A. (1995). Contributions of anterior cingulate cortex to behaviour. *Brain, 118(pt 1),* 279–306.

Diamond, A. & Goldman-Rakic, P.S. (1989). Comparison of human infants and rhesus monkeys on Piaget's AB task: Evidence for dependence on dorsolateral prefrontal cortex. *Experimental Brain Research, 74(1),* 24–40.

Eccles, J.C. (1992). Evolution of consciousness. *Proceedings of the National Academy of Sciences, 89(16),* 7320–7324.

Edwards-Lee, T., Miller, B.L., Benson, D.F., Cummings, J.L., Russell, G.L., Boone, K. & Mena, I. (1997). The temporal variant of frontotemporal dementia. *Brain, 120,* 1027–1040.

Farrer, C., Franck, N., Georgieff, N., Frith, C.D., Decety, J. & Jeannerod, M. (2003). Modulating the experience of agency: A positron emission tomography study. *Neuroimage, 18(2)*, 324–333.

Farrer, C. & Frith, C.D. (2002). Experiencing oneself vs another person as being the cause of an action: The neural correlates of the experience of agency. *Neuroimage, 15(3)*, 596–603.

Finn, S.E. (1986). Stability of personality self-ratings over 30 years: evidence for an age/cohort interaction. *Journal of Personality and Social Psychology, 50(4)*, 813–818.

Fisher, C.M. (1963). Symmetrical mirror movements and left ideomotor apraxia. *Transactions of the American Neurological Association, 88*, 214–216.

Fisher, C.M. (2000). Alien hand phenomena: a review with the addition of six personal cases. *Canadian Journal of Neurological Science, 27(3)*, 192–203.

Forstl, H., Besthorn, C., Burns, A., Geiger-Kabisch, C., Levy, R. & Sattel, A. (1994). Delusional misidentification in Alzheimer's disease: A summary of clinical and biological aspects. *Psychopathology, 27(3–5)*, 194–199.

Fossati, P., Hevenor, S.J., Graham, S.J., Grady, C., Keightley, M.L., Craik, F. & Mayberg, H. (2003). In search of the emotional self: An FMRI study using positive and negative emotional words. *American Journal of Psychiatry, 160(11)*, 1938–1945.

Gallagher, I.I. (2000). Philosophical conceptions of the self: Implications for cognitive science. *Trends in Cognitive Science, 4(1)*, 14–21.

Gallup, G.G. (1970). Chimpanzees: Self-recognition. *Science, 167*, 86–87.

Gallup, G.G., Jr. (1987). Toward a comparative psychology of self-awareness: Species limitations and cognitive consequences. In: G.R. Goethals & J. Strauss (Eds.) *The Self: An Interdisciplinary Approach* (pp. 121–135). New York: Springer.

Gregory, C.A. (1999). Frontal variant of frontotemporal dementia: A cross-sectional and longitudinal study of neuropsychiatric features. *Psychological Medicine, 29(5)*, 1205–1217.

Greicius, M.D., Krasnow, B., Reiss, A.L. & Menon, V. (2003). Functional connectivity in the resting brain: A network analysis of the default mode hypothesis. *Proceedings of the National Academy of Science, 100(1)*, 253–258.

Gusnard, D.A., Akbudak, E., Shulman, G.L. & Raichle, M.E. (2001). Medial prefrontal cortex and self-referential mental activity: relation to a default mode of brain function. *Proceedings of the National Academy of Science, 98(7)*, 4259–4264.

Gusnard, D.A. & Raichle, M.E. (2001). Searching for a baseline: functional imaging and the resting human brain. *National Review of Neuroscience, 2(10)*, 685–694.

Hart, D. & Whitlow, J.W., Jr. (1995). The experience of self in the bottlenose dolphin. *Consciousness and Cognition, 4(2)*, 244–247.

Hodges, J.R., Patterson, K., Oxbury, S. & Funnell, E. (1992). Semantic dementia. Progressive fluent aphasia with temporal lobe atrophy. *Brain, 115(Pt 6)*, 1783–1806.

Hof, P.R., Vogt, B.A., Bouras, C. & Morrison, J.H. (1997). Atypical form of Alzheimer's disease with prominent posterior cortical atrophy: A review of lesion distribution and circuit disconnection in cortical visual pathways. *Vision Research, 37(24)*, 3609–3625.

Joffe, T.H. & Dunbar, R.I. (1997). Visual and socio-cognitive information processing in primate brain evolution. *Proceedings of the Royal Society of London B Biological Sciences, 264(1386)*, 1303–1307.

Johnson, S.C., Baxter, L.C., Wilder, L.S., Pipe, J.G., Heiserman, J.E. & Prigatano, G.P. (2002). Neural correlates of self-reflection. *Brain, 125(Pt 8)*, 1808–1814.

Kagan, J. (1982). The emergence of self. *Journal of Child Psychology and Psychiatry and Allied Disciplines, 23(4)*, 363–381.

Keenan, J.P., Wheeler, M.A., Gallup, G.G., Jr. & Pascual-Leone, A. (2000). Self-recognition and the right prefrontal cortex. *Trends in Cognitive Science, 4(9)*, 338–344.

Kelley, W.M., Macrae, C.N., Wyland, C.L., Caglar, S., Inati, S. & Heatherton, T.F. (2002). Finding the self? An event-related fMRI study. *Journal of Cognitive Neuroscience, 14(5)*, 785–794.

Kompoliti, K., Goetz, C.G., Boeve, B.F., Maraganore, D.M., Ahlskog, J.E., Marsden, C.D., Bhatia, K.P., Greene, P.E., Przedborski, S., Seal, E.C., Burns, R.S., Hauser, R.A., Gauger, L.L., Factor, S.A., Molho, E.S. & Riley, D.E. (1998). Clinical presentation and pharmacological therapy in corticobasal degeneration. *Archives of Neurology, 55(7)*, 957–961.

Kuniecki, M., Urbanik, A., Sobiecka, B., Kozub, J. & Binder, M. (2003). Central control of heart rate changes during visual affective processing as revealed by fMRI. *Acta Neurobiologiae Experimentalis (Wars), 63(1)*, 39–48.

Levine, B. (2004). Autobiographical memory and the self in time: Brain lesion effects, functional neuroanatomy, and lifespan development. *Brain and Cognition, 55(1)*, 54–68.

Levine, B., Black, S.E., Cabeza, R., Sinden, M., McIntosh, A.R., Toth, J.P., Tulving, E. & Stuss, D.T. (1998). Episodic memory and the self in a case of isolated retrograde amnesia. *Brain, 121(Pt 10)*, 1951–1973.

Lewis, M. (1997). The self in self-conscious emotions. *Annals of the New York Academy of Science, 818*, 118–142.

Lewis, M. & Brooks-Gunn, J. (1979). *Social Cognition and the Acquisition of Self.* New York: Plenum Press.

Lorenz, J., Minoshima, S. & Casey, K.L. (2003). Keeping pain out of mind: The role of the dorsolateral prefrontal cortex in pain modulation. *Brain, 126(Pt 5)*, 1079–1091.

Markus, H. (1977). Self-schemata and processing information about the self. *Journal of Personality & Social Psychology, 35(2)*, 63–78.

Marten, K. & Psarakos, S. (1995). Using self-view television to distinguish between self-examination and social behavior in the bottlenose dolphin (Tursiops truncatus). *Consciousness and Cognition, 4(2)*, 205–224.

McGuire, P.K., Paulesu, E., Frackowiak, R.S. & Frith, C.D. (1996). Brain activity during stimulus independent thought. *Neuroreport, 7(13)*, 2095–2099.

Mesulam, M.M. (1981). A cortical network for directed attention and unilateral neglect. *Annals of Neurology, 10(4)*, 309–325.

Mesulam, M.M. (1982). Slowly progressive aphasia without generalized dementia. *Annals of Neurology, 11(6)*, 592–598.

Miller, B.L., Boone, K., Cummings, J.L., Read, S.L. & Mishkin, F. (2000). Functional correlates of musical and visual ability in frontotemporal dementia. *British Journal of Psychiatry, 176*, 458–463.

Miller, B.L., Cummings, J.L., Villanueva-Meyer, J., Boone, K., Mehringer, C.M., Lesser, I.M. & Mena, I. (1991). Frontal lobe degeneration: Clinical, neuropsychological, and SPECT characteristics. *Neurology, 41(9)*, 1374–1382.

Miller, B.L., Ponton, M., Benson, D.F., Cummings, J.L. & Mena, I. (1996). Enhanced artistic creativity with temporal lobe degeneration. *Lancet, 348(9043)*, 1744–1745.

Miller, B.L., Seeley, W.W., Mychack, P., Rosen, H.J., Mena, I. & Boone, K. (2001). Neuroanatomy of the self: Evidence from patients with frontotemporal dementia. *Neurology, 57(5)*, 817–821.

Nauta, W.J.H. (1971). The problem of the frontal lobe: A reinterpretation. *Journal of Psychiatry Research 8*, 167–187.

Neary, D., Snowden, J.S., Gustafson, L., Passant, U., Stuss, D., Black, S., Freedman, M., Kertesz, A., Robert, P.H., Albert, M., Boone, K., Miller, B.L., Cummings, J. & Benson,

D.F. (1998). Frontotemporal lobar degeneration: A consensus on clinical diagnostic criteria. *Neurology, 51(6),* 1546–1554.

Neisser, U. (1988). Five kinds of self-knowledge. *Philosophy and Pscychology, 1,* 35–59.

Nimchinsky, E.A., Gilissen, E., Allman, J.M., Perl, D.P., Erwin, J.M. & Hof, P.R. (1999). A neuronal morphologic type unique to humans and great apes. *Proceedings of the National Academy of Science, 96(9),* 5268–5273.

Nimchinsky, E.A., Vogt, B.A., Morrison, J.H. & Hof, P.R. (1995). Spindle neurons of the human anterior cingulate cortex. *Journal of Comparative Neurolology, 355(1),* 27–37.

Parker, S.T. (1997). A general model for the adaptive function of self-knowledge in animals and humans. *Consciousness and Cognition, 6(1),* 75–86.

Patterson, F. (1984). Self-recognition by gorilla (Gorilla gorilla). *Gorilla, 7,* 2–3.

Peyron, R., Laurent, B. & Garcia-Larrea, L. (2000). Functional imaging of brain responses to pain. A review and meta-analysis (2000). *Neurophysiologie Clinique, 30(5),* 263–288.

Piolino, P., Desgranges, B., Belliard, S., Matuszewski, V., Lalevee, C., De la Sayette, V. & Eustache, F. (2003). Autobiographical memory and autonoetic consciousness: Triple dissociation in neurodegenerative diseases. *Brain, 126(Pt 10),* 2203–2219.

Platek, S.M., Keenan, J.P., Gallup, G.G., Jr. & Mohamed, F.B. (2004). Where am I? The neurological correlates of self and other. *Brain Research Cognitive Brain Research, 19(2),* 114–122.

Potts, R. (2004). Paleoenvironmental basis of cognitive evolution in great apes. *American Journal of Primatology, 62(3),* 209–228.

Povinelli, D.J. & Cant, J.G. (1995). Arboreal clambering and the evolution of self-conception. *Quarterly Review of Biology, 70(4),* 393–421.

Povinelli, D.J. & Simon, B.B. (1998). Young children's understanding of briefly versus extremely delayed images of the self: Emergence of the autobiographical stance. *Developmental Psychology, 34(1),* 188–194.

Raichle, M.E., MacLeod, A.M., Snyder, A.Z., Powers, W.J., Gusnard, D.A. & Shulman, G.L. (2001). A default mode of brain function. *Proceedings of the National Academy of Science, 98(2),* 676–682.

Rinne, J.O., Lee, M.S., Thompson, P.D. & Marsden, C.D. (1994). Corticobasal degeneration. A clinical study of 36 cases. *Brain, 117(Pt 5),* 1183–1196.

Rochat, P. (1998). Self-perception and action in infancy. *Experimental Brain Research, 123(1–2),* 102–109.

Rosen, H.J., Gorno-Tempini, M.L., Goldman, W.P., Perry, R.J., Schuff, N., Weiner, M., Feiwell, R., Kramer, J.H. & Miller, B.L. (2002). Patterns of brain atrophy in frontotemporal dementia and semantic dementia. *Neurology, 58(2),* 198–208.

Ross, S.J., Graham, N., Stuart-Green, L., Prins, M., Xuereb, J., Patterson, K. & Hodges, J.R. (1996). Progressive biparietal atrophy: An atypical presentation of Alzheimer's disease. *Journal of Neurology, Neurosurgery, and Psychiatry, 61(4),* 388–395.

Rosso, S.M., Roks, G., Stevens, M., de Koning, I., Tanghe, H.L.J., Kamphorst, W., Ravid, R., Niermeijer, M.F. & van Swieten, J.C. (2001). Complex compulsive behaviour in the temporal variant of frontotemporal dementia. *Journal of Neurology, 248(11),* 965–970.

Schmitz, T.W., Kawahara-Baccus, T.N. & Johnson, S.C. (2004). Metacognitive evaluation, self-relevance, and the right prefrontal cortex. *Neuroimage, 22(2),* 941–947.

Scoville, W.B. & Milner, B. (1957). Loss of recent memory after bilateral hippocampal lesions. *Journal of Neurochemistry, 20(1),* 11–21.

Seeley, W.W., Bauer, A.M., Miller, B. L., Gorno-Tempini, M.L., Kramer, J.H., Weiner, M., & Rosen, H.J. (2004). First symptoms and compulsions in temporal variant frontotemporal dementia: Behavioral and linguistic distinctions. *56th Annual Meeting of the American Academy of Neurology, Neurology 62(7, Suppl 5),* A322.

Seeley, W.W., A.M. Baur, B.L. Miller, M.L. Gorno-Tempini, J.H. Kramer, M. Weiner, & H.J. Rosen (in press). The natural history of temporal variant frontotemporal dementia. *Neurology*.

Seger, C.A., Stone, M. & Keenan, J.P. (2004). Cortical activations during judgments about the self and another person. *Neuropsychologia, 42(9)*, 1168–1177.

Singer, T., Seymour, B., O'Doherty, J., Kaube, H., Dolan, R.J. & Frith, C.D. (2004). Empathy for pain involves the affective but not sensory components of pain. *Science, 303(5661)*, 1157–1162.

Snow, C. (1990). Building memories: The ontogeny of autobiography. In: D.C.M. Beeghly (Ed.) *The Self in Transition* (pp. 213–242). Chicago: University of Chicago Press.

Snowden, J.S., Bathgate, D., Varma, A., Blackshaw, A., Gibbons, Z.C. & Neary, D. (2001). Distinct behavioural profiles in frontotemporal dementia and semantic dementia. *Journal of Neurology, Neurosurgery, and Psychiatry, 70(3)*, 323–332.

Thompson, S.A., Patterson, K. & Hodges, J.R. (2003). Left/right asymmetry of atrophy in semantic dementia: Behavioral-cognitive implications. *Neurology, 61(9)*, 1196–1203.

Tulving, E., Kapur, S., Craik, F., Moscovitch, M. & Houle, S. (1994). Hemispheric encoding/ retrieval asymmetry in episodic memory: positron emission tomography findings. *Proceedings of the National Academy of Science, 91(6)*, 2016–2020.

Victoroff, J., Ross, G.W., Benson, D.F., Verity, M.A. & Vinters, H.V. (1994). Posterior cortical atrophy. Neuropathologic correlations. *Archives of Neurology, 51(3)*, 269–274.

Vogeley, K., Bussfeld, P., Newen, A., Herrmann, S., Happe, F., Falkai, P., Maier, W., Shah, N.J., Fink, G.R. & Zilles, K. (2001). Mind reading: Neural mechanisms of theory of mind and self-perspective. *Neuroimage, 14(Pt 1)*, 170–181.

Von Economo, C. (1926). Eine neue Art Spezialzellen des Lobus cinguli und Lobus insulae. *Zeitschrift für die Gesamte Neurologie und Psychiatrie, 100*, 706–712.

Wheeler, M.A., Stuss, D.T. & Tulving, E. (1997). Toward a theory of episodic memory: The frontal lobes and autonoetic consciousness. *Psychological Bulletin, 121(3)*, 331–354.

Zysset, S., Huber, O., Ferstl, E. & von Cramon, D.Y. (2002). The anterior frontomedian cortex and evaluative judgment: An fMRI study. *Neuroimage, 15(4)*, 983–991.

11

Autism—"Autos": Literally, a Total Focus on the Self?

SIMON BARON-COHEN

The idea that as a result of neurological factors one might lose aspects of the self is scientifically important, in that it offers the promise of teaching us more about what the self is. In this chapter I do not tackle the thorny question of how to define the self (though this is attempted in other chapters in this book). Rather, I accept that this word refers to something we recognize and instead raise the question: are people with autism trapped—for neurological reasons—to be totally self-focused?

Autism

Autism is a neurodevelopmental condition diagnosed on the basis that a child or adult has difficulties with social relationships and communication, alongside strongly repetitive behavior and unusually narrow interests ("obsessions"). The term *autism* literally means "self"-ism, derived from the Greek word *autos* ("self"). It was first coined by Bleuler to describe the social withdrawal characteristic of someone with schizophrenia, but Kanner (1943) co-opted the term as more fitting for the group of children he saw in his clinic who (he wrote) paid as little attention to people in the room as they did to the furniture. It is testimony to Kanner's insight that although across the subsequent 60 years there have been changes in the diagnostic criteria for autism, and although theories about its cause have come and gone, his focus on the self as abnormal in autism has remained essentially applicable to these children and adults.

Today we recognize a spectrum of autistic conditions, with Kanner's autism (also referred to as "classic autism") being the more severe form. In the case of Kanner's autism, the total focus on the self is (forgive the pun) self-evident. The child has his or her interests (usually his, since this condition affects males more often than females) and tends to focus totally on these. To the extent that other people figure in the child's life, it tends to be if the other person is interested to join in with the child's interests. If there is any invitation by another person for the child to join in with someone else's interests, typically the child will simply turn away. Other people's behavior and other people's minds are of no interest to children with autism. Typically, this is because the child with autism is interested in phenomena that are controllable, and, of course, other people's behavior is difficult to control. That is not to say that children with autism do not try to control others' behavior, for example, through tantrums when others introduce change, or by being very bossy, or by insisting that people perform a scripted sequence of behaviors. Some children with autism also appear to be interested in others, such as by asking them questions, but typically the children are amassing information relevant to their own interests, rather than this being a genuine interest in the other person for its own sake.

Part of this autistic spectrum is a subgroup known as Asperger syndrome (Asperger, 1944). We will return to this later, but for now it is worth summarizing the argument made in this chapter. My proposal is this: that what drives a nonautistic person to be interested in another self (not just his or her own) is *empathy,* and that what drives a person with autism (be it classic autism or the milder Asperger syndrome) to be relatively disinterested in other selves and primarily focused on his or her own interests, knowledge, goals, and projects is an impairment in empathy. But to understand this, we have to start by examining what is meant by empathy.

Empathizing

Empathizing is the drive to identify another person's emotions and thoughts and to respond to these with an appropriate emotion (Davis, 1994). Empathizing does not just entail the cold calculation of what someone else thinks and feels (what is sometimes called mind reading). Psychopaths can do that much. Empathizing is also about having an appropriate emotional reaction inside, an emotion triggered *by* the other person's emotion. And empathizing is done in order to understand other people, predict their behavior, and connect or resonate with them emotionally. Imagine you could recognize that "Jane is in pain," but this left you cold, or detached, or happy, or preoccupied. This would not be empathizing. Now imagine you do not just see Jane's pain, but you also automatically feel concern, wince yourself, and feel a desire to run over and help alleviate her pain. That is empathizing. And empathizing extends to recognizing and responding to any emotion or state of mind, not just the more obvious ones, such as pain. For me, empathy arises out of a natural desire to *care* about others.

Empathy is a skill (or a set of skills). As with any other skill, such as athleticism or mathematical or musical ability, we all vary in it. In the same way that we can think about why someone is talented or average or even disabled in these other areas, so we can think about individual differences in empathy. One can even think of empathy as a trait, like height, since that is also something in which we all differ. And in the same way that you can measure someone's height, so you can measure differences in empathizing between individuals. The strange thing about empathizing is that, by definition, you would have a hard time realizing that you were short of it, if indeed you were a few points lower on the Empathy Quotient (EQ) than other people (Baron-Cohen et al., 2003; Baron-Cohen & Wheelwright, 2004). Empathizing requires you to be aware of how others see you, and you might *believe* that they see you as the most sensitive being on the planet. But none of us can ever really know how we are coming across to others (we can only do our best). The reality may be that our own evaluation of ourselves falls short of how others *actually* perceive us.

Most of us have some *awareness* of our empathizing skills, but may not have any awareness of when we hit our limits. In this sense empathizing is not like athletic ability, for which you get direct feedback during your performance of whether you are any good or not. With empathy you might aim to be very empathic during a conversation and walk away from it believing that you were truly empathic. The person you were just interacting with might never tell you how limited your empathy was—they may have been too hurt or too diplomatic to tell you.

Empathizing is about spontaneously and naturally tuning in to the other person's thoughts and feelings, whatever these might be. It is not just about reacting to a small number of emotions in others, such as their pain or sadness. It is about reading the emotional atmosphere between people. It is about effortlessly putting yourself into another's shoes. It is about sensitively negotiating an interaction with another person so as not to hurt or offend him or her in any way. It is about caring about another's feelings. A good empathizer can immediately sense when an emotional change has occurred, and what might cause an emotional change and can rapidly anticipate what might make this particular person feel better or worse. A good empathizer responds intuitively to a change in another person's mood with concern, appreciation, understanding, comforting, or whatever the appropriate emotion might be.

Empathizing leads you to pick up the phone and tell someone you are thinking about them and their current situation, even when your own life demands are equally pressing. Empathizing leads you to constantly search people's tones of voice and scan people's faces, especially their eyes, so as to pick up how they might be feeling or what they might be thinking. You use the "language of the eyes" and intonation as windows to their minds. Empathizing drives you to do this because you start from the position that your view of the world may not be the only one or the true one and that their views and feelings matter.

The natural empathizer can perceive fine shifts of mood, all the intermediate shades of an emotion in another person that might otherwise go unnoticed. Take hostility, for example. Some people notice only a small number of shades of hostility (such as aggression, hate, and threat). In contrast, a good empathizer might recognize 50 different shades of hostility (such as contempt, cruelty, condescension, and superciliousness). It is like color vision. Some people notice just a few shades of blue, while others notice 100. My colleagues Jacqueline Hill, Sally Wheelwright, Ofer Golan, and I recently completed an emotion taxonomy (an encyclopedia of emotions, if you like) and discovered that there are actually 412 discrete (mutually exclusive, semantically distinct) human emotions. Some people find it easy to define the subtle differences between such shades of emotion, and for others the differences can be very hard to see (Baron-Cohen et al., 2004).

A natural empathizer not only notices others' feelings, he or she is constantly thinking about what people might be feeling, thinking, or intending. He or she empathizes with people who are present and with those who are not present but whose thoughts and feelings have a bearing on the present in some way. They read the emotional weather in this way *not* because they want to manipulate people. A psychopath or a businessman might think of a person as an object to be exploited. This is not empathizing (Blair, 1995). Rather, an empathizer continually cares how the other might be feeling.

Why Do We Empathize?

Empathy is a defining feature of human relationships. For example, empathy stops you from doing things that would hurt another person's feelings. Empathy makes you bite your lip rather than saying something that might offend someone or make him or her feel hurt or rejected. Empathy also stops you from inflicting physical pain on a person or animal. You may feel angry toward your dog for barking, but you do not hit it because you know it would suffer. Empathy helps you tune into someone else's world, setting aside your own world—your perceptions, knowledge, assumptions, and feelings. It allows you to see another side of an argument easily. Empathy drives you to care for or offer comfort to another person, even if they are unrelated to you and you stand to gain nothing in return. Imagine you are a bystander witnessing a car crash, and you are the first on the scene. Empathy propels you to sit with the victim of the crash, checking how they are, and reassuring them that someone is there for them. Seconds before, you had never met each other. Minutes later, you might never see that person again, but you still care.

Empathy also makes real communication possible (Baron-Cohen, 1988). Talking "at" a person is not real communication. It is a monologue. If you talk for significantly more than 50% of the time every few sentences, it is not a conversation. It is venting, or storytelling, or lecturing, or indoctrinating, or controlling, or persuading, or dominating, or filling silence. There is, in any conversation, a risk that one party will hijack the topic in an undemocratic manner, not that his or her intention is necessarily to be undemocratic. But in hijacking the conversation, the speaker does not stop to consider that if he or she is doing all the talking, this is only fulfilling his or her *own* needs, not the listeners'. Empathy ensures this risk is minimized by enabling the speaker to check how long to carry on and to be receptive to the listener's wish to switch to a different topic.

Real conversation is sensitive to *this* listener at *this* time. Empathy leads you to ask the listener how he or she feels and to check if he or she wants to enter the dialogue or what he or she thinks about the topic. It leads you to check not just once and then ignore the other's thoughts and feelings while you focus on your own but rather to keep asking, frequently, in the dialogue. Why check? You check because otherwise you might be pouring words all over your listener without them being interested.

Empathy leads you not just to check, but to be able to follow through on what others say, so they do not feel it was insincere, shallow interest you showed in them.

Empathy allows for a reciprocal dialogue because you are constantly making space in the conversation for others, through turn-taking. Empathy allows you to adjust your conversation to be attuned to theirs. Empathy involves a leap of imagination into someone else's headspace. While you can try to figure out other persons' thoughts and feelings by reading their faces, their voices, and their postures, ultimately their internal worlds are not transparent, and to climb inside their heads requires imagining what it must be like to be them.

But empathy is not just doing all of the above in order to *appear* appropriate or as an intellectual exercise. You do it because you cannot help doing it, because you *care* about the other person's thoughts and feelings, and because it matters. For someone who is poor at empathizing, she may be able to do it when she is reminded or if she discovers that people will include her more often if she does or says the right thing, and she may even rehearse how to empathize so as to get the benefits. But she may not do it spontaneously. For her, other people's feelings matter less, and it takes an effort to maintain empathic appearances. For the natural empathizer, it is easy.

Empathy ensures you see a person as a person with feelings, rather than as a thing to be used to satisfy your own needs and desires. For example, an empathic father decides not to smack his child, even if he is feeling outraged at the child's obstinate refusal to cooperate. The parent's own feelings of frustration are set aside in the face of the hurt that could be caused to another. Or an empathic boss appreciates that her employees are not production slaves but have personal lives that need their own private time and space, even within working hours.

Empathy also provides a framework for the development of a moral code. Moral codes are built by people out of natural empathy, fellow feeling, and compassion. Some people think that it is legal systems that determine how we should act. There is no doubt that it is a great achievement to produce a legal system that underpins a moral code. Just look at what happens in countries where the legal code has collapsed. It would be marvelous if systemetizing, the pure process of logic, could give us a sense of justice and injustice, but there are plenty of instances in history in which logic and legal systems have been used to defend autocratic, even genocidal, regimes, Nazism being one of the clearest of recent examples. One can be an excellent logician, but without a full quotient of empathy, one's morality can end up being quite harmful. So it is good that we do not have to depend on pure logic as a guide to moral behavior. Rather, it is our feelings of empathy that help us choose between one set of laws and another. This is not a complete list of the reasons why empathy is so important, but it highlights the fact that empathy is central to what it is to be a person, as distinct from any other kind of animal.

Two Elements to Empathy

There are basically two major elements to empathy (Baron-Cohen & Wheelwright, 2004). The first is the "cognitive" component: *understanding* others' feelings and switching to take their perspectives. Swiss developmental psychologist Jean Piaget referred to empathy as "decentering," or responding nonegocentrically, which are both nice ways of capturing this cognitive component (Piaget & Inhelder, 1956). More recent developmental psychologists refer to this aspect of empathy in terms of using a "theory of mind," or "mindreading" (Astington, Harris, & Olson, 1988; Whiten, 1991) . Essentially, the cognitive component entails setting aside your own current perspective, attributing a mental state (sometimes called an "attitude") to other persons, and then inferring the likely contents of their mental states, given their experiences. The cognitive element also allows you to *predict* others' behavior or mental state.

The second aspect to empathy is the "affective" component (Hobson, 1993). This is an appropriate emotional response in the observer to the emotional state of another person. Sympathy is just one such type of empathic response, in which you feel both an emotional response to someone else's distress and a desire to alleviate his suffering. (You may not actually act on this desire, but at least you feel you want to reduce the other's distress.) Sympathy is perhaps the clearest case of empathy. You walk past a homeless person in the winter, and you are moved to want to help her out of her misfortune. This counts as sympathy. You may do nothing about it, as you may also feel that your action would be futile given the many other homeless people in the same neighborhood and the difficulty of helping all of them, so you walk past. Your reaction was still sympathetic because you felt the desire to alleviate the other person's suffering. It was still sympathy whether or not you took the appropriate action and gave the poor woman your gloves. But in other empathic reactions, there is a different, still appropriate, emotional response to someone else's feelings. Perhaps you feel anger (at the system) in response to the homeless person's sadness, or fear (for her safety), or guilt (over not being able to help), and so on. All of these are empathy. Feeling pleasure, or smugness, or hatred toward the poor woman would not count as empathy, as none of these emotions are appropriate to *her* emotion.

If we accept that there are these two aspects to empathizing (the cognitive and the affective), can this be formalized? Alan Leslie suggests the cognitive aspect involves what he calls an "M-Representation" (M for mental state) (Leslie, 1987). Here is how he characterises it:

Agent-*Attitude*-Proposition

For example:

John-*thinks*-Sarah is beautiful

Here, the attitude (in the mind of the agent, in this case John), is highlighted in italics. This tripartite structure captures the cognitive aspect of empathizing, but this leaves out the extra element, namely, that the observer experience an emotion triggered by the other person's emotion or mental state. To capture this second aspect would require a longer formulation, along the lines of

Self-**Emotion** (Agent-*attitude*-proposition)

Here, the Emotion term is within the observer and is highlighted in bold. It is an appropriate affective reaction to everything that follows in parentheses, and the Agent is always another person or animal. For example:

Jane-**is concerned** (John-*feels sad*- his mother died)

This notation suggests that empathy is really quite complex, involving long chains of information embedded in highly specific ways. But this notational description of empathizing fails to convey how immediate and automatic empathy is, that is, Jane does not have to grind through laborious cognitive reasoning to feel concern at John's sadness. You just feel it, as clearly as you feel fear if you look over a cliff edge or disgust if you see half a worm in your half-eaten apple. These are emotions triggered by physical situations, and in empathy you simply have an emotion triggered by someone else's emotion. As we all know, when we get a lump in the throat and tears well up in our eyes during a movie or when reading a book, such emotions can be very powerful, even if all we are reacting to is the imagined emotion of the imaginary character.

Asperger Syndrome: A Disability of Empathy?

Let us go back to autism and Asperger syndrome. There is little doubt that classic autism involves a total focus on the self and little if any apparent interest in the emotional states of others. It is not out of some sense of cruelty, but purely a result of a complete failure to understand another person's emotions and thoughts resulting from a neurologically based "mindblindness" (Baron-Cohen, 1995). But the challenge in this essay is to ask if this total focus on the self—"autos"—also applies to everyone on the autistic spectrum, even those with Asperger syndrome (AS). A brief description of AS follows.

These are people (mostly men) who may talk to others only at work for the purposes of work alone, or talk only to obtain something they need, or talk only to share factual information. They may answer with "just the facts" when you ask them a question, but otherwise they do not ask questions of others because they do not naturally consider what others might think. These are people who cannot see the point of social chit-chat. They do not mind having a discussion (note, not a chat) on a particular issue in order to establish the truth of the matter (mostly persuading you of their views). But just a casual, superficial chat? Why bother? And what on earth about? How? For these people, it is both too hard and pointless.

These are people who, in the first instance, think of solving tasks *on their own* by figuring it out for themselves. The object or system in front of them is all that is in their minds, and they do not stop for a moment to consider another person's knowledge of it. Present them with a system, and they become interested in spotting the underlying factual regularities. They tune in to the tiny details to such a great degree that in their fascination with cracking the system, they may become oblivious to all those around them. The spotlight of attention onto a tiny variable becomes all that matters, and the fact that a person is standing next to them with tears rolling down his cheeks is irrelevant information that is passed over. All that they focus on is determining the unvarying if-then rules, which allow them to control and predict the system, in principle completely. Present them with some speculation about what someone might think or feel or with a topic that is ultimately not factual, and they switch off or even avoid it because of its unknowability and therefore unpredictability.

Diagnostic, Historical, and Etiological Issues

Autism is diagnosed when a person shows abnormalities in social development and communication and displays unusually strong obsessional interests from an early age. Even as recently as the 1980s, autism was thought of as the most *severe* childhood psychiatric condition, and it was thought of as *rare*. It was thought of as severe because half of these children did not speak, and most (75%) had below-average intelligence (IQ). Their poor language skills and low IQ predicted great difficulties later (Rutter, 1978).

In addition, they displayed the core features of autism: poor social skills, limited imagination, and obsessive interests in unusual topics, such as collecting types of stones or traveling to every railway station in Britain just to look at each depot. And autism was thought of as rare because only 4 children in every 10,000 seemed to be affected in this severe way. But an interesting shift occurred during the early 1990s. It had always been known that a small portion (25%) of children with autism had normal, or even above-average, intelligence, but slowly such "high-functioning" cases started being identified more frequently. By the late 1990s it seemed that the high-functioning children with autism were no longer in the minority. It is part of the diagnosis of autism that such children are late to start talking. But in these high-functioning cases of autism, the late start in language does not seem to stop them from developing good or even talented levels in mathematics, chess, mechanical knowledge, and other factual, scientific, technical, and rule-based subjects.

In the 1990s clinicians and scientists also started talking about a group of children who were just a small step away from high-functioning autism. They called this Asperger syndrome (AS) (Frith, 1991). AS was proposed as a variant of autism. The child with AS has the same difficulties in social and communication skills and has the same obsessional interests, but such children (like those with high-functioning autism) not only have normal or high IQ, they also start speaking on time. And their problems are not all that rare. Today, approximately 1 in 200 children have one of the autistic spectrum conditions, which include AS, and many of them are in mainstream schools (Scott et al., 2002). So now we have to radically reconceptualize autism. Cases rose from 4 in 10,000 in the 1970s to 1 in 200 at the start of this millenium. That is more than a tenfold increase in prevalence. This is most likely a reflection of better awareness and broader diagnosis to include AS.

In people with AS, the problems are not as obviously severe as are seen in the mute and learning-disabled children with autism. But most children with AS are nevertheless often miserable at school because they cannot make friends. It is hard to imagine what this must be like. Most of us just take it for granted that we will fit in well enough to have a mix of friends, but for people with AS, the sad realization is that they are surrounded by acquaintances or strangers but not friends as we understand the word. Many of them are teased and bullied because they do not manage to fit in or have no interest in fitting in. Their lack of social awareness means they may not even try to camouflage their oddities.

Autism spectrum conditions are strongly genetic in origin. The evidence for this comes from twin and family studies. If an identical twin has autism, the chance of his or her co-twin also having an autism spectrum condition is very high (between 60% and 90%) (Bailey, 1993). If a nonidentical twin has an autism spectrum condition, the equivalent risk for his or her co-twin is much less (about 20%). Autism spectrum conditions are also neurodevelopmental. That is to say, they start early—probably prenatally—and affect the development and functioning of the brain. There is evidence of brain dysfunction (such as epilepsy in a percentage of cases). There is also evidence of structural and functional differences in regions of the brain (such as the amygdala being abnormal in size and less responsive to emotional cues) (Baron-Cohen et al., 2000; Baron-Cohen et al., 1999).

Empathy Deficit in Adults with Asperger Syndrome

In our clinic in Cambridge we meet adults who suspect they may have AS but whose problems went undetected in their childhood. AS simply was not recognized when they were in school. Hence, they have limped through childhood, adolescence, and young adulthood, but slowly the accumulated difficulties have piled up until they reach a clinic such as ours, where they are desperate for a way to make sense of a lifetime of not fitting in. Many of them struggle to work out a huge set of rules of how to behave in each and every situation and expend enormous effort into consulting a sort of mental look-up table for how to behave and what to say from minute to minute. It is as if they are trying to write a manual for social interaction made of if-then rules. It is as if they are trying to "systemize" social behavior whereas the natural approach to socializing should be via empathizing.

Imagine Victorian books on social etiquette for dinner parties (which fork to use, how to reply to questions such as "would you like some more dessert?" etc.) but writ large, to cover every eventuality in social intercourse. Of course, it turns out to be impossible to be fully prepared, but some of these individuals do a brilliant job in getting close to this goal. Even so, it is physically exhausting. By the time they get home from work, where they have been "pretending to be normal" (Willey, 1999), the last thing they want to do is socialize. They just want to close the door on the world and say the words or perform the actions that they had to censor all day. They do not know why they cannot say what they think, wish that others would do the same, and cannot see why saying what they think could cause offence or lead them into social difficulties.

One man with AS put it very clearly to me. "What I say is what I believe. How someone else perceives what I say has nothing to do with me." This shows that this man (who had an IQ in the superior range) could not appreciate that people have feelings that we have a responsibility not to hurt. Nevertheless, many people with AS learn to stay silent rather than make a personal comment about someone. They do this not out of any empathic understanding or concern, but because that way they avoid getting into trouble. Once again, they learn a rule rather than being motivated by empathy. Hence, many adults with AS have to train themselves through trial and plenty of error to learn what can be said and done and what cannnot. The typical set of characteristics we see in our clinic for adults with AS (they are almost all male) are as follows.

In Childhood

When we look back at the childhoods of people with AS, we find a common picture. They almost always tended to be loners. Even though they saw the other children in the playground, many of them did not know how to interact with them. Some of them describe the experience as like being "a Martian in the playground" (Sainsbury, 2000). Instead, many preferred to talk to adults, such as teachers, than to other children.

Sadly, it was the case that as children they were rarely invited to play at other children's houses or to their birthday parties. If they were invited once, they tended not to be invited back. When we ask their parents what kind of play their child participated in, we find they did not produce much varied, social pretend play. Instead, they were far more focused on constructional play (building things) or reading factual books (such as encyclopedias). If another child did come around to play, the child with AS was often described as "bossy," trying to control the other person, not just choosing the game, but directing the other child in what to say and what to do. Many of them as children were content to spend long, solitary hours playing with jigsaw puzzles, Lego, Meccano, and other constructional systems. Some also built houses out of boxes around the home or dens outside. Some enjoyed miniature systems, such as model-making or setting up armies of tiny figures of knights in armor, soldiers, or fantasy figures.

Typically, they pursued their own intellectual interests to high levels, such as learning books of facts, or studying the movement of the sun and shadows around their bedroom, or attempting to breed tropical fish, becoming very knowledgeable on these subjects. But many also did not hand in the required schoolwork, so that they failed in some academic subjects. Having no drive to please the teacher, they simply followed their own interests rather than the whole curriculum. Throughout childhood there were those signs of obsessional or deep interest in narrow topics, such as collecting a complete set of wildlife picture cards, or carrying around mathematical equations in their pockets, or learning language after language, as part of a collection of knowledge. As for the female patients with AS, many of them recall being described as "tomboys" in their behaviors and interests.

As Teenagers

When we asked our patients with AS to recall their adolescences, most recalled that they did best at factual subjects, such as mathematics, science, history, and geography, or at the vocabulary and syntax aspects of foreign languages. Many (but not all) were weakest in literature, in which the task was to *interpret* a fictional text, or write pure fiction, or enter into a character's emotional life. Some learned rules to systemize the analysis of fiction and obtained good grades in this way. In an extreme example a young woman with AS bought exam preparation books and learned literary criticisms about texts without actually reading the texts herself.

Many became acutely aware that they were low in social popularity and were failing at making friends, especially girlfriends for the boys with AS. Their obsessions continued, changing topic when the last one was fully exhausted every few years. The female patients found their adolescent peer groups particularly confusing and impossible to join: "All that giggling in lifts, and talk about fashion and hair. I couldn't understand why they did it." Some got into trouble for pursuing unusual interests (such as the chemistry of poisons and the construction of explosives). Most at one time or another had said things that had hurt others' feelings, often on a frequent basis, yet could not understand why the other persons took offence if their statement was true.

As Adults

We see them now as adults. Many have held a series of jobs and have experienced social difficulties leading to clashes with colleagues and employers, so that they have had to leave. In their work they are often considered technically expert and thorough but may never get promoted because their "people skills" are so limited. Some have had a series of short-term sexual relationships. Such relationships usually flounder, in part because the other person feels he or she is being over-controlled or used or because he or she feels his or her partner is not emotionally supportive or communicative. Other people recognize they are socially odd (though this is harder to detect in the female patients), and their few friends are also usually somewhat odd. Typically, their friendships drop away because they do not maintain them. A significant percentage of adults with AS experience clinical levels of depression, and some even feel suicidal through not belonging and feelings of social failure.

Many continue to say things that offend others, even though they do not intend any offence. They may learn to avoid obvious statements such as reference to someone's weight and instead commit faux pas of a more subtle kind. For example, at his sister's second wedding, sitting at the reception dinner table with the new husband, one adolescent with AS turned to his sister and asked: "How's David [the first husband]? Do you see much of him these days?" Almost invariably, they are disinterested in small talk and do not know how to do it or what it is for. They frequently feel they cannot say what they think, as people often seem shocked by their independent, extreme, unempathic, and sometimes offensive views. For example, one man with AS described his politics as "green fascism," the belief that anyone spoiling nature should be shot. Another said he believed in "meritocratic misogyny," the belief that women have not achieved equally high positions in society because they are less able. Most have no time for political correctness or spin. They believe in saying what they think, seeing no point in sugaring the pill or spin-doctoring.

Frequently they hate crowds, or people dropping in, as they find people unpredictable and annoying when things are moved around. If people are invited over for supper by a partner, the person with AS might just walk into the next room and read a book while the guests are at the table. Politically or in other ways, their views are often held very strongly and are black or white. They are typically convinced by the rightness of their beliefs, and, given the chance, will spend hours relentlessly trying to convince other people to change their view. They feel their beliefs are not beliefs in the sense of being "just one point of view," a matter of subjectivity. Rather, they believe their own beliefs are a true reflection of the world, and as such, correct. Coming up against others' beliefs therefore can mean them trying to persuade the others that they are right and the others wrong.

Sitting next to them at dinner can begin to feel like being pinned to the wall while they go too far in explaining their views. Or, in response to a polite question about his or her weekend, a person with AS might go into too much detail about the technicalities of a hobby, not picking up that the listener has long since become bored. In other individuals with AS, the conversation might be too brief and strictly factual, giving too little information, as if they cannot judge what is expected by or interesting to another mind.

One patient I met watched news reports of buildings collapsing after terrorist bombings on video over and over again in order to understand the differences among types of architecture and the consequences. He could give statistics on how many people were killed in each building collapse, the materials that the buildings were made of, and of the physics of each type of material but admitted that he did not find himself spontaneously stopping to think about the victims or their families.

Some marry but remain married only if their partners are patient to the point of saintliness, and are able to accommodate family life to the rigidity of the autistic routines and systems, and can accept an eccentric, remote, often controlling partner. Some marry partners of different ethnicity, possibly because their social oddness and communication abnormality are less apparent to nonnative speakers. Their partners often learn to avoid asking friends over because their spouses with AS are so socially embarrassing. Their social lives may be restricted to that which is structured for them such as through the church or by others. I should stress that the above symptoms are typical only of those people with AS who are suffering enough that they have sought the help of a clinic, but now you have a picture of AS.

Experimental Evidence for Impaired Empathizing— An Extreme of the Male Brain?

On the Empathy Quotient (EQ) women score higher than men, but people with AS, or high-functioning autism, score even lower than men (Baron-Cohen & Wheelwright, 2004). On social tests such as the Reading the Mind in the Eyes Test and the Facial Expressions Test, women score higher than men, but people with AS score even lower than men (Baron-Cohen et al., 1997; Baron-Cohen el al., 2001; Baron-Cohen, Wheelwright, & Jolliffe, 1997). In terms of eye contact, women make more eye contact than do men, and people with autism or AS make less eye contact than men (Lutchmaya, Baron-Cohen, & Raggett, 2002; Swettenham, 1996). In terms of language, girls develop vocabulary faster than do boys, and children with autism are even slower than are boys to develop vocabulary (Lutch-maya, Baron-Cohen, & Raggatt, 2002).

Women tend to be superior to men in terms of chatting and the pragmatics of conversation, and it is precisely this aspect of language that people with AS find most difficult (Baron-Cohen, 1988). Women are also better than men at the Faux Pas Test, and people with autism or AS have even lower scores than men do (Baron-Cohen et al., 1999). Girls also tend to be better than boys on standard "theory of mind" tests (involving thinking about others' thoughts and feelings), and people with autism or AS are even worse than are normal boys (Baron-Cohen, Leslie, & Frith, 1985; Happe, 1995). Finally, women score higher on the Friendship Questionnaire (FQ) which assesses empathic styles of relationships. Adults with AS score even lower than do normal men on the FQ (Baron-Cohen & Wheelwright, 2003).

Conclusion

What gets one out of one's own self and into someone else's is the rare and special resource of empathy. In this chapter I have argued that people on the autistic spectrum, even the high-functioning individuals, such as those with AS, are essentially wholly focused on their own concerns, through a neurologically based inability to empathize to normal levels. Some can empathize with others and in this way overcome their self-focus—by supreme effort and reminding themselves constantly—but most would wish just to relax and revert to their essentially self-centred world. That is not to say that they are inward-focused, as many enjoy hobbies and interests that are outside of themselves, but because they are self-chosen interests, they are essentially self-focused. I have also argued that people with AS are not cruel or bad people, in that they have no wish to hurt others, even if they inadvertently do so through their lack of awareness of the effects of their actions on others' emotions. In this critical regard they are not callous psychopaths whose empathy deficit is accompanied by a moral deficit. People with AS may have trouble empathizing, which imprisons them inside their own selves, but they are frequently highly moral individuals who think deeply about how—in novelist Nick Hornby's words—to be good. Through their good logic, they typically have a strong sense of justice for others as well as for themselves.

Acknowledgments
I am grateful to the MRC UK for support during the period of this work. Parts of this chapter are taken from *The Essential Difference* (New York: Basic Books, 2004).

References:

Asperger, H. (1944). Die "autistischen psychopathen" im kindesalter. *Archiv fur Psychiatrie und Nervenkrankheiten, 117,* 76–136.

Astington, J., Harris, P., & Olson, D. (1988). *Developing Theories of Mind.* New York: Cambridge University Press.

Bailey, A. (1993). The biology of autism. Editorial. *Psychological Medicine, 23,* 7–11.

Baron-Cohen, S. Joliffe, T., Mortimore, C., & Robertson, M. (1997). Another advanced test of theory of mind: Evidence from very high functioning adults with autism or Asperger Syndrome. *Journal of Child Psychology and Psychiatry, 38,* 813–822.

Baron-Cohen, S. (1988). Social and pragmatic deficits in autism: Cognitive or affective? *Journal of Autism and Developmental Disorders, 18,* 379–402.

Baron-Cohen, S. (1995). *Mindblindness: An Essay on Autism and Theory of Mind.* Boston: MIT Press/Bradford Books.

Baron-Cohen, S., Golan, O., Wheelwright, S., & Hill, J.J. (2004). *Mindreading: The Interactive Guide to Emotions.* London: Jessica Kingsley.

Baron-Cohen, S., Leslie, A.M., & Frith, U. (1985). Does the autistic child have a "theory of mind"? *Cognition, 21,* 37–46.

Baron-Cohen, S., O'Riordan, M., Jones, R., Stone, V., & Plaisted, K. (1999). A new test of social sensitivity: Detection of faux pas in normal children and children with Asperger syndrome. *Journal of Autism and Developmental Disorders, 29,* 407–418.

Baron-Cohen, S., Richler, J., Bisarya, D., Gurunathan, N., & Wheelwright, S. (2003). The Systemising Quotient (SQ): An investigation of adults with Asperger syndrome or high functioning autism and normal sex differences. *Philosophical Transactions of the Royal Society, Series B, Special issue on "Autism : Mind and Brain," 358,* 361–374.

Baron-Cohen, S., Ring, H., Bullmore, E., Wheelwright, S., Ashwin, C., & Williams, S. (2000). The amygdala theory of autism. *Neuroscience and Behavioural Reviews, 24,* 355–364.

Baron-Cohen, S., Ring, H., Wheelwright, S., Bullmore, E.T., Brammer, M.J., Simmons, A., et al. (1999). Social intelligence in the normal and autistic brain: An fMRI study. *European Journal of Neuroscience, 11,* 1891–1898.

Baron-Cohen, S. & Wheelwright, S. (2003). The Friendship Questionnaire (FQ) : An investigation of adults with Asperger syndrome or high functioning autism, and normal sex differences. *Journal of Autism and Developmental Disorders, 33,* 509–517.

Baron-Cohen, S. & Wheelwright, S. (2004). The Empathy Quotient (EQ). An investigation of adults with Asperger syndrome or high functioning autism, and normal sex differences. *Journal of Autism and Developmental Disorders, 34,* 163–175.

Baron-Cohen, S., Wheelwright, S., Hill, J., Raste, Y., & Plumb, I. (2001). The "Reading the Mind in the Eyes" test revised version: A study with normal adults, and adults with Asperger syndrome or high-functioning autism. *Journal of Child Psychiatry and Psychiatry, 42,* 241–252.

Baron-Cohen, S., Wheelwright, S., & Jolliffe, T. (1997). Is there a "language of the eyes"? Evidence from normal adults and adults with autism or Asperger syndrome. *Visual Cognition, 4,* 311–331.

Blair, R.J. (1995). A cognitive developmental approach to morality: Investigating the psychopath. *Cognition, 57,* 1–29.

Davis, M.H. (1994). *Empathy: A Social Psychological Approach.* Madison, WI: Brown & Benchmark.

Frith, U. (1991). *Autism and Asperger's Syndrome.* Cambridge: Cambridge University Press.

Happe, F. (1995). The role of age and verbal ability in the theory of mind task performance of subjects with autism. *Child Development, 66,* 843–855.

Hobson, R.P. (1993). *Autism and the Development of Mind.* Hove: Lawrence Erlbaum Associates.

Kanner, L. (1943). Autistic disturbance of affective contact. *Nervous Child, 2,* 217–250.

Leslie, A.M. (1987). Pretence and representation: The origins of "theory of mind." *Psychological Review, 94,* 412–426.

Lutchmaya, S., Baron-Cohen, S., & Raggatt, P. (2002). Foetal testosterone and vocabulary size in 18- and 24-month-old infants. *Infant Behavior and Development, 24(4),* 418–424.

Lutchmaya, S., Baron-Cohen, S., & Raggett, P. (2002). Foetal testosterone and eye contact in 12-month-old infants. *Infant Behavior and Development, 25,* 327–335.

Piaget, J. & Inhelder, B. (1956). *The Child's Conception of Space.* London: Routledge & Kegan Paul.

Rutter, M. (1978). Diagnosis and definition. In: M. Rutter & E. Schopler (Eds.), *Autism: A Reappraisal of Concepts and Treatment* (pp. 1–26). New York: Plenum Press.

Sainsbury, C. (2000). *Martian in the Playground.* Bristol, UK: Lucky Duck Publishing.

Scott, F., Baron-Cohen, S., Bolton, P., & Brayne, C. (2002). Prevalence of autism spectrum conditions in children aged 5–11 years in Cambridgeshire, UK. *Autism, 6(3),* 231–237.

Swettenham, J. (1996). Can children with autism be taught to understand false belief using computers? *Journal of Child Psychology and Psychiatry, 37,* 157–165.

Whiten, A. (1991). *Natural Theories of Mind.* Oxford: Basil Blackwell.

Willey, L.H. (1999). *Pretending to be Normal.* London: Jessica Kingsley.

12

Recognizing the Sensory Consequences of One's Own Actions and Delusions of Control

SARAH-JAYNE BLAKEMORE

Delusions of control are symptoms associated with schizophrenia in which people misattribute self-generated actions to an external source (Schneider, 1959). The actions in question can be mundane, such as picking up a cup or combing one's hair. Auditory hallucinations are common in schizophrenia and normally consist of hearing spoken speech or voices (Johnstone, 1991). Both delusions of control and auditory hallucinations are considered "first rank" features in schizophrenia (Schneider, 1959; Mellors, 1970).

Normally, we are readily able to detect whether a movement is self-generated or externally caused. It has been proposed that an internal predictor, or forward model, uses information about intentions to enable this distinction between self-generated and externally generated sensory events (Miall & Wolpert, 1996; Wolpert, Ehahramani, & Jordon, 1995, Wolpert, Ehahramani, Flanagan, 2001). Forward models use an "efference copy" of the motor command (von Holst, 1954) to make a prediction of the consequences of a motor act. A *forward dynamic model* makes predictions about the next state of the system and compares this with the desired state. A *forward output model* makes predictions about the sensory consequences of a movement, and this prediction is compared with the actual sensory consequences of a movement (Figure 12–1). This comparison can be used to cancel the sensory effect of the motor act, attenuating it perceptually compared with identical stimulation that is externally produced.

This predictive system is useful because it can be used to filter incoming sensory signals, picking out sensory information caused externally, such as touch produced by an external object or agent, and distinguishing it from sensory stimulation that occurs as a necessary consequence of self-produced movement. An impairment in such a predictive system could cause a lack of attenuation of the sensory consequences of self-produced actions, which would therefore be indistinguishable from externally generated sensations. This would result in the interpretation of one's own movements as being externally caused—a delusion of control (Frith, 1992; Frith, Blakemore, & Wolpert, 2000).

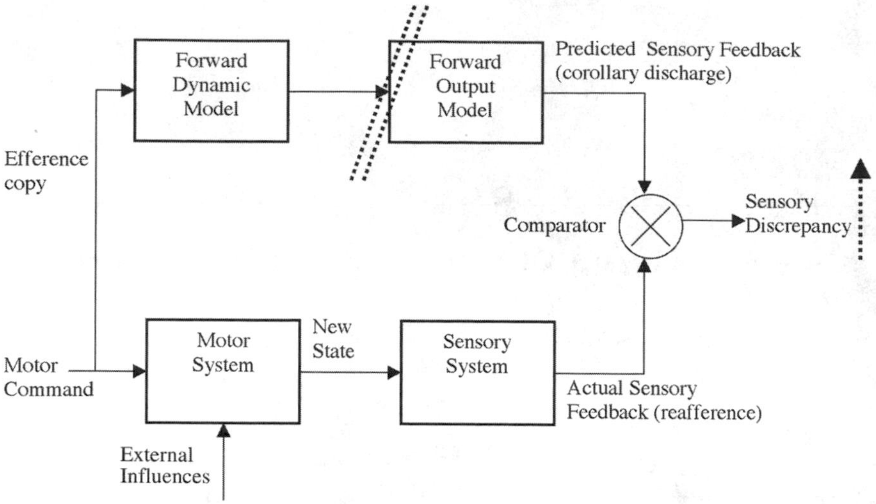

Figure 12–1. The forward model of motor control, as proposed by Miall et al. (1993). A forward dynamic model predicts the consequences of motor commands, and these are compared with the desired state. The forward output model makes a prediction of the sensory consequences of motor commands, which is compared with the actual consequences of movement (reafference). Discrepancies resulting from this comparison can be used to cancel reafferent inputs and to distinguish self-produced and externally produced signals. The dashed lines indicate the proposed underlying disorder leading to delusions of control and a possible mechanism by which hypnotic suggestion can alter the experience of a self-produced movement. In both delusions of control and hypnotic suggestion the subject can formulate the action appropriate to his or her intention, and the action is successfully performed. The forward output model is dysfunctional such that it cannot make an accurate prediction of the sensory consequences of the movement based on the efference copy. This might be because the efference copy signals do not reach the forward output model, or because the forward output model cannot make accurate predictions based on the efference copy it receives. This results in a high level of sensory discrepancy (indicated by the dashed arrow) and no cancellation of the reafference, so that the (self-produced) movement feels externally produced.

Perception of the Sensory Consequences of Actions

Evidence suggests that the sensory consequences of some self-generated movements are perceived differently from identical sensory input when it is externally generated. An example of such differential perception is the phenomenon that people cannot tickle themselves (Weiskrantz, Elliot, & Darkington, 1971). It has been argued that efference copy produced in parallel with the motor command underlies this phenomenon. To investigate this proposal, we asked participants to rate the sensation of a tactile stimulus on the palms of their hands, and examined the perceptual effects of altering the correspondence between self-generated movement and its sensory (tactile) consequences.

A robotic interface was employed to produce the delays and trajectory rotations. Participants moved a robotic arm with their left hands, and this movement caused a foam-tipped robotic arm to move across their right palms. Thus, motion of the left hand determined the tactile stimulus on the right palm. By using this robotic interface so that the tactile stimulus could be delivered under remote control by the participant, *delays* of 100 ms, 200 ms and 300 ms were introduced between the movement of the left hand and the tactile stimulus on the right palm. In a further condition *trajectory rotations* of 30°, 60°, and 90° were introduced between the direction of the left hand movement and the direction of the tactile stimulus on the right palm. The result of increasing the delay or trajectory rotation was that the sensory stimulus no longer corresponded to that normally expected based on the efference copy produced in parallel with the motor command. Therefore, as the delay or trajectory rotation increased, the sensory prediction became less accurate.

The results demonstrated that participants rated the self-produced tactile sensation as being significantly less tickly, intense, and pleasant than an identical stimulus produced by the robot (Blakemore, Frith, & Wolpert, 1999a). Furthermore, participants reported a progressive increase in the tickly rating as the delay was increased between 0 ms and 200 ms, and as the trajectory rotation was increased between 0° and 90°. These results support the hypothesis that the perceptual attenuation of self-produced tactile stimulation is due to precise sensory predictions. As the sensory feedback deviates from the prediction of the forward model (by increasing the delay or trajectory rotation), the sensory discrepancy between the predicted and actual sensory feedback increases, which leads to a decrease in the amount of sensory attenuation.

Do Patients with Delusions of Control Predict the Sensory Consequences of Their Own Actions?

To test the hypothesis that delusions of control and auditory hallucinations occur due to a defect in self-monitoring, we investigated whether individuals with auditory hallucinations and/or passivity experiences are abnormally aware of the sensory consequences of their own movements. Individuals with a diagnosis of schizophrenia, bipolar affective disorder and depression were divided into two groups on the basis of the presence or absence of auditory hallucinations and/or passivity experiences. These patient groups and a group of age-matched healthy control participants were asked to rate the perception of a tactile sensation (a piece of soft foam) on the palms of their left hands. The tactile stimulation was either self-produced by movement of the participant's right hands or externally produced by the experimenter.

The results demonstrated that healthy control participants and participants with neither auditory hallucinations nor passivity symptoms experienced self-produced stimuli as less intense, tickly, and pleasant than identical externally produced tactile stimuli. In contrast, participants with these symptoms did not show a decrease in their perceptual ratings for tactile stimuli produced by themselves as

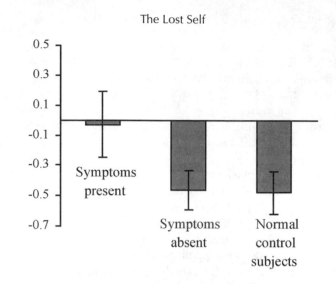

Figure 12–2. Graph showing the mean (tickly, pleasant, and intense combined) perceptual rating difference between self-produced and externally produced tactile stimulation conditions for the three participant groups: patients with auditory hallucinations and/or passivity, patients without these symptoms, and normal control participants. There was no significant difference between the perceptual ratings in the two conditions for participants with auditory hallucinations and/or passivity, hence the mean rating difference was close to 0. In contrast, there was a significant difference between the perceptual ratings in the two conditions for patients without these symptoms and in normal control participants: both groups rated self-produced stimulation as less tickly, intense, and pleasant than externally produced stimulation.

compared to those produced by the experimenter (Blakemore et al., 2000). Figure 12–2 shows the difference between the ratings for self-produced and externally produced tactile stimulation for the three participant groups. These results support the proposal that auditory hallucinations and passivity experiences are associated with an abnormality in the forward model mechanism that normally allows us to distinguish self-produced from externally produced sensations. It is possible that the neural system associated with this mechanism, or part of it, operates abnormally in people with such symptoms.

The Physiological Basis of the Perceptual Modulation of Self-Produced Sensory Stimuli

Neurophysiological data demonstrate that neuronal responses in the somatosensory cortex are attenuated by self-generated movement. Active touch is attenuated in the primary somatosensory cortex of animals (Chapman, 1994) compared to passive and external touch of an identical tactile stimulus. It is possible that this movement-induced somatosensory attenuation is the physiological correlate of the decreased sensation associated with self-produced tactile stimuli in humans. In order for somatosensory cortex activity to be attenuated to self-produced sensory stimuli, these stimuli need to be predicted accurately. The cerebellum is a possible site for a forward model of the motor apparatus that provides predictions of the sensory consequences of motor commands. This proposal has been supported by computational (Miall et al., 1993; Wolpert, Miall, & Kawato, 1998), neurophysiological (Simpson, Wylie, & De Zeeuw, 1995), and functional neuroimaging data (Imamizu et al., 2000).

To investigate the hypothesis that the somatosensory cortex and the cerebellum are involved in modulating the sensation of a self-produced tactile stimulation, we used functional magnetic resonance imaging (fMRI) to examine the neural basis of self- versus externally produced tactile stimuli in humans (Blakemore, Wolpert, & Frith, 1998). Healthy participants were scanned while a tactile stimulation device allowed a tactile stimulus (a piece of soft foam) to be applied to the participants' left palms. The tactile stimulus was produced either by the participants' right hands or by the experimenter.

The results showed an increase in activity of the secondary somatosensory cortex (SII) and the anterior cingulate cortex (ACC) when participants experienced an externally produced tactile stimulus relative to a self-produced tactile stimulus. The reduction in activity in these areas to self-produced tactile stimulation might be the physiological correlate of the reduced perception associated with this type of stimulation. The activity in the ACC in particular may have been related to the increased tickliness and pleasantness of externally produced compared to self-produced tactile stimuli. Previous studies have implicated this area in affective behavior and positive reinforcement (Vogt & Gabriel, 1993). Alternatively the activity in the ACC might be related to the requirement to monitor the sensations the participants were experiencing (Lane et al., 1997; Frith & Frith, 2003).

While the decrease in activity in the SII and ACC might underlie the reduced perception of self-produced tactile stimuli, the pattern of brain activity in the cerebellum suggests that this area is the source of the SII and ACC modulation. In the SII and ACC activity was attenuated by all movement: these areas were equally activated by movement that did and that did not result in tactile stimulation. In contrast, the right anterior cerebellar cortex was selectively deactivated by self-produced movement that resulted in a tactile stimulus, but not by movement alone, and significantly activated by externally produced tactile stimulation. This pattern suggests that the cerebellum distinguishes between movements depending on their specific sensory consequences.

A second experiment supported the proposal that the cerebellum distinguishes between movements depending on their specific sensory consequences (Blakemore, Frith, & Wolpert, 2001). In this experiment participants were scanned using positron emission tomography (PET) while generating a tactile stimulus on the palms of their hands, as before. This time, however, the tactile stimulation was produced under remote control via a robotic interface. Participants moved a robotic arm with their left hands, and this movement caused a second foam-tipped robotic arm to move across their right palms. By using this robotic interface so that the tactile stimulus could be delivered under remote control by the participants, delays of 0 ms, 100 ms, 200 ms, and 300 ms were introduced between the movement of the left hand and the tactile stimulus on the right palm. Under all delays the left hand made the same movements, and the right hand experienced the tactile stimulus. Only the temporal correspondence between the movement of the left hand and the sensory effect on the right palm was altered. Blood flow in the right cerebellar cortex significantly correlated with delay. This suggests that activity in this region increases as the actual feedback from movement deviates from the predicted sensory feedback. On the basis of these results we proposed that the cerebellum is involved in signalling discrepancies between the predicted and actual consequences of action.

The Role of the Parietal Cortex in the Distinction Between the Self and the Other

There is accumulating evidence that in addition to the cerebellum, the parietal cortex is involved in distinguishing self-produced actions and actions generated by others (see Chapter 16, this volume). Activity in the parietal operculum (secondary somatosensory cortex) is attenuated during self-initiated movements compared with passive movements (Weiller et al., 1996), and, as discussed in the previous section, during self-produced compared with external sensory stimulation (Blakemore, Wolpert, & Frith, 1998).

There is evidence from neurological patients that the parietal cortex plays a role in the distinction between the self and the other. Patients with left parietal lesions tend to confuse the ownership of hand movements when they are shown someone else's hand making movements similar to those they are making themselves (Sirigu et al., 1999). A case study reported a patient with a right-hemisphere lesion in which the white matter underlying cortex including the parietal operculum had been damaged. This patient suffered from the delusional belief that her left limb belonged to her niece (Bottini et al., 2002).

Parietal lesions impair the ability to use mental motor imagery, a process believed to involve an internal model of action. Parietal patients are unable to predict the time necessary to perform finger movements and visually guided pointing gestures using their imagination. Normally, imagined and executed movement times are highly correlated, Fitts's Law accounting equally well for both types of movement (Sirigu et al., 1995; Decety & Jennerod, 1995). This was found to be true for a patient with motor cortex damage, whereas in patients with parietal lesions actual movement execution was modulated by target size, but motor imagery was not (Sirigu et al., 1996). More recently, using similar tasks, a patient with a right temporoparietal lesion was tested on his ability to imagine and perform visually guided hand movements. It was found that unlike his performance for visually guided actions, there was no relationship between accuracy and speed for imagined movements (Danckert et al., 2002).

Functional neuroimaging studies have also demonstrated that the parietal cortex is involved in the distinction between self and other. The right inferior parietal cortex is activated when subjects simulate actions or beliefs from someone else's perspective but not from their own (Ruby & Decety, 2000; 2003). This region is activated when subjects observe their own actions being imitated by someone else compared with when they imitate someone else's action (Decety et al., 2002). The inferior parietal cortex is differentially activated according to whether subjects attend to someone else's actions or their own (Farrer & Frith, 2002) and whether they lead or follow another person's actions (Chaminade & Decety, 2002).

Delusions of Control and the Cerebellum and Parietal Cortex

Overactivity of the parietal cortex appears to contribute to the feeling that active movements are externally controlled in delusions of control (Spence et al., 1997). In this PET study patients with delusions of control were scanned while they performed a simple motor task in which they were required to move a joystick in one of four directions chosen at random. This "willed action" task was compared with a similar task in which the joystick movements were paced. The patients with delusions of control showed overactivity in the superior parietal cortex and in the cerebellum relative to normal controls and to patients who did not have delusions of control. Normally, activity in the parietal cortex is more typical of passive movements than active ones. Thus, at the experiential level, when the patient makes an active movement, it can feel like a passive movement. It is this feeling that leads to the belief about alien control. Further support for this suggestion came from the finding that parietal activity had returned to "normal" levels when, some months later, the same patients who were scanned in the initial study and whose symptoms had now subsided were rescanned performing the same task.

Inducing Delusions of Control in the Normal Brain

Further evidence that overactivity of the parietal cortex and cerebellum is involved in generating the feeling that a movement is externally produced comes from a recent study in which experiences of control were induced in healthy control subjects (Blakemore et al., 2003). In this study hypnosis was used as a cognitive tool to create delusions of control in normal, healthy subjects. "Ideomotor movement" is a frequently demonstrated hypnotic phenomenon in which self-produced actions are attributed to an external source (Heap & Aravind, 2002). A typical example involves suggesting to the hypnotized subject that her arm is being raised upward passively by an external device, such as a helium balloon attached to her wrist. This suggestion causes highly hypnotizable subjects to produce an appropriate movement. Despite generating the movement herself, the subject describes the raising and lowering of her arm as being involuntary and typically claims that it was caused by the helium balloon.

In our study PET was used to scan highly hypnotizable participants during a similar "alien control" experience. In an active movement condition each participant was instructed to move his left arm up and down, which he correctly attributed to himself. In another condition (the deluded passive movement condition), the participant was told that his left arm would be moved up and down by the pulley, but in fact the pulley did not move and resulting arm movements were self-generated. This suggestion induced the participants, who were all highly hypnotizable according to the Harvard Hypnotizability Scale (Shor & Orne, 1962), to move their arm up and down in the suggested manner. However, crucially, participants misattributed this movement to the pulley. All conditions were performed while participants were hypnotized. Thus, movements in the active movement and deluded passive conditions were identical—participants made the same self-generated arm movements in both conditions. The only difference between these two conditions was the source to which the movement was attributed.

Using this paradigm we were able to compare brain activation during active movements that were correctly attributed to the self with identical active movements that were misattributed to an external source. The results demonstrated the cerebellum and parietal operculum were differentially activated depending on whether an active movement was experienced as truly active or as passive. Parietal-opercular and cerebellar activity was significantly higher and more widespread in the deluded passive condition, in which movements were misattributed to an external source, than in the active movement condition, in which identical movements were correctly attributed to the self.

In terms of the forward model (Figure 12–1), which is believed to be stored in the cerebellum (Miall et al., 1993; Imamizu et al., 2000), the abnormality in the deluded passive condition might lie in the forward output model and not the forward dynamic model. The forward dynamic model compares the estimated state with the desired state, and the results of this comparison are used to adjust motor commands in order to optimize motor control and learning. Participants produced the same smooth arm movements in the deluded passive and active movement conditions. Therefore, the motor system appears to be functioning normally in terms of motor control in the deluded passive condition. In contrast, the forward output model compares the predicted consequences of motor commands with the actual consequences of movement (reafference), and discrepancies resulting from this comparison can be used to cancel reafferent inputs and to distinguish self-produced and externally produced sensory signals.

We have tentatively suggested that hypnotic suggestion in the deluded passive condition prevents the motor intentions from reaching the forward output model. In this case the forward output model would no longer be able to make an accurate prediction of the sensory consequences of the movement. This would lead to a discrepancy between predicted and actual sensory feedback, which would result in no attenuation of the sensory feedback, making the (self-produced) movement feel externally produced. If the cerebellum signals sensory discrepancies between predicted sensory feedback of movements and their actual sensory consequences (Andersson & Armstrong, 1985; Blakemore, Frith, & Wolpert, 2001), increased cerebellar activation would be expected in the deluded passive condition.

According to evidence from patient and neuroimaging studies described above, the parietal cortex appears to be involved in inducing the feeling that an action or sensory event is external. Activity in the parietal cortex seems to be required for an arm movement to feel as if it is externally generated. The inferior parietal lobe is the direct target of output from the cerebellum (Clower et al., 2001) and parietal-opercular cortex activity can be influenced by cerebellar activity (Blakemore, Wolpert, & Frith, 1999). In the deluded passive condition, if the cerebellum signals a discrepancy between predicted and actual sensory feedback, then no parietal-opercular attenuation would occur, which is what normally occurs during externally produced sensory stimulation.

There is an alternative—or additional—explanation for the parietal activity in the deluded passive condition. It is well established that attention to a particular sensory modality or feature increases activity in the brain region that processes that feature, even in the absence of a sensory signal (Driver & Frith, 2000). It has also been suggested that hypnotic suggestion, by focussing attention, can produce increased activity in specific brain areas, which causes a modulation of sensory experience (Rainville et al., 1997). Rainville and colleagues have shown that the hypnotic suggestion to increase or decrease the affective components of constantly applied experimental pain are accompanied by a modulation of activity in the anterior cingulate cortex, an area previously shown to be involved in the experience of pain. Activity in this region increased as the experience of pain increased in response to suggestion even though the painful stimulus itself did not change. It is possible that in our study, participants' attention was more highly focused on the sensations associated with passive movement in the deluded passive condition than in the active movement condition. This increased attention produces activation in brain regions that process such sensations (the parietal operculum). It is the activation in this region that causes the movement to feel external.

A similar mechanism may underlie the disorder leading to delusions of control in schizophrenia and other clinical conditions. In particular, it has been proposed that delusions of control are caused by an impairment in the forward model system that predicts the sensory consequences of one's own actions (Frith, Blakemore, & Wolpert, 2000). This could cause a lack of attenuation of the sensory consequences of self-produced actions, which would therefore be indistinguishable from externally generated sensations, hence causing a confusion between the self and the other (Frith, 1992; Frith, Blakemore, & Wolpert, 2000). A similar theory that attempts to account for delusions of control posits that these symptoms reflect a disruption of the cognitive processes that normally produce a sense of agency or volitional control (Jeannerod, 1999). Jeannerod has suggested that conscious judgment about a movement requires a different form of representation from that needed for unconscious comparisons of predictions and outcomes within the motor system, specifically that conscious judgments about movements require "third-person" information, while control of movement depends on private "first-person" information, on this basis Jeannerod proposes that patients with delusions of control fail to monitor the third-person signals that enable them to make judgments about their own actions. Spence (1996), on the other hand, has suggested that the problem underlying delusions of control has to do with the timing of awareness. The awareness of the actual outcome of the movement precedes the awareness of the predicted outcome, which is contrary to the normal experience of our own agency.

The ability to distinguish between active and passive movements is an important part of a "who" system, which allows one to link an action with its cause (Georgieff & Jeannerod, 1998). The data reviewed in this chapter suggest that overactivation of a cerebellar-parietal network during self-generated actions is associated with the misattribution of those actions to an external source. Overactivity of the parietal cortex and cerebellum occurs during self-generated movements in patients with delusions of control and subsides when the same patients are in remission (Spence et al., 1997). It is possible that malfunctioning in this network leading to overactivity produces the feeling of "otherness" associated with self-produced movements in delusions of control.

Acknowledgment
The research decribed in this chapter was supported by the Wellcome Trust UK and carried out with Chris Frith and Daniel Wolpert.

References

Andersson, G. & Armstrong, D.M. (1985). Climbing fibre input to b zone Purkinje cells during locomotor perturbation in the cat. *Neuroscience Letters Supplement, 22,* S27.

Blakemore, S.-J., Wolpert, D.M., & Frith, C.D. (1998). Central cancellation of self-produced tickle sensation. *Nature Neuroscience, 1(7),* 635–640.

Blakemore, S.-J., Frith, C.D., & Wolpert, D.W. (1999). Spatiotemporal prediction modulates the perception of self-produced stimuli. *Journal of Cognitive Neuroscience, 11,* 551–559.

Blakemore, S.-J, Wolpert, D.M., & Frith, C.D. (1999). The cerebellum contributes to somatosensory cortical activity during self-produced tactile stimulation. *NeuroImage, 10 (4),* 448–459.

Blakemore, S.-J., Smith, J., Steel, R., Johnstone, E., & Frith, C.D. (2000). The perception of self-produced sensory stimuli in patients with auditory hallucinations and passivity experiences: Evidence for a breakdown in self-monitoring. *Psychological Medicine, 30,* 1131–1139.

Blakemore, S.-J., Frith, C.D., & Wolpert, D.W. (2001). The cerebellum is involved in predicting the sensory consequences of action. *NeuroReport, 12(9),* 1879–1885.

Blakemore, S.-J., Oakley, D.A. & Frith, C.D. (2003). Delusions of alien control in the normal brain. *Neuropsychologia, 41(8),* 1058–1067.

Bottini, G., Bisiach, E., Sterzi, R., & Vallar, G. (2002). Feeling touches in someone else's hand. *NeuroReport, 13(2),* 249–252.

Chaminade, T. & Decety J. (2002). Leader or follower? Involvement of the inferior parietal lobule in agency. *NeuroReport 13(15),* 1975–1978.

Chapman, C.E. (1994). Active versus passive touch: Factors influencing the transmission of somatosensory signals to primary somatosensory cortex. *Canadian Journal of Physiology and Pharmacology, 72,* 558–570.

Clower, D.M., West, R.A., Lynch, J.C., & Strick, P.L. (2001). The inferior parietal lobule is the target of output from the superior colliculus, hippocampus, and cerebellum. *Journal of Neuroscience, 21(16),* 6283–6291.

Decety, J. & Jeannerod M. (1995). Mentally simulated movements in virtual reality: Does Fitts's law hold in motor imagery? *Behavior and Brain Research, 14,* 127–134.

Danckert, J., Ferber, S., Doherty, T., Steinmetz, H., Nicolle, D., & Goodale, M.A. (2002). Selective, non-lateralized impairment of motor imagery following right parietal damage. *Neurocase 8(3),* 194–204.

Decety, J., Chaminade, T., Grezes, J. & Meltzoff, A.N. (2002). A PET exploration of the neural mechanisms involved in reciprocal imitation. *Neuroimage, 15(1),* 265–272

Driver, J. & Frith, C. (2000). Shifting baselines in attention research. *Nature Reviews Neuroscience, 1(2),* 147–148.

Farrer, C. & Frith, C.D. (2002). Experiencing oneself vs another person as being the cause of an action: The neural correlates of the experience of agency. *Neuroimage, 15(3),* 596–603.

Frith, C.D. (1992). *The Cognitive Neuropsychology of Schizophrenia.* Hove, Sussex, UK: Lawrence Erlbaum Associates.

Frith, C.D., Blakemore, S-J., & Wolpert, D.M. (2000). Abnormalities in the awareness and control of action. *Philosophical Transactions of the Royal Society of London: Biological Sciences, 355(1404),* 1771–1788.

Frith, U. & Frith, C. (2003). Development and neurophysiology of mentalizing. *Proceedings of the Royal Society of London, Biological Sciences, 358,* 459–473.

Georgieff, N., & Jeannerod, M. (1998). Beyond consciousness of external reality. A "who" system for consciousness of action and self-consciousness. *Consciousness and Cognition, 7,* 465–477.

Heap, M. & Aravind, K.K. (2002). *Hartland's Medical and Dental Hypnosis,* 4th ed. Edinburgh: Churchill Livingston.

Imamizu, H., Miyauchi, S., Tamada, T., Sasaki, Y., Takino, R., Püutz, B., Yoshioka, T., & Kawato, M. (2000). Human cerebellar activity reflecting an acquired internal model of a new tool. *Nature, 403,* 192–195.

Jeannerod, M. (1999). To act or not to act: Perspectives on the representation of actions. *Quarterly Journal of Experimental Psychology A, 52,* 981–1020.

Johnstone, E.C. (1991). Defining characteristics of schizophrenia. *British Journal of Psychiatry Supplement, (13),* 5–6.

Lane, R.D., Fink, G.R., Chua, P.M., & Dolan, R.J. (1997). Neural activation during selective attention to subjective emotional responses. *NeuroReport, 8,* 3969–3972.

Mellors, C.S. (1970) First-rank symptoms of schizophrenia. *British Journal of Psychiatry, 117,* 15–23.

Miall, R.C., Weir, D.J., Wolpert, D.M., & Stein, J.F. (1993). Is the cerebellum a Smith predictor? *Journal of Motor Behaviour, 25,* 203–216.

Miall, R.C. & Wolpert, D.M. (1996). Forward models for physiological motor control. *Neural Networks, 9,* 1265–1279.

Rainville, P., Duncan, G.H., Price, D.D., Carrier, B., & Bushnell, M.C. (1997). Pain affect encoded in human anterior cingulate but not somatosensory cortex. *Science, 277,* 968–971

Ruby, P. & Decety, J. (2001). Effect of subjective perspective taking during simulation of action: A PET investigation of agency. *Nature Neuroscience, 4(5),* 546–550.

Ruby, P. & Decety, J. (2003). What you believe versus what you think they believe: A neuroimaging study of conceptual perspective-taking. *European Journal of Neuroscience, 17(11),* 2475–2480.

Schneider, K. (1959). *Clinical Psychopathology.* New York: Grune & Stratton.

Shor, R.E. & Orne, E.C. (1962). *Harvard Group Scale of Hypnotic Susceptibility.* Palo Alto, CA: Consulting Psychologists Press.

Simpson, J.L., Wylie, D.R., & De Zeeuw, C.I. (1995). On climbing fiber signals and their consequence(s). *Behavioural and Brain Sciences, 19(3),* 384.

Sirigu, A., Cohen L., Duhamel J.R., Pillon B., Dubois B., Agid Y., & Pierrot-Deseilligny, C. (1995). Congruent unilateral impairments for real and imagined hand movements. *NeuroReport, 6,* 997–1001.

Sirigu, A., Duhamel J.R., Cohen, L., Pillon, B., Dubois, B., & Agid, Y. (1996). The mental representation of hand movements after parietal cortex damage. *Science, 273,* 1564–1568.

Sirigu, A., Daprati, E., Pradat-Diehl, P., Franck, N., & Jeannerod, M. (1999). Perception of self-generated movement following left parietal lesion. *Brain, 122,* 1867–1874.

Spence, S.A., Brooks, D.J., Hirsch, S.R., Liddle, P.F., Meehan, J., & Grasby, P.M. (1997). A PET study of voluntary movement in schizophrenic patients experiencing passivity phenomena (delusions of alien control). *Brain, 120,* 1997–2011.

Spence, S.A. (1996). Free will in the light of neuropsychiatry. *Philosophy, Psychiatry and Psychology, 3,* 75–90.

Vogt, B.A. & Gabriel, M., eds. (1993). *Neurobiology of Cingulate Cortex And Limbic Thalamus.* Boston: Birkauser.

von Holst, E. (1954). Relations between the central nervous system and the peripheral organs. *British Journal of Animal Behaviour, 2,* 89–94.

Weiller, C., Juptner, M., Fellows, S., Rijntjes, M., Leonhardt, G., Kiebel, S., Muller, S., Diener, H.C., & Thilmann, A.F. (1996). Brain representation of active and passive movements. *Neuroimage, 4(2),* 105–110.

Weiskrantz, L., Elliot, J., & Darlington, C. (1971). Preliminary observations of tickling oneself. *Nature, 230,* 598–599.

Wolpert, D.M., Ghahramani, Z., & Jordan, M.I. (1995). An internal model for sensorimotor integration. *Science, 269,* 1880–1882.

Wolpert, D.M., Miall, R.C., & Kawato, M. (1998). Internal models in the cerebellum. *Trends in Cognitive Science, 2(9),* 338–347.

Wolpert, D.M., Ghahramani, Z., & Flanagan, R. (2001). Perspectives and problems in motor learning. *Trends in Cognitive Science, 5(11),* 487–494.

13

The Neural Correlates
of Depersonalization:
A Disorder of Self-Awareness

HEDY KOBER, ALYSA RAY, SUKHVINDER OBHI,
KEVIN GUISE, AND JULIAN PAUL KEENAN

Depersonalization can be understood, at least in part, as a disorder involving disruptions of self-awareness. Recent neuroimaging evidence indicates that the right hemisphere is likely essential to self-related processing, such as self-recognition, autobiographical retrieval, self-evaluation, and autonoetic consciousness. Disorders of self-awareness caused by focal lesions, such as asomatognosia and mirror sign, have also implicated the right hemisphere (see Chapter 8, Feinberg, this volume and Chapter 9, Postal, this volume). Although early studies were inconclusive, we review the most recent literature and suggest that as imaging techniques improve, right hemisphere dysfunction may be implicated in dissociative processing and particularly in depersonalization.

The Self and the Right Hemisphere

For centuries philosophers have considered the concept of self-awareness as central to human existence. Many attempts have been made to elucidate the nature of self-awareness, most recently by cognitive neuroscientists seeking to identify possible neural correlates of this most fundamental of human capabilities (for a review, see Keenan, Gallup, & Falk, 2003). Over the past few years the rise of modern neuroimaging techniques has led a number of researchers independently to speculate that the right hemisphere, particularly in prefrontal areas, may be dominant for self-related processing. Such self-related processing includes self-recognition, self-face recognition, self-voice recognition, autobiographical/episodic retrieval, self-evaluation, first-person perspective, and autonoetic consciousness (Keenan et al., 2001; Sugiura et al., 2000; Breen, Caine & Coltheart, 2001; Nakamura, Kawashima, Sugiura, Kato, Nakamura et al., 2001; Markowitsch, 1995; Miller et al.,

2001; Spangenberg, Wagner & Bachmnan, 1998; Fink et al., 1996; Levine et al., 1998; Craik et al., 1999; Vogeley et al., 2001; Stuss, 1991; Wheeler, Stuss, & Tulving 1997), as both self-related processing and self-recognition may be considered markers of self-awareness (Keenan et al., 2003).

Over the past few years many studies have found greater right-hemisphere involvement in tasks involving self-face recognition, especially in prefrontal areas. Whereas the fusiform gyrus has been implicated in general face recognition (Kanwisher, Stanley, & Harris, 1999; Kanwisher, McDermott, & Chun, 1997), investigations examining self-face versus other face recognition have found that recognition of the self-face is often correlated with greater activity in the right hemisphere. For example, in a neuroimaging study employing functional magnetic resonance imaging (fMRI), Keenan, McCutcheon, and Pascual-Leone (2001) contrasted subjects' brain activity when they viewed their own faces with the activity when they viewed the face of another individual (Bill Clinton). The results showed that when subjects viewed their own faces there was significantly more activation within the right inferior frontal gyrus than when they viewed the nonself face. In a different study Keenan and coworkers (2001) employed the WADA test to further investigate the role of the right hemisphere in self-face recognition. In this procedure, (named after the neurologist Juhn A. Wada) typically used to find the language-dominant hemisphere before surgery, one hemisphere at a time is anesthetized following administration of amobarbital (a strong barbiturate) to the intracarotid artery. Keenan and colleagues used a morphing procedure to create pictures that were a combination of patients' own faces and that of a famous person. While anesthetized, the patients were shown a picture of the morphed face and were instructed to remember it. After recovery from the anesthesia, the patients were asked to choose the picture they saw while anesthetized, from the two original pictures used to construct the morphed face. Following anesthesia to the left hemisphere, all five patients selected the self-face, suggesting that self-recognition does not depend on the left hemisphere. In contrast, following anesthesia to the right hemisphere, four of the five patients selected the famous face, suggesting that the right hemisphere is essential for self-face recognition. To ensure that this effect was not due to a simple biasing of naming (i.e., the left hemisphere is needed to name famous faces), 10 normal subjects were presented with similar morphed images. The authors used transcranial magnetic stimulation (TMS) to determine the cortical excitability of the left and right hemispheres and found that excitability in the left hemisphere did not differ significantly between self- and other morphs. This suggests that the level of cortical activation in the left hemisphere was similar for self- and other processing. Interestingly, however, there was significantly greater activation of the right hemisphere for self-morphs compared to familiar morphs. Consistent with these findings, Keenan and colleagues (2003) have recently found evidence in split-brain patients for a right-hemisphere bias in self-related processing. In addition, when peripheral physiological data are collected (e.g., skin resistance), it has been found that the right hemisphere of split-brain patients is significantly more active in response to the self-face even when emotionality is controlled for (Preilowski, 1977). Again, the left hemisphere shows no such differentiation between self and other (but see Turk et al., 2002, for contradictory evidence).

In addition to the experimental evidence suggesting a right-hemisphere dominance for tasks involving self-recognition, there is also considerable evidence for a right-lateralized bias from clinical studies examining deficits in self-recognition, known as "mirror sign" (see Chapters 8 and 9, this volume).

Other deficits in self-awareness have also been linked to right-hemisphere dysfunction (Feinberg, 2000; Stuss 1991). Feinberg in Chapter 8 in this volume details a number of delusional misidentifications, all of which which seem to involve right-hemisphere disorders. Further support for the preferential involvement of the right hemisphere compared to the left in delusional misidentification comes from the WADA test. In a study by Meador et al., 2000, the right hemispheres of 32 patients were anesthetized, and it was found that only 8 of these patients were able to correctly recognize their own hands, while the other 24 patients claimed their hands were someone else's. This study clearly suggests that the right hemisphere is important for self-related processing and that this processing is not limited to self-face recognition but extends to other aspects of self-identity.

Drawing another link between self-processing and right-lateralized activation, Ruby and Decety (2003) recently used PET to investigate the neural correlates of first-person perspective-taking versus third-person perspective-taking. In the experiment participants were asked to answer questions from both their own perspectives and from the perspective of a third person. The authors concluded that the right inferior parietal lobe was critical for distinguishing self and other, along with frontopolar and somatosensory regions. These results confirmed previous results reported in the motor domain in which activation in the right somatosensory cortex was associated with a "preservation of the sense of self" (Iacoboni et al., 1999). In a recent review article Decety and Sommerville (2003) argued that the inferior parietal cortex and the prefrontal cortex in the right hemisphere play a special role in interpersonal awareness, such that they are critical for understanding and separating self from other. In addition, Decety and coworkers have suggested that the right parietal cortex is important for self-representation (Decety et al., 2002).

The experimental studies and clinical cases reviewed thus far seem to suggest a dominant role for areas in the right hemisphere in self-awareness and self-related processing. If this is indeed the case, then it is reasonable to suppose that other disorders of self-awareness and self-related processing may involve dysfunction in similar or related areas. Thus, findings from previous studies can be used as a platform from which to investigate and interpret data concerning the neural mechanisms of other self-related disorders, such as dissociative disorders and particularly depersonalization disorder (DPD). The dissociative disorders, of which DPD is an example, are characterized by two main deficits: a disruption in the usually integrated sense of self or identity, and a dissociation of mental processes (DSM IV, APA). By their very nature these disorders are concerned with the experience of self and with the mechanisms of self-awareness. Indeed, it has been argued that depersonalization is always associated with altered levels of awareness (Mayer-Gross, 1935). Despite great interest and decades of research, the neural correlates and biological mechanisms underlying these disorders remain poorly understood.

Many factors complicate the study of such disorders as well as the interpretation of results. Among these complicating factors are the dynamic nature of the symptoms, differential diagnoses, presence of medication in many patient populations, insufficient sample sizes, poor controls, and the frequent presence of comorbid disorders. As might be expected, these problems are especially evident in earlier studies.

Due to the overwhelming complexity of each of the dissociative disorders and the variation among different disorders within the dissociative cluster, only DPD and the depersonalized states will be considered here.

Depersonalization

As the name suggests, depersonalization disorder (DPD) is characterized by persistent or recurrent episodes of depersonalization, a state that is, in itself, characterized by a distortion in self-awareness. Depersonalization often includes an altered, detached, or estranged subjective experience of one's self, one's mental processes, and one's surroundings while reality testing remains intact. Transient experiences of depersonalization have been reported by nearly 50% of college students (Dixon, 1963), and such states can be induced in normal individuals following temporal lobe stimulation (Penfield & Rasmussen, 1950), or administration of tetrahydrocannabinol (THC; Mathew et al., 1999; Mathew et al., 1993; Johnson, 1990; Melges et al., 1970b; Moran 1986; Herman & Szymanski 1981), alcohol (Raimo et al., 1999), amphetamines (Vollenweider et al., 1998), the partial serotonin agonist m-CPP (Simeon et al., 1995), and the 5-HT1a and 5-HT2a receptor agonist Psilocybin (Vollenweider et al., 1999; see also Chapter 5, this volume).

In the presence of symptoms, a diagnosis of DPD is made only if the symptoms are severe enough to cause marked distress or to impair normal functioning. Furthermore, although DPD is diagnosed only when symptoms are not secondary to any other disorder, it is often found in association with other syndromes such as temporal lobe epilepsy and complex partial seizures (Shorvon et al., 1946; Kenna & Sedman, 1965; Greenberg, Hochberg, & Murray, 1984), anxiety disorders and depression (Simeon & Hollander 1993; Nuller, 1982), head trauma (Grigsby & Kaye, 1993; Grigsby, 1986; Ackner, 1954), extreme stress and posttraumatic stress disorder (PTSD) (Bremner & Brett 1997; Lanius et al., 2002), and others.

Early Studies

Early investigations of the neural correlates of depersonalization often did not focus on the disorder per se but rather on depersonalized states, often as part of a comorbid disorder. Moreover, these studies frequently reported mixed or inconsistent results regarding regions of activation and laterality. Shorvon and colleagues (1946) examined records of the electrical activity over the scalp as measured by electroencephalography (EEG). Specifically, the EEGs of 23 patients for whom depersonalization was the leading symptom were examined, and it was found that 13 of them displayed minor and diffused abnormalities. Only one patient, who reported a history of migraines, had a focal abnormality, but unfortunately the focus of this abnormality was not specified. Although more than 50% of the sample was found to have mildly abnormal EEGs, the authors concluded that EEG abnormalities were not directly related to the mechanism of depersonalization. Similarly, Kenna and Sedman (1965) were unable to show an association between depersonalization and any particular focal disturbance. Of 32 epileptic patients reviewed, 11 patients reported depersonalization, all of whom had abnormal EEGs. The authors reported that no focal activity was found in the EEGs of 4 patients, whereas 4 had a left-sided focus, and 3 had a right-sided focus. In addition, only 5 of 64 patients with organic psychoses reported depersonalization. EEGs were recorded in only 4 of those patients, and 3 of those were found normal. The authors concluded that the data did not implicate any particular brain area, "though the total functioning of the limbic system and/or temporal lobe may be involved" (p. 298). These conclusions regarding possible temporal lobe dysfunction implicated in dissociation have been echoed elsewhere (Penfield & Jasper, 1947; cited in Ackner, 1954).

After the somewhat equivocal findings from early studies, more informative results have been reported in later investigations. For example, Devinsky and colleagues (1989) reviewed cases of 71 epileptic patients and reported that those with left-hemisphere foci had higher depersonalization scores on the Dissociative Experience Scale (DES), although the median score for this group was lower than that of psychiatric patients diagnosed with multiple personality disorder. In a single case study described by Hollander and coworkers (1992), a young male with primary DPD was found to have a normal EEG and a normal MRI scan, although results from brain electrical mapping, evoked potentials, and Single Photon Emission Computed Tomography (SPECT) suggested a left-hemisphere frontotemporal dysfunction. The authors interpreted these findings as suggesting a common neurobiological underpinning for DPD and obsessive-compulsive disorder (OCD), including left-hemisphere lateralization of dysfunction.

Modern Neuroimaging Studies

Recent studies employing advanced functional neuroimaging techniques have attempted to resolve some of the findings that emerged from earlier studies and have directly addressed DPD per se although only with mild success. In a pioneering PET study Simeon and colleagues (2000) attempted to localize abnormalities in eight subjects diagnosed with DPD as they performed a variant of the California Verbal Learning Test. Unfortunately, the comorbidity profiles of the subjects in this study were not reported. Compared to normal controls, those with DPD had significantly lower metabolic rates in the right superior temporal gyrus and right middle temporal gyrus (Brodmann's Areas [BA] 22 and 21, respectively). Conversely, these same subjects showed significantly higher metabolic rates in parietal association areas (BA 7B and 39—the angular gyrus) bilaterally, and in left occipital BA 19. Dissociation and depersonalization ratings on the DES scale correlated positively with activation in area 7B. The authors stated that these findings may be consistent with the perceptual alterations reported in DPD, as differences in activity were marked in areas whose known function is association and integration, although they are inconsistent with much of the previous literature on temporal lobe epilepsy, for example.

In the first study to employ fMRI in the investigation of DPD, Phillips and colleagues (2001) compared neural responses of patients diagnosed with DPD or OCD and normal control subjects to emotional stimuli (aversive scenes). For this purpose they recruited 6 DPD patients (5 males, 1 female), 10 OCD patients (8 men, 2 women), and 6 normal volunteers (4 men, 2 women). Again, the comorbidity and pharmacological profile of the participants was not specified. Compared to normal control subjects and those with OCD, subjects with DPD failed to show activation of the insula in response to aversive stimuli and showed lower activation in the middle and superior temporal gyri (BA 22 and 37) and inferior parietal regions (BA 40). Both patient groups showed significantly more activation in the right ventral prefrontal cortex (BA 47) in response to the aversive scenes compared to healthy controls subjects, although only DPD patients showed this activation in the absence of insula activation, indicating an inverse functional relationship in DPD between these neural regions during presentation of emotional stimuli potentially reflecting attempts at emotion regulation. The lower activation found in DPD patients in temporal regions is consistent with the findings of Simeon and coworkers (2000), although the activation in the right ventral prefrontal cortex is inconsistent with the same findings, as is the inverse relationship suggested between the insula and the right ventral prefrontal cortex. This latter finding regarding activation in the right ventral prefrontal cortex is consistent, however, with the right lateralization of self-related dysfunction and with findings regarding cerebral blood flow in the THC-induced depersonalization state (see below).

Another recent study that employed fMRI determined the neural activation underlying dissociative responses to traumatic script-driven imagery in sexual abuse–related PTSD patients who were also diagnosed with dissociative disorder, not otherwise specified (but not DPD). In the study Lanius and colleagues (2002) compared 7 female patients who suffered from PTSD as a result of childhood abuse to 10 control subjects who suffered abuse but did not meet the criteria for PTSD. Subjects were scanned while a traumatic script was read and were encouraged to remember any sensations related to the traumatic events. After each script was read to them, they were assessed for dissociative symptoms using the Clinician-Administered Dissociative State Scale (CADSS) and the DES scale. The dissociated PTSD group showed greater bilateral activation in inferior frontal gyrus (BA 47) and greater occipital lobes activation (BA 19) compared to control subjects. However, they also showed greater activation that was right-lateralized in the superior and middle temporal gyri (BA 38), anterior cingulate (BA 24, 32), medial parietal lobe (BA 7), medial frontal gyrus (BA 10), and medial prefrontal cortex (BA 9).

Although the results of Lanius and coworkers (2002) and Phillips and coworkers (2001) lend some support in favor of a greater involvement of right-lateralized circuitry in the dissociative symptoms compared to left-lateralized mechanisms, the interpretation of these results, along with the results of Simeon and coworkers

(2000), is difficult. First, the results from the three studies are somewhat inconsistent. For example, although DPD patients in both Simeon and coworkers (2000), and Phillips and coworkers (2001) showed lower activation in superior and middle temporal regions, patients in Lanius and coworkers (2002), showed greater activation in the same areas during a depersonalized state. These inconsistencies stem from several problems: the patient profile in each study is different, sample sizes are insufficient, comorbid disorders are unspecified, it is unknown whether patients were medicated, each study used entirely different procedures, and in some cases different neuroimaging techniques were used as well. As a result of these serious methodological inequalities and concerns, it is useful to identify alternative approaches to the search for the neural correlates of depersonalization. One example of such an alternative approach is studies that employ temporarily induced states of depersonalization.

Manipulating Depersonalization

Studies concerned with induced states of depersonalization provide an alternate line of evidence regarding the possible neural mechanisms of depersonalization. This is especially important in light of the limitations of studies investigating patients suffering from DPD. Although the depersonalization symptoms reported following THC (Delta-9-tetrahydrocannabinol—the main psychoactive ingredient of marijuana) intoxication do not constitute a disorder such as that seen in DPD patients, the phenomenology of the experience is similar, as measured, for example, by the DES scale. Furthermore, these experiences do constitute a disturbance of self-awareness and an alteration in the experience of self as seen in DPD as exemplified by an estranged or detached sense of one's self.

The effects of THC administration on depersonalization have been known for quite some time. Indeed, Melges and colleagues (1970a) first reported that THC induces temporal disintegration, or an impairment of one's ability to plan sequential adjustment during goal pursuit. Melges and colleagues (1970b) reasoned that a fundamental component of one's sense of self is one's sense of subjective time. On this premise they investigated the relationship between temporal disintegration and the possibility of THC-induced depersonalization. Eight subjects were administered oral doses of THC and were asked to perform the Goal-Directed Serial Alteration (GDSA) task and to respond to the Temporal Integration Inventory (TTI) and the Depersonalization Inventory (DPI). The results showed that THC did induce temporal disintegration and that the degree of depersonalization was positively correlated with the degree of temporal disintegration. Hence, Melges and colleagues (1970b) provided the first evidence for a link between THC intoxication and the depersonalized state.

Another early report by Herman and Szymanski (1981) reviewed four cases of prolonged depersonalization following marijuana abuse. Of the four cases, three had normal EEGs, while one showed right-lateralized frontal temporal slowing. Consistent with these findings are those described by Moran (1986), who reported occurrences of depersonalization following marijuana use in six subjects, and by

Mathew and colleagues (1993), who reported similar findings in 35 healthy volunteers during marijuana intoxication. In their study marijuana smoking but not placebo smoking induced significant depersonalization that peaked 30 minutes after administration of the drug.

In an attempt to identify the neural correlates of the administration of THC, Mathew and colleagues (1992) investigated regional cerebral blood flow (rCBF) using the ^{133}Xe inhalation technique. No significant changes were found following placebo administration, whereas THC administration was associated with bilateral CBF increase, with greater increase marked in frontal areas, and in the right hemisphere compared to the left. To extend these findings, Mathew and colleagues (1997) studied brain activation following THC administration using PET. IV infusions of low-dose THC, high-dose THC, or placebo in a double blind procedure were given to 32 subjects. Levels of intoxication reached a peak 30 minutes after administration in the drug groups. CBF significantly increased following THC administration, with more marked increases in the right hemisphere compared to the left, and in anterior regions compared to posterior. In the high-dose group increased activation was found bilaterally in frontal, temporal, and parietal areas and the cingulate, basal ganglia, insula, and thalamus at 30 minutes and at 60 minutes. More specifically, the right hippocampus and amygdala were significantly more active at 30 minutes, but not at 60 minutes. The low-dose group displayed a similar pattern, with activation peaking at 60 minutes post administration. Levels of intoxication were measured using the Analogue Intoxication Scale (AIS), and scores correlated significantly with global CBF, with the strongest correlation marked with levels of activation in the right frontal lobe and left cingulate gyrus. Depersonalization was reported significantly more in the drug groups, but no specific correlations between depersonalization and activation were reported.

In a follow-up study Mathew and colleagues (1999) used PET to directly investigate a possible direct relationship between global CBF and depersonalization during THC intoxication and to further examine the involvement of subcortical structures. CBF was measured before and during intravenous administration of low-dose or high-dose THC or placebo in a paradigm similar to Mathew and colleagues (1997). As predicted, THC infusion induced depersonalization compared to placebo, with ratings reaching a maximum at 30 minutes after infusion. In both dosage groups THC administration was associated with a significant increase in global CBF, most markedly in the right hemisphere, the frontal lobes, and anterior cingulate. In this study depersonalization scores (as measured using the DPI and AIS) were positively correlated with increased CBF in most regions. particularly significant correlations were found between depersonalization and activation of the right frontal lobe and right anterior cingulate. These studies, taken together, may lend support to an account of depersonalization suggestive of right-hemisphere dominance.

Treatment

DPD is considered refractory to most pharmacological treatments (Simeon, Stein, & Hollander, 1998; see also Steinberg, 1991). In recent years a few very prelimi-

nary reports have emerged that suggest a possible role for selective serotonin reuptake inhibitors (SSRIs) in the treatment of DPD, although, to our knowledge, no
major clinical trial has been published that could be taken as evidence that such
treatment is indeed effective for DPD. For example, Hollander and colleagues
(1990) reported substantial improvement in six of eight patients who suffered from
either DPD or depersonalization symptoms following treatment with fluoxetine.
However, seven of the reported patients suffered from comorbid OCD, obsessive-
compulsive symptoms, panic disorder, or panic symptoms, which are known to be
ameliorated by SSRI therapy. The one patient who did not suffer from any comorbid disorders, a 26-year-old woman, was one of the two who showed little or
no improvement in symptoms following treatment. Similarly, Simeon, Stein, and
Hollander (1998) reported on eight adult subjects who entered a double-blind
crossover trial of clomipramine versus desipramine. Again, every subject in the
study suffered from comorbid disorders such as dysthymia, panic disorder, generalized anxiety disorder, OCD, and social phobia. The authors themselves stated
that the small sample size did not lend itself to statistical analysis but described
improvement in two of the cases.

Relevant to this discussion, Keenan, Freund, and Fascual-Leone (1999) described a case study of a single woman suffering from DPD, who was treated with
administration of inhibitory 1 Hz repetitive transcranial magnetic stimulation
(rTMS) to her right prefrontal cortex. After the second day of stimulation, her depersonalization symptoms dramatically subsided. In her posttreatment journal the
patient described herself compellingly: "I was me again; awake and feeling what's
around me. I was looking through freed eyes. God has reopened my eyes, and not
just a little, but wide open. I don't feel unsure and afraid of myself any longer. I
feel like _____ [patient's name]."

The patient's reactions noted here occurred within the first two days of a two-
week treatment for depression. Over the course of the next two weeks, the patient
slipped back into her depersonalized state. For example, in the second week of
treatment, the patient indicated, "I'm disappointed about todays [sic] results from
the treatment. Although things are appearing clearer and more real to me, I still
feel as though I'm on the outside of myself." The patient returned for further
treatment, and the initial positive results were never replicated. Again, while these
data initially suggested an important role for the right hemisphere, the fact that
there was no replication makes it extremely difficult to establish the true role of
the right hemisphere in the depersonalized state. That is, it is unclear whether the
subjective experience of the patient was a direct result of right-hemisphere TMS
specifically or a more general result of experiencing TMS; the initial reaction may
have occurred if stimulation was applied to the left frontal region or even if sham
TMS had been administered.

Conclusion

Right-hemisphere dysfunction has been implicated in self-related processing and
in deficits in the perception or recognition of self, as seen in mirror sign and

asomatognosia. Similarly, several converging lines of investigation provide some support to the notion that the depersonalized state and DPD, characterized by a distorted sense of self, are associated with right-lateralized dysregulation. However, to date there have been very few rigorous and well-designed neuroimaging studies that attempted to identify the neural underpinnings of DPD. It is, however, encouraging that as research continues the limitations of earlier studies are being addressed and amended. Although much progress has been made in recent years compared to earlier periods of investigation, findings are still contradictory, and it is too early to draw bold conclusions regarding the neural circuitry underlying self-related processing. Nevertheless, it is abundantly clear that studies that seek to investigate these phenomena can contribute to our understanding of self-awareness and self-processing in general. In doing do, they will surely help to unravel the exact role of both frontal and parietal regions of the right hemisphere in self-related processing and self-related dysfunction.

However, in order to improve our understanding of, among other things, lateralization of function in self-related processing, several recommendations are in order. Ideally, future research on dissociative conditions and depersonalization should seek to use advanced high-resolution neuroimaging techniques, employ larger sample sizes, and include carefully designed control and experimental conditions in the case of empirical studies, and well-matched control groups in the case of patient studies. Furthermore, more detailed patient profiles would assist in comparing results across different studies. Neuroscientific investigation of DPD and related states is still very much in its infancy, but it promises to aid in not only our understanding of such disorders, but also the development of possible treatments. Finally, there is no doubt that it will also contribute a great deal to the identification of the neural correlates of self-awareness in general.

References

Ackner, B. (1954). Depersonalization: Aetiology and phenomenology. *Journal of Mental Science, 100,* 838–853.

American Psychiatric Association (1994). *Diagnostic and Statistical Manual of Mental Disorders (DSM IV).* Washington, DC: American Psychiatric Association.

Breen, N., Caine, D., & Coltheart, M. (2001). Mirrored-self misidentification: Two cases of focal onset dementia. *Neurocase, 7,* 239–254.

Bremner, D.J. & Brett, E. (1997). Trauma-related dissociative states and long-term psychopathology in posttraumatic stress disorder. *Journal of Traumatic Stress, 10,* 37–49.

Craik, F.I.M., Moroz, T.M., Moscovitch, M., Stuss, D.T., Winocur, G., Tulving, E., & Kapur, S. (1999). In search of the self: A positron emission tomography study. *Psychological Science, 10,* 26–34.

Decety J., Chaminade, T., Grezes J., & Meltzoff, A.N. (2002). A PET exploration of the neural mechanisms involved in reciprocal imitation. *Neuroimage, 15,* 265–272.

Decety, J. & Sommerville, J.A. (2003). Shared representations between self and other: A social cognitive neuroscience view. *Trends in Cognitive Science, 7,* 527–533.

Devinsky, O., Putnam, F., Grafman, J., Bromfield, E., & Theodore, W.H. (1989). Dissociative states and epilepsy. *Neurology, 30,* 835–840.

Dixon, J.C. (1963). Depersonalization phenomena in a sample population of college students. *British Journal of Psychiatry, 109,* 371–375.

Feinberg, T.E., Haber, L.D., & Leeds, N.E. (1990). Verbal asomatognosia. *Neurology, 40,* 1391–1394.

Feinberg, T.E. & Shapiro, R. (1989). Misidentification-reduplication and the right hemisphere. *Neuropsychiatry, Neuropsychology, and Behavioral Neurology, 2,* 39–48.

Fink, G.R., Markowitsch, H.J., Reinkemeier, M., Bruckbauer, T., Kessler, J., & Heiss, W.D. (1996). Cerebral representation of one's own past: Neural networks involved in autobiographical memory. *Journal of Neuroscience, 16,* 4275–4282.

Greenberg, D.B., Hochberg, F.H., & Murray, G.B. (1984). The theme of death in complex partial seizures. *American Journal of Psychiatry, 141,* 1587–1589.

Grigsby, J.P. (1986). Depersonalization following minor closed head injury. *International Journal of Clinical Neuropsychology, 8,* 65–68.

Grigsby, J.P. & Kaye, K. (1993). Incidence and correlates of depersonalization following head trauma. *Brain Injury, 7,* 507–513.

Herman, V. & Szymansky, M.D. (1981). Prolonged depersonalization after marijuana use. *American Journal of Psychiatry, 138,* 231–233.

Hollander, E., Carrasco, J.L., Mullen, L.S., Trungold, S., DeCaria, C.M., & Towey, J. (1992). Left hemispheric activation in depersonalization disorder: A case report. *Biological Psychiatry, 31,* 1157–1162.

Hollander, E., Liebowitz, M.R., DeCaria, C., Faibanks, J., Fallon, B., & Klein, D.F. (1990). Treatment of depersonalization with serotonin reuptake blockers. *Journal of Clinical Psychopharmacology, 10,* 200–203.

Iacoboni, M., Woods, R.P., Brass, M., Bekkering, H., Mazziotta, J.C., & Rizzolatti, G. (1999). Cortical mechanisms of human imitation. *Science, 286(5449),* 2526–2528.

Johnson, B.A. (1990). Psychopharmacological effects of cannabis. *British Journal of Hospital Medicine, 43,* 114–122.

Kanwisher, N., McDermott, J., & Chun, M.M. (1997). The fusiform face area: A module in human extrastriate cortex specialized for face perception. *Journal of Neuroscience, 17,* 4302–4311.

Kanwisher, N., Stanley, D., & Harris, A. (1999). The fusiform face area is selective for faces not animals. *Neuroreport, 10,* 183–187.

Keenan, J.P., Freund, S., & Pascual-Leone, A. (1999). Repetitive transcranial magnetic stimulation and depersonalization disorder: A case study. *Proceedings and Abstracts of the Eastern Psychological Association, 70,* a78.

Keenan, J.P., Gallup, G.G., Jr., & Falk, D. (2003). *The Face in the Mirror: The Search for the Origins of Consciousness.* New York: HarperCollins/Ecco.

Keenan, J.P., McCutcheon, N.B., & Pascual-Leone, A. (2001). Functional magnetic resonance imaging and event related potentials suggest right prefrontal activation for self-related processing. *Brain and Cognition, 47,* 87–91.

Keenan, J.P., Nelson, A., O'Connor, M., & Pascual-Leone, A. (2001). Self-recognition and the right hemisphere. *Nature, 409,* 305.

Keenan, J.P., Wheeler, M., Platek, S., Lardi, G. & Lassonde, M. (2003). Self-face processing in a callosotomy patient. *European Journal of Neuroscience, 18,* 2391–2395.

Kenna, J.C. & Sedman, G. (1965). Depersonalization in temporal lobe epilepsy and the organic psychoses. *British Journal of Psychiatry, 111,* 293–299.

Lanius, R.A., Williamson, P.C., Boksman, K., Densmore, M. Gupta, M., Neufeld, R.W.J., Gati, J.S., & Menon, R.S. (2002). Brain activation during script-driven imagery induced dissociative response in PTSD: A functional magnetic resonance imaging investigation. *Biological Psychiatry, 52,* 305–311.

Levine, B., Black, S.E., Cabeza, R., Sinden, M., McIntosh, A.R., Toth, J.P., Tulving, E., & Stuss, D.T. (1998). Episodic memory and the self in a case of isolated retrograde amnesia. *Brain, 121,* 1951–1973.

Markowitsch, H.J. (1995). Which brain regions are critically involved in the retrieval of old episodic memory? *Brain Research and Brain Research Reviews, 21,* 117–127.

Mathew, R.J., Wilson, W.H., Humphreys, D., Lowe, J.V., & Weithe, K.E. (1993). Depersonalization after marijuana smoking. *Biological Psychiatry, 33,* 431–441.

Mathew, R.J., Wilson, W.H., Humphreys, D., Lowe, J.V., & Weithe, K.E. (1992). Regional cerebral blood flow after marijuana smoking. *Journal of Cerebral Blood Flow and Metabolism, 12,* 750–758.

Mathew, R.J., Wilson, W.H., Coleman, E. Turkington, T.G., & DeGrado, T.R. (1997). Marijuana intoxication and brain activation in marijuana smokers. *Life Sciences, 60,* 2075–2089.

Mathew, R.J., Wilson, W.H., Chiu, N.Y., Turkington, T.G., DeGrado, T.R., & Coleman, R.E. (1999). Regional cerebral blood flow and depersonalization after tetrahydrocannabinol administration. *Acta Psychiatrica Scandinavica, 100,* 67–67.

Mayer-Gross, W. (1935). On depersonalization. *British Journal of Medical Psychology, 15,* 103–122.

Meador, K.J., Loring, D.W., Feinberg, T.E., Lee, G.P., & Nichols, M.E. (2000). Anosognosia and asomatognosia during intracarotid amobarbital inactivation. *Neurology, 55,* 816–820.

Melges, F.T., Tinklenberg, J.R., Hollister, L.E., & Gillespie, H.K. (1970a). Marihuana and temporal disintegration. *Science, 168,* 1118–1120.

Melges, F.T., Tinklenberg, J.R., Hollister, L.E., & Gillespie, H.K. (1970b). Temporal disintegration and depersonalization during marihuana intoxication. *Archives of General Psychiatry, 23,* 204–210.

Miller, B.L., Seeley, W.W., Mychack, P., Rosen, H.J., Mena, I., & Boone, K. (2001). Neuroanatomy of the self: Evidence from patients with frontotemporal dementia. *Neurology, 57,* 817–821.

Moran, C. (1986), Depersonalization and agoraphobia associated with marijuana use. *British Journal of Medical Psychology, 59,* 187–196.

Nakamura, K., Kawashima, R., Sugiura, M., Kato, T., Nakamura, A., Hatano, K., Nagumo, S., Kubota, K., Fukuda, H., Ito, K., & Kojima, S. (2001). Neural substrates for recognition of familiar voices: A PET study. *Neuropsychologia, 39,* 1047–1054.

Nuller, Y.L. (1982). Depersonalization—symptoms, meaning, therapy. *Acta Psychiatrica Scandinavica, 66,* 451–458.

Penfield, W., & Rasmussen, T. (1950). *The Cerebral Cortex of Man: A Clinical Study of Localization of Function.* New York: Macmillan.

Preilowski, B. (1977). Self-recognition as a test of consciousness in left and right hemisphere of 'split-brain' patients. *Acta Nerv Super (Praha), 19, (Suppl 2),* 343–344.

Phillips, M.L., Medford, N., Senior, C., Bullmore, E.T., Suckling, J., Brammer, M.J., Andrew, C., Sierra, M., Williams, S.C.R., & Davis, A.S. (2001). Depersonalization disorder: Thinking without feeling. *Psychiatry Research: Neuroimaging Section, 108,* 145–160.

Raimo, E.B., Roemer, R.A., Moster, M., & Shan, Y. (1999). Alcohol-induced depersonalization. *Biological Psychiatry, 45,* 1523–1526.

Ruby, P., & Decety, J. (2003). How would *you* feel versus how do you think *she* would feel? A neuroimaging study of perspective-taking with social emotions. *Journal of Cognitive Neuroscience, 16,* 988–999.

Shorvon, H.J, Hill, J.D.N., Burkitt, E., & Halstead, H. (1946). The depersonalization syndrome. *Proceedings of the Royal Society of Medicine, 39,* 779–792.

Simeon, D., Guralnik, O., Hazlett, E.A., Spiegel-Cohen, J., Hollander, E., & Buchsbaum, M.S. (2000). Feeling unreal: A PET study of depersonalization disorder. *American Journal of Psychiatry, 157,* 1782–1788.

Simeon, D., & Hollander, E. (1993). Depersonalization disorder. *Psychiatric Annals, 23,* 382–388.

Simeon, D., Hollander, E., Stein, D.J., DeCaria, C., Cohen, L.J., Saoud, J.B., Islam, N., & Hwang, M. (1995). Induction of depersonalization by the serotonin agonist meta-chlorophenylpiperazine. *Psychiatry Research, 58,* 161–164.

Simeon, D., Stein, D.J., & Hollander, E. (1998). Treatment of depersonalization disorder with clomipramine. *Biological Psychiatry, 44,* 302–303.

Spangenberg, K., Wagner, M., & Bachman, D. (1998). Neuropsychological analysis of a case of abrupt onset following a hypotensive crisis in a patient with vascular dementia. *Neurocase, 4,* 149–154.

Steinberg, M. (1991). The spectrum of depersonalization: Assessment and treatment. In: A. Tasman & S.M. Goldfinger, (Eds). *Psychiatric Update,* Vol 10. Washington, DC: American Psychiatric Press.

Stuss, D. (1991). Disturbance of self-awareness after frontal lobe damage. In: G. Prigatano & D. Schachter (Eds). *Awareness of Deficit after Brain Injury.* New York: Oxford University Press.

Sugiura, M., Kawashima, R., Nakamura, K., Okada, K., Kato, T., Nakamura, A., Hatano, K., Itoh, K., Kojima, S., & Fukuda, H. (2000). Passive and active recognition of one's own face. *Neuroimage, 11,* 36–48.

Turk, D.J., Heatherton, T.F., Kelley, W.M., Funnell, M.G., Gazzaniga, M.S., & Macrae, C.N. (2002). Mike or me? Self-recognition in a split-brain patient. *Nature Neuroscience, 5,* 841–842

Vollenweider, F.X., Maguire, R.P., Leenders, K.L., Mathys, K., & Angst, J. (1998). Effects of high amphetamine dose on mood and cerebral glucose metabolism in normal volunteers using positron emission tomography (PET). *Psychiatry Research: Neuroimaging Section, 83,* 149–162.

Vollenweider, F.X., Vontobel, P., Hell, D., & Leenders, K.L. (1999). 5-HT modulation of dopamine release in basal ganglia in psilocybin-induced psychosis in man—A PET study with [11C]raclopride. *Neuropsychopharmacology, 20,* 424–433.

Wheeler, M.A., Stuss, D.T., & Tulving, E. (1997). Toward a theory of episodic memory: The frontal lobes and autonoetic consciousness. *Psychological Bulletin, 121,* 331–354.

Vogeley, K., Bussfeld, D., Newein, A., Herrmann, S., Happé, F., Falkai, P., Maier, W., Shah, N.J., Fink, G.R., & Zilles, K. (2001). Mind reading: Neural mechanisms of theory of mind and self-perspective. *Neuro Image, 14,* 170–181.

14

The Self in Dreams

ANTTI REVONSUO

Would you agree with the following statements: "I *have* my own dreams"; "I am *present* in my own dream world while the dream unfolds"? My guess is that you would. When we wake up we have no doubts that the dreams we vividly remember were our *own* dreams. We personally experienced them just the same way we personally experience our waking lives. We would hardly consider saying that "*There was* a dream during the night, but I have no idea *whose* dream it was." We feel a sense of *ownership* toward our dream experiences, no different from our waking experiences.

Hence, it seems that the self must be continuous throughout the sleep–wake cycle. The self retains its sense of identity even when in the dream world. Yet, in dreams our own self sometimes appears in strange guises. In the dream world our actions may be ludicrous or morally suspect. As long as the dream lasts we are not even aware of these radical discrepancies between our dreaming and waking selves. Therefore, it is justified to say that although dreaming itself is a perfectly normal, nonpathological state of the mind–brain, our self may be altered during dreaming. In dreams the self-character with whom the dreamer identifies him- or herself does not necessarily represent the dreamer faithfully.

But do we really know what kind of person we are in our dream world? In what ways exactly does our self become altered? We spend years of our subjective personal lives in the dream world, yet we do not really know much about the life we lead there or even about the person we are in our dreams. Thus, in the present chapter I explore the nature of the self's secret life in the dream world by drawing together the results that systematic studies of the phenomenological content of dreams have revealed.

What Is Dreaming?

We shall start by clarifying some of the central concepts in this chapter. First, we need to have a clear idea of the definition of *dreaming*. Dreaming consists of internally generated, hallucinatory *subjective experiences during sleep,* but not just any subjective experience arising during sleep counts as a dream. Dream experience includes *multisensory content* rather than a single sensory modality. Visual, auditory, and tactile experiences, bodily feelings, emotions, taste, smell, pain, or any combination of the above appear in dreams. Furthermore, these multisensory experiences do not constitute a chaotic kaleidoscope of disorganized patterns, but instead they form a carefully organized *sensory-perceptual world,* or dream setting. Dream experience is not like a still photograph. By contrast, genuine dreaming includes temporal progress, sequences of experiences that unfold in time and form continuous dream events. Subjective experiences during sleep that do not fulfil the above requirements are not regarded as dreams. Unimodal, static, or disorganized experiences during sleep are called 'sleep mentation' rather than dreaming. Dreaming is a full-scale *simulation* of the perceptual world. Sleep mentation consists of more fragmentary sensory-perceptual content not bound together to form a simulated world. (For a detailed analysis about dreaming as a simulated world, see Revonsuo, in press).

What Is the "Self" in Dreams?

The self in the dream is the character who represents the dreamer. This character, the dream self, usually possesses a *body image* much like the one experienced during wakefulness. The dream self is positioned in the center of the dream world. The dream setting and events are seen and experienced from his or her point of view. The dreamer feels as if he or she were *embodied* inside the dream self's body, more or less the same way we feel our own embodiment inside our bodies during wakefulness. Thus, the dream self has a bodily existence and location in the dream world. In this respect the dream self is not all that different from the waking self.

Cognitively, the dream self may be somewhat distant from its counterpart in the waking world. Certainly, the dream self has *some* access to her long-term autobiographical memory, but often the access is rather limited. While immersed in the dream world, the dreamer may remember some facts concerning her waking life correctly, yet many, if not most, facts about her waking life the dreamer has little access to, although the same facts would be easily accessible in a comparable situation during wakefulness. Therefore, the dream self suffers from transient *amnesia,* reversed immediately on awakening.

Amnesia may occur when the dream self encounters other dream persons, for example (Revonsuo & Tarkko, 2002). The dream self may run into an old friend or a close relative in the dream and behave as if nothing special had happened to the person in real life, yet the person may have moved away or died years ago. If one should unexpectedly come across the same person in the waking world, the first thing one would remember would be that this just cannot be true: he is dead, or he now lives in North Korea—he just cannot suddenly be back here. In the dream world even our long-dead parents and grandparents may still be around, as if that was just business as usual.

Furthermore, the dreamer may *confabulate* false memories that she believes to be accurate. In the dream world a family member may suddenly have a profession that he or she has nothing to do with in the real world, yet the dream self does not access the correct information during the dream and reject the confabulation. Even more radical cases of confabulation emerge in the form of impostor relatives and friends. Sometimes there are characters in the dream who do not correspond to anyone we know from real life, yet in the dream the person may be posed as our "sister" or "brother" or "cousin" or "uncle" or just a vague "good friend," and we have no problem in fully accepting that interpretation. During wakefulness we know perfectly well that we have no such relatives or friends. There should be no basis in our long-term memory for such a peculiar interpretation attached to some person we have met in the dream. In the waking world, should someone we have never seen or heard about before pose him- or herself as a family member, we would be extremely skeptical about such information.

As far as long-term memory is concerned, we tend to be both amnesiac and confabulatory in dreams. Furthermore, during dreaming we seem to have no insight into these memory deficits. We are totally unable to reflect upon the credibility of our own beliefs, in the light of previous knowledge and rational judgement. Hobson (1997) goes so far as to describe our mental state during dreaming as a specific type of madness: delirium. Memory disorders, confabulation, and lack of insight into our own deficient cognition implies that we are out of our minds while dreaming.

Be that as it may, the dream self is in any case largely disengaged from the waking self when it comes to being aware of accurate memories of the past and of future plans. The dream self largely lacks the capacity for self-reflection or full self-awareness. The dream self lives only in the present moment of the dream events. She does not know much about what has happened to her waking counterpart the previous day or what the waking self is supposed to do the next day. The dream self cannot freely engage in "mental time-traveling"—the hallmark of self-awareness—in the same way as during wakefulness. The dream self cannot become aware of her past as a coherent autobiographical story that led to the present moment, or about the plans that lay a path for the future. Yet, when we wake up we identify ourselves with the dream self: it was *me* who was in the dream, rather than somebody else.

In dream research the mysterious life of the dream self has been probed systematically and in great detail. The results reviewed below are based on a large number of dream reports systematically collected from several subjects. Hence, they tell us what *typically* happens to the self during dreaming. Let us first explore whether the dream self is present in the dream world without exception, or is it possible to have a dream without any dream self at all.

Presence of Self in Dreams

Laboratory studies of REM dreams confirm the everyday observation that the dream self is present in the vast majority of dreams. A particularly detailed study of 198 REM dreams from 22 subjects (Strauch & Meier, 1996) indicates that the dream self is *present* in about 90% of dreams. Thus, the dream self is totally absent in only about 10% of dreams. Furthermore, in the same study the dreamer was an *active participant* in the dream events in a little more than 70% of the dreams and passive or uninvolved in less than 20% of dreams. Hence, the dream self is typically not only present in the dream but also actively doing something, not just watching. Other studies support these conclusions: The dreamer feels that he or she belongs to the scene in about 90% of the dream reports in a database of 800 dreams collected in the laboratory (Cicogna & Bosinelli, 2001). The dream self was the central actor in 95% of dreams in a database of 285 REM dream reports (more than 150 words long) reported by 50 subjects (Snyder, 1970; reviewed in Farthing, 1992). It seems that the longer the dream, the more likely it is that the dream self will be present and active in the dream.

Although the dream self is present in most dreams, it is not present in *every* single dream. If one collects, say, 100 REM dream reports, it is probable that there will be a few reports in which no character identifiable as the dream self will be present. This finding may be theoretically quite significant. There are theories of consciousness that regard the self (or a representation of the self) as a *necessary* condition for subjective conscious experience. In other words, the self is believed to be a *constituent* of consciousness. Therefore, consciousness without self ought to be outright impossible. A case in point is Antonio Damasio's theory of consciousness: "The neural patterns and images necessary for consciousness to occur are those which constitute proxies for the organism, for the object, and for the relationship between the two" (Damasio, 1999, p. 20). Damasio holds that consciousness arises from the interrelation between representations of the organism (self) and representations of external objects. If it follows from this theoretical concept that an experience of a world without any simultaneous experience of the self is impossible, then dream experiences without any dream self are in conflict with Damasio's theory. In dreams without a dream self, there is a simulation of the world unfolding in subjective consciousness. There are objects, persons, and events, but there is no representative of the dreamer present in that world simulation. Any plausible theory of consciousness must accommodate the possibility of a world of subjective experiences devoid of an explicit representation of the self.

Who Is the Self That *Has* the Dreams?

Even dreams without any self-representation are *my* dream experiences, not someone else's. I feel a sense of *ownership* toward those dreams; there is no doubt that *I* had the dream. This may seem puzzling at first: who is the "I" that *has* the dreams when there is nobody to represent the dreamer within the dream? The phenomenological tradition in philosophy invokes an entity called the *prereflective self* that is believed to underlie all subjective experiences and to account for the sense of ownership. It remains somewhat unclear, however, what sort of entity the prereflective self is supposed to be, as it seems to be something not directly experienced. I would rather explain the sense of ownership of dreams in the following way. The simulated world of dreams is realized by the very same neurophysiological mechanisms as the sensory-perceptual world we experience during wakefulness. Regardless of whether there is any representation of self present, dream experiences are continuous with waking experiences realized in the same brain. Both dreaming and waking experiences are patterns of activity at a higher neurophysiological level of organization, the *phenomenal* level (Revonsuo, 2000a). Hence, they are experienced by the same system, the same brain, the same *subject,* if you like. However, they become *my* experiences if and only if they leave a memory trace behind that can be accessed at some later time when self-awareness is enabled, say, immediately upon waking up from the dream. With the help of the memory trace it is possible to reconstruct the dream experience and feel that *this* experience originally took place in the same system of conscious experience in which my current experiences take place. Thus, it becomes *my* experience, part of the waking person's autobiographical memory, only after the original experience is already long gone.

Conversely, if it were possible to obtain a record of all the dreams I have had during my lifetime, there would be thousands of dreams that I would have no idea of ever having experienced. Hence, it would be impossible to have any sense of ownership for those dreams: they would appear totally alien to me. From the subjective point of view, they could be someone else's experiences just as well. I would have to admit that those experiences took place in my brain; they were patterns of activation in my brain's world simulation system at the phenomenal level, but they never left any traces behind that *I* (or my long-term autobiographical self) could have accessed. Therefore, they did not become *my* experiences. They were experiences *in my brain,* but only potentially *my* experiences.

Point of View in Dreaming

In an interesting study Foulkes and Kerr (1994) attempted to determine the perspective from which dreams are typically experienced. They collected 64 laboratory dream reports from four subjects and asked them not only to describe their dreams but also to specify whether the visual dream imagery was experienced from own-eyes perspective (as if the dreamer were embodied in the dream self) or whether they could see themselves (that is, whether they could see the dream self) the way another person might see him or her (from an external, or disembodied, point of view). The result was that about 90% of the dreams were experienced from an embodied perspective and about 10% from an external perspective. Dreams with an external perspective rarely contained movielike (kinematic) imagery but tended to be static. Thus, most of them would not fulfill the definition of dreaming as temporally progressive simulation of the perceptual world. Furthermore, most of the disembodied dreams were reported by a single subject, which suggests that such dreams are probably even less frequent in the general population than in this study.

Cicogna and Bosinelli (2001) found that in about 3% of dream reports, a *double* representation of the dreamer's presence or image can be observed. In such dreams the dreamer is represented, on the one hand, as a participant in the dream action and, on the other hand, as a more or less external observer. Thus, it seems that in some dreams there may be shifts between two or more perspectives: the own-eyes perspective and the camera eye perspective. Here is one REM report that displays multiple perspectives and self-representations (from Cicogna & Bosinelli, 2001, p. 32):

> "I was in a sort of South-American country, two hundred years ago, I was mounting a horse: with me there were two more persons riding a horse, and other people on foot. We were pursuing a man, who was myself, we were pursuing him because he had some money, and I was observing the whole scene."

The overwhelming majority of dreams are experienced from an embodied, first-person point of view in which the dream self is actively engaged in a full-scale simulation of the world. It is a theoretically and philosophically significant observation that disembodied, selfless, and double-perspective dream experiences are possible at all. However, the available data indicate that such experiences are relatively rare and appear to be somewhat incompatible with a fully animated dream world.

Role of the Dream Self in Dream Events

Because of the high involvement of the dream self, dreams have been characterized as highly personal or narrowly self-centered experiences (Strauch & Meier, 1996; Foulkes, 1985), but this characterization may not be entirely accurate. A colleague and I conducted a study in which the semantic content of 217 dream reports from 32 subjects was analysed in great detail (Revonsuo & Salmivalli, 1995). An interesting discrepancy emerged in the results: As expected, the dream self was present in the vast majority of the dreams, indicated by the first-person pronoun used to describe the subject or observer of the dream events. Yet the reports contained almost no further information about the dream self or its features. Most of the semantic content of the dream reports described such things as objects (23%), action (20%), persons (13%), and places (11%). The dream self occupied the last position out of 10 different categories: only 3% of the informative semantic content in the dream reports described the dream self. This result suggests that although the dream self is almost invariably present in the dream world, it is totally immersed into the surrounding environment and fully occupied by acting in it. The dream self does not pay very much attention to itself—perhaps a further indication of the diminished self-awareness during dreaming.

Strauch and Meier (1996) analysed 140 REM dreams in which the dream self was present, according to the relations among the dream self and the other dream characters. In only 13% of the reports did the dream self act all by itself, whereas in almost 70% of the dreams the dream self interacted with other characters or at least acted together with them.

Thus, typical dreams are not solipsistic but highly social and interactive experiences. Although the dream characters we interact with in the dream world are only simulated or virtual persons invented by our own brain, they appear to inhabit the dream world as if they were real and totally independent of the dream self.

The Dream Self and the Bizarreness of Dreams

In dream research the term *bizarreness* refers to features of the dream world that significantly deviate from corresponding features of the waking world. Objects, persons, places, events, actions, and other dream contents that appear in a form or combination that would be highly improbable or totally impossible in the real world are defined as bizarre. Bizarreness may be conceptualized by using the notion of "binding," because in bizarre dream contents discrepant information sources are bound together, or the formation of coherent and continuous representations in consciousness flounders in some other way (Revonsuo & Tarkko, 2002).

There is no doubt that bizarreness is a pervading feature of our dreams, regularly distorting and recombining contents of consciousness in peculiar ways (Revonsuo & Salmivalli, 1995; Revonsuo & Tarkko, 2002). The question that interests us here is whether and to what extent dream bizarreness touches the dream self. Is the dream self significantly different from its waking counterpart? If so, in what ways precisely is it different? The Revonsuo & Salmivalli (1995) study sheds some light on this question. First, we divided bizarreness into three different categories: incongruity (a dream element with mismatching features), vagueness (a dream element whose nature is unclear, indeterminate, or obscure), and discontinuity (a dream element that suddenly appears, disappears, or is transformed in the dream). Incongruity was found to be the most common form of bizarreness in all dream contents. Furthermore, it was the only type of bizarreness that was manifested in the dream self to a sufficient degree to allow quantitative analysis. Even so, the dream self seems to be particularly well protected from bizarre, incongruous features. Only about 8% of the information that described the dream self in the reports was judged as deviating from the real self. This was the lowest percentage of incongruity in any dream content that was analyzed by Revonsuo and Salmivalli (1995). The other dream characters perceived in the dream included incongruous features much more frequently (15%). Thinking and language were the most incongruous contents: more than 30% of their occurrences in dreams deviated from what would be expected in the real world.

Because the category of dream thinking (or cognition) refers to the internal intellectual or mental functions of the dream self, the overall picture that emerges suggests that the dream self is in one respect *less* bizarre than any other dream contents but in another respect *more* bizarre than any other contents. During sleep, when we find ourselves in the dream world, we tend to pay little attention to our own outlook, or body image, or other external self-related features—they just form a kind of phenomenal background or perspectival center from which we observe and act in the dream world. For the most part the external features of ourselves appear to be just the same as they are during wakefulness. But what goes on inside the mind of the dream self—our thinking, beliefs, and other cognitive functions—quite often deviate from our waking cognition.

One explanation for this curious pattern has been found in the patterns of brain activation during REM sleep (Schwartz & Maquet, 2002). Large areas in the prefrontal cortex show a lowered level of activation during REM sleep. The same areas are known to be critical for planning, decision making, critical thinking, and voluntary direction of attention. Thus, the pattern of cortical deactivation in REM would predict deficits in exactly the cognitive functions that have been found to flounder in the dream self.

Examples of Bizarre Dream Self

Although the dream self in most dreams appears much the same as during wake-fulness, there is a small percentage of dreams in which the self appears in an al-tered form. In the dream database we have used in our earlier studies (Revonsuo & Salmivalli, 1995; Revonsuo & Valli, 2000; Revonsuo & Tarkko, 2002), several alterations of the self appeared, from relatively mild to extremely radical. The milder variations include cases in which the dreamer is the same person but appears in strange clothing or is of a different age, say, a small child in the dream. The more radical ones include cases in which the dreamer appears as a completely different person, sometimes of the opposite sex or different race. In the most radical case the dream self was not a person at all but an animal.

Let us look at a few examples from the dream reports written by Finnish stu-dents. This one was reported by a 25-year-old, blond female student:

> It's the Second World War and *I am a dark-haired, strongly built, Finnish male sol-dier.* The enemies are probably German. . . . [Later in the same dream]: I could see myself in a mirror. *Now I was a blond, strongly built woman.*

Here we witness a clear discontinuity in the nature of the self: the sex and the color of the hair change during the course of the dream. This dreamer shows an unusual degree of self-awareness during the dream, as she is capable of describing herself and even observing herself in a mirror within the dream. Yet this dream was expe-rienced from an own-eyes perspective; the dreamer was embodied in the dream as those persons who did not externally look much like her real self.

The next excerpts show that although discontinuity of the self is rare in dreams, sometimes it does happen. The first sample is from the dream diary of a 21-year-old woman the second from a 22-year-old man:

> I was on my way to the campus, it was late in the evening. On my way I stopped off at a nearby shop. They had a sale. I remember buying at least some lettuce. Suddenly my mother was working in this shop, and somehow *I was my mother.* The boss gave me permission to go home. When I was biking home, the road was full of wet snow. Somehow my big brother also came to the shop and then with me. When I got to my place at the campus, *I was myself again.*

> I was walking (*apparently it was me*) in a suburban area, past a house whose yard was about one and a half meters above the street level. In the yard a girl I know from medical school was leading a big bearlike dog. I was leading a dog that actually was my female classmate from medical school. The girl suddenly attacked the bear-dog

and they fought. *The person in the dream that so far had been me, now was suddenly my classmate J. Somehow I became (physically) detached from myself and I noticed that I was not me but him.* This was accompanied by a funny feeling.

The last dream exemplifies the dissociation of the dreamer's point of view from a specific frame of embodied reference; in fact, it seems to be an out-of-body experience of some sort. It is interesting that after detachment from the perspective (and presumably from proprioceptive awareness) of the body, *the subject construes "himself" as being the detached disembodied point of view* rather than the person from whose body image the perspective had detached. The perspective itself seems to entail a disembodied subject who observes the world, and "me" is automatically associated with *that* point of view, rather than with any of the characters externally observed. This dream seems to have suddenly switched from an "own-eyes-perspective," or "first-person perspective," to a "third-person perspective." After the switch there is no dream self present in the dream anymore, but another person has taken the place of the person who used to be the dream self.

The most radical departure from the waking self in this dream database was reported by a 22-year-old female student. She described a dream in which she was "a dog or some other animal." The dream consisted of events experienced from the animal's point of view; the dream self was embodied as a doglike predator that was running in a dark forest with another animal, hunting for prey. Eventually, she caught a rabbit, but something larger than herself took it away from her.

These radical transformations of the self show that it is not impossible for the self to appear in almost any form or guise in the dream world. Although such transformations are rare, they do happen every now and then. And into whatever creature our own-eyes perspective is embodied, that is the character who we are in the dream, no matter how different from the waking self it may be (for more about dream self and bizarreness, see Revonsuo, in press).

Self-Awareness and Lucidity in Dreams

Reflective consciousness involves the ability to focus on some particular aspect of the content of consciousness and pass a judgment about it, or explicitly categorize or name it, or wonder about its causes or significance. Self-awareness involves the ability to connect a current self-related experience (say, my own actions or my body image as experienced) with the enduring self-representation in long-term memory and thus to become aware of the experiences as *my own* experiences, experiences that belong to an enduring person or self (Revonsuo, in press).

The traditional view has it that dreams are devoid of reflective consciousness and self-awareness. Dream events just happen to us; we are incapable of reflecting upon them, becoming aware of ourselves, or controlling the events or even our own actions voluntarily. This "deficiency" view of dreaming may be true of some dream experiences, but certainly not all of them. During dreaming our ability to critically reflect upon the events we witness is surely diminished, but it is not completely wiped out. McCarley and Hoffman (1981) found that in 16% of 104 REM dreams, the dreamer explicitly noticed some bizarre feature of the dream. That is, reflective awareness of something not being quite right was present, at least for a fleeting moment. In the same study, in only 2 dreams of 104 did the dreamer halt and start to think it over or became fully aware that it must be a dream.

Similar figures of spontaneous lucidity have been found in other studies. Purcell, Moffitt, and Hoffman (1993) reported that lucid awareness of dreaming while dreaming occurs spontaneously in about 1% of dreams of university students. Cicogna and Bosinelli (2001) found that in a database of 800 dreams from different sleep stages collected in the laboratory, about 3% of dreams contain lucidity. Although spontaneous lucidity is a relatively rare phenomenon, lesser degrees of reflective awareness occur with considerable frequency according to Purcell and colleagues:

> [S]elf reflection and intentional action occur naturally and substantially in the dream state. . . . Spontaneous and uninfluenced dreaming demonstrated a range of self-reflectiveness from none to fully lucid awareness of state . . . In the vast majority of spontaneous dreams the dreamer is moderately self-reflective and moderately effective in his or her actions. (Purcell, Moffitt, & Hoffmann 1993, p. 240)

The Function of Dreaming

The overall picture that emerges suggests that the self is usually present in dreams in an embodied form similar to wakefulness and surrounded by a simulation of the perceptual world. The self is active in its physical and social dream environment but pays relatively little attention to itself. Its higher cognitive functions and autobiographical memory are not working as well as during wakefulness. Therefore, the dream self is isolated from full self-awareness, although moderate amounts of reflective thought and self-reflectiveness may occur.

The inevitable question arises: *Why* should our brain go through all the trouble of simulating this elaborate self-in-a-world experience during sleep? Why do we not just sleep in an entirely selfless and nonconscious state and let our brains do their night shift job in restoring neurochemical balance and consolidating new memory traces without our personal subjective involvement? In other words, what possible function could the adventures of a dream self in the virtual reality of dreams serve? Most cognitive neuroscientists seem to think that it does not serve any function whatsoever (for a review, see Revonsuo, 2000b). Dreaming reflects some nonfunctional lower-level noise arising as the side effect of purely neurophysiological processes. The dream world and the dream self are just a neural coincidence: they serve no independent biological or psychological function whatsoever.

Contrary to this view that admits no independent function for dreams, perhaps there is a good reason why our selves are resurrected in the dream world and have to go through a variety of adventures in a simulated world during sleep. The answer should be found, first, by conducting a careful analysis of dream content and of the real experiences that seem to have the greatest impact on dreams and, second, by placing the dreaming brain in the context in which it evolved. In the ancestral environment it would have been useful to simulate and rehearse events that were the most crucial to the survival and the future reproductive success of the self. Thus, according to the threat simulation theory of dreaming (Revonsuo, 2000b) the dreaming brain is originally *a threat simulation mechanism* that selects emotionally charged memory traces from autobiographical memory. Consequently, it composes nightmarish simulations of real threats—and how to deal with them— during the idle time that is spent in behavioral inactivity during sleep. In the ancestral environment the nocturnal simulation of threatening events in dreams may have led to a greater likelihood of survival when similar threats were encountered in reality. The biological function of dreaming—the explanation for why dreaming was selected for during evolution—is the ability to mentally rehearse threat perception and threat avoidance in a perfectly safe place, the virtual reality of dream consciousness.

Do you remember ever having had nightmares in which an evil person or an aggressive animal chases you or an intruder tries to enter your home? What about dreams in which you are desperately late for important social events, fail miserably in studies or work, or you and your close ones have to face dangerous forces of nature—storms, hurricanes, tidal waves, floods, fires—or life-threatening car accidents and plane crashes? These and other types of unpleasant themes are very frequent in dreams universally, and the threat simulation theory explains why: They are simulations either of the types of threats that our ancestors had to face continuously during hundreds of thousands of years, or the kinds of threats that we ourselves often see, and hear about, and think about in our waking lives. The threat simulation mechanism in the brain uses the memory traces of threat-related content and constructs dreams in which we have to face these threats in order to be better prepared to cope with them in our waking lives.

In posttraumatic nightmares the threat simulation mechanism manifests itself in the clearest form. Anyone who has ever encountered an extremely frightening, life-threatening event in real life has probably experienced afterward a sequence of forceful threat simulations based on the experience, sometimes replaying the original event more or less as it occurred. War veterans, victims of crime and violence, and survivors of major natural catastrophes regularly suffer from persistent posttraumatic nightmares that often last throughout life. However, the threat simulation theory accurately applies only to the evolutionary context. In the ancestral environment the threat avoidance skills rehearsed during dreaming were directly related to the probability of reproductive success. In the modern world our reproductive success hardly depends on the kinds of dreams we tend to have. Thus, although the original biological function of dreaming is still clearly *reflected* in the content of our dreams, it is doubtful whether dreaming truly contributes to our survival or reproductive success anymore. Furthermore, most of us never encounter the kinds of threats our ancestors dealt with on a daily basis. Thus, our dream production mechanisms are mostly in a resting state, often also producing mundane and nonthreatening dreams. If the threat simulation theory of dreaming has any truth to it, we are the descendants of those ancestral humans whose brains were particularly good at simulating the threats abundant in the environment in which the human brain evolved.

The Dream Self in Nightmares and Threatening Dreams

In our recent studies we have looked more carefully at threatening events in dreams. We define threatening dream events in this way: *an event such that, should it occur in real life, someone or someone's important resources would be placed in danger.*

The definition does not give the dream self any special role in dream threats. Thus, movielike dream threats in which the self is not involved in any way are in principle possible. However, the data from several studies now reveal that the dream self plays the starring role in threatening dream events. When a threat occurs in a dream, it is very likely to place the dream self in danger, whereas other dream characters are threatened much less often. In a study of dream threats reported by university students, 73% of the threats were targeted at the dream self (Revonsuo & Valli, 2000). In children's dreams the dream self was the target of the threat in more than 80% of dream threats (Valli et al., 2005). Other dream characters that often come under threat in dreams are people significant for the dream self such as family members and friends, yet they are much less often threatened (in about 25% to 40% of threatening events in different groups).

The dream self is furthermore the most active character in reacting to the threatening events. The dream self is explicitly reported to do something about the threat, say, defend itself or attempt an escape, in about 35% to 55% of dream threats. Interestingly, a significant interaction between the severity of the threat and the reaction of the dream self has been observed. The dream self was significantly more likely to do something about the threat if the situation was life threatening than if it was not (67% versus 47%) (Revonsuo & Valli, 2000). Hence, the dream self was likely to engage its threat avoidance reactions in mortal threats but tended to ignore some of the less dangerous threats. The dream self rarely experienced any serious consequences (such as death or serious injury) from the threat—it seems that dreams are not "eager" to simulate the events that take place after the threat is over (Revonsuo & Valli, 2000).

Our recent unpublished results suggest that when threat simulations are constructed, the dreaming brain has access to the emotionally charged memory traces in autobiographical memory. The content of threatening dreams as revealed by dream diaries resembles the content of the most emotionally charged memories relating to real dangers during a person's entire lifetime. By contrast, dream threats do not reflect to any detectable degree the life events that happened to take place concurrently with the reported dreams. The strongest emotional memory traces from the more remote past are being used for threat simulation rather than recent traces. Thus, during dreaming we will most likely relive simulations of the worst dangers of our whole lives, even if they took place in the distant past. The only mildly irritating events from yesterday or last week do not enter our dream worlds with very high frequency.

Summary: The Adventures of a Simulated Self in a Simulated World

In a nutshell, the self in our dreams is a bodily representation of our waking self. It is a behaviorally active self that shows a regular pattern of cognitive deficits. The dream self suffers from amnesia and diminished critical thinking but is unaware of its own deficits. It is immersed into the center of a simulated world where dangerous, threatening events appear with considerable frequency. Those events are mostly based on emotionally charged memory traces from real-life experiences of threats. The biological function of this nocturnal simulation remains controversial: Some believe that the dream world arises in the sleeping brain for no particular reason at all. By contrast, the threat simulation theory suggests that perhaps the dream self was forced to face simulated threats during dreaming so that the brain would be prepared to face real threats during wakefulness. Threat simulation during dreaming may have increased the survival fitness of our distant ancestors. This might explain why we still find our simulated selves roaming the simulated world every night.

Acknowledgment
The writing of this article was supported by the Academy of Finland (project 45704).

References

Cicogna, P.C. & Bosinelli, M. (2001). Consciousness during dreams. *Consciousness and Cognition, 10,* 26–41.

Damasio, A.R. (1999). *The Feeling of What Happens.* New York: Harcourt Brace.

Farthing, W.G. (1992). *The Psychology of Consciousness.* New York: Prentice Hall.

Foulkes, D. (1985). *Dreaming: A Cognitive-Psychological Analysis.* Hillsdale, NJ: Lawrence Erlbaum.

Foulkes, D. & Kerr, N.H. (1994). Point of view in nocturnal dreaming. *Perceptual and Motor Skills, 78,* 690.

Hobson, J.A. (1997). Dreaming as delirium: A mental status exam of our nightly madness. *Seminars in Neurology, 17,* 121–128.

McCarley, R.W. & Hoffman, E. (1981). REM sleep dreams and the activation-synthesis hypothesis. *American Journal of Psychiatry, 138,* 904–912.

Purcell, S., Moffitt, A., & Hoffman, R. (1993). Waking, dreaming, and self-regulation. In: A. Moffitt, M. Kramer, & R. Hoffmann (Eds) *The Functions of Dreaming* (pp. 197–260). Albany, NY: SUNY Press.

Revonsuo, A. (2000a). Prospects for a scientific research program on consciousness. In: T. Metzinger (Ed.). *Neural Correlates of Consciousness* (pp. 57–75). Cambridge, MA: MIT Press.

Revonsuo, A. (2000b). The reinterpretation of dreams: An evolutionary hypothesis of the function of dreaming. *Behavioral and Brain Sciences, 23(6),* 877–901.

Revonsuo, A. (in press) *Inner Presence.* Cambridge, MA: MIT Press.

Revonsuo, A. & Salmivalli, C. (1995). A content analysis of bizarre elements in dreams. *Dreaming, 5(3),* 169–187.

Revonsuo, A. & Tarkko, K. (2002). Binding in dreams. *Journal of Consciousness Studies, 9(7),* 3–24.

Revonsuo, A. & Valli, K. (2000). Dreaming and consciousness: Testing the threat simulation theory of the function of dreaming. *Psyche, 6,* http://psyche.cs.monash.edu.au/v6/psyche-6-08-revonsuo.html

Schwartz, S. & Maquet, P. (2002). Sleep imaging and the neuro-psychological assessment of dreams. *Trends in Cognitive Sciences, 6,* 23–30.

Snyder, F. (1970). The phenomenology of dreaming. In: L. Madow & L.H. Snow (Eds), *The Psychodynamic Implications of the Physiological Studies on Dreams* (pp. 124–151). Springfield, IL: Charles S. Thomas.

Strauch, I. & Meier, B. (1996). *In Search of Dreams. Results of Experimental Dream Research.* Albany, NY: SUNY Press.

Valli, K., Revonsuo, A., Pälkäs, O., Ismail, K.H., Ali, K.J., & Punamäki, R.L. (2005). The threat simulation theory of the evolutionary function of dreaming: Evidence from dreams of traumatized children. *Consciousness and Cognition.* 14(1): 188–218.

15

Psychoactive Agents and the Self

ROY J. MATHEW

The self represents one's perception of oneself. It can be experienced only by the individual in question and nobody else. Since the experience cannot be translated into language in full, it cannot be shared. Thus, the self is predominantly, if not exclusively, subjective and does not fall within the objective realm of scientific inquiry. Devoid of spatial or temporal bounds, the subjective self is difficult to define and to describe. It may be small or large depending upon one's perceptual style, philosophy of life, and worldview.

For example, the argument may be made that perception of the external world is an event that takes place within one's mind. Neuropsychologists hold that the image that falls on the retina and what is seen by the mind's eye are different (Gazzaniga, 1998). In fact, it is well understood that a great deal of trimming, twisting, and stretching take place in the brain to give form and structure to the electrical impulses that reach the brain from the eye. In other words, perception is as much a mental as a peripheral sensory activity. This would put both the external world and the self within the realm of mental activity, blurring the distinction between self and not self.

Ancient philosophers of India put forward the argument that only the self is reality and that the rest is phantasmal (Gupta, 1995). Some support for this view is provided by the fact that dreams and wakefulness have identical contents. Dreams consist of subjects and objects, and while dreaming the contents are as real as they are during wakefulness. Brain function and electrical activity of the brain during the two are also very similar (Hobson, 1989; Madsen & Vorstrup, 1991). This clearly shows that the mind is capable of constructing a reality out of thin air that is as real as any other reality. This approach adds strength to the view that the phenomenal world may be a creation of the mind. Thus, both the external world and the self may be generated by the mind. The point I am trying to make is that the self can be a galactically broad concept.

Alternatively, one may take the more commonly held narrow approach. According to this view the self is whatever an individual considers him- or herself, distinct from the external world. The body is usually regarded as an integral part of the self. However, even this definition lacks the precision it may seem to have at first glance. The body may be distinct from the mind, but what about the image of the body that is carried in the mind? The well-known phantom limb that represents persisting mental imagery of the physical body even after a limb is surgically removed provides some scientific basis for this (Ramachandran & Blakeslee,1998). The main source of confusion is whether body image is part of the mind or of the body. If body image is part of the self, then while trimming one's nails one is also trimming one's self-image. Pieces of nail before they were cut were part of the self, but once they were cut they leave the image of self. The same may be said about haircuts or the detachment of any part of a person's anatomy.

Although difficult to define and existing on the outer fringes of science, there is general consensus that the self is an important part of mental processes. It has even found its way into such scientific documents as the *Diagnostic and Statistical Manual* (DSM IV) of the American Psychiatric Association. According to DSM IV, depersonalization disorder (300.6) is characterized as "a feeling of detachment or estrangement from one's self" (American Psychiatric Association, 1994). The description that follows leads one to conclude that the self includes one's mental processes, one's body, and the parts of the body. It may also be linked to affective responses and control over one's actions, including speech. Such a definition is too vague to be of use here.

Since science is of limited help, we may have to turn to philosophy. Not being a philosopher, I am at a serious disadvantage in considering the philosophy of the self. However, being of Indian extraction, I am somewhat familiar with certain Indian philosophical concepts. Although several descriptions of the self can be found in the highly varied schools of philosophical thought in India, the system put forward in *Taittriya Upanishad,* composed sometime between 500 B.C. and 200 A.D., seems most useful here (Radhakrishnan, 1994).

According to the *Taittriya Upanishad,* the central core of the mind is Atman. Derived from the Sanskrit word *an* meaning "to breathe," Atman means life or soul. It is linked to the scientific term *consciousness* (Crick & Koch, 1992; Hogan & Kaiboriboon, 2003) and the theological term *divine spark* (of Christianity). Most Indian philosophical documents (with the notable exception of Buddhist) accept Atman as the fundamental life-giving principle, bereft of time, space, and causation. Atman is surrounded by vestures, or sheaths (*kosas* in Sanskrit). This type of ensheathing is strictly functional and not anatomic. The *kosas* represent the body (*annamaya kosa*), vital functions (*pranamaya kosa*), mind (*manomaya kosa*), intelligence (*vijnanamaya kosa*), and bliss (*anandamaya kosa*). The sum total of Atman with the surrounding sheaths is what most ordinary people regard as the self. To the enlightened, the self is just Atman divested of the sheaths.

According to DSM IV, in depersonalization disorder "there may be a sensation of being an outside observer of one's mental processes, one's body, or parts of one's body." This would seem to imply that the core sense of self can be independent of mental processes and the body, and that means that the core self is not the mind or body. Thus, strangely enough, DSM IV seems to agree with the *Taittiriya Upanishad* description of the self, in particular the concept of a core self, which may be rendered independent of one's mental processes and one's body. DSM IV does not give any clue as to if or how the brain produces the core sense of self.

Thus, there appear to be two ways of conceptualizing the self, one that includes the mental processes and body image and a second that excludes the mental processes and body. For the sake of clarity, we shall call the former composite self and the latter, core self.

Drugs and the Self

If we accept the *Taittriya Upanishad*'s mundane concept of composite self, then in this chapter we will have to consider every pharmacological agent that affects the body, vital functions, mind, intelligence, and emotions. That would include most of general pharmacology, and it would clearly be an unrealistic goal.

Drugs That Influence the Composite Self

Perhaps it is more realistic to confine our attention to the drugs that disrupt the sense of self (Sedman, 1966; Mellor, 1988), as happens during what DSM IV calls depersonalization. From ancient days a variety of drugs have been used with the specific purpose of accomplishing precisely this, that is, detaching the self from the mind and body. Most of these drugs have strong associations with religions. Many alter the sense of time and space in addition to inducing depersonalization, and several of them produce perceptual distortions. This chapter is limited primarily to this group of drugs that produce dissociation and depersonalization (Stafford, 1978; Good, 1989; McKim, 1991; Schultes & Hofmann, 1992, Mathew, 2001).

Many drugs from all over the world fit this description, but only a few of them with possible uses in medicine have been subjected to scientific inquiry. Most are too toxic even for experimental use in human subjects, and animal research is of little help here. Most regulatory and funding agencies are not very excited about research on the self, and permission and funding to study the effects of such drugs are hard to come by. Thus, our sources of information about many drugs of this class are limited to anecdotal reports and descriptions by the laity.

Drugs that produce dissociation are loosely known as hallucinogens. They bring about changes in perception, thought, and mood, but they seldom produce mental confusion, memory loss, or disorientation for person, place, or time. They do not induce sedation or stimulation, with few exceptions, but they do alter the quality of the conscious experience, that is, the experience of self. Most of these compounds are present in plants, although a few have been found in animals. Information is available on about 150 of them, but pharmacologists estimate that about 500,000 such plant species exist (Stafford, 1978; McKim, 1991; Schultes & Hofmann, 1992; Mathew, 2001).

Cannabis
Today the single most popular dissociative drug in the world is marijuana. In all probability, it is as old as alcohol since even the most ancient civilizations seem to have known the drug. According to some, records of its earliest use originated

from the island of Taiwan more than 10,000 years ago (Abel, 1980). Marijuana, a member of the hemp family, was useful to the ancients as medicine and fiber and in religious ceremonies.

The Chinese seem to have been the first people to note the intoxicating effects of the drug. The Chinese word for cannabis is *Ma.* Emperor Fu Hsi (2900 B.C.) noted that marijuana was endowed with both Yin and Yang, the opposing principles that constitute the universe. Taoists, who permeated China, knew about marijuana intoxication but condemned it as the liberator of sin. During the early part of the Common Era, the Chinese were using cannabis seeds in their incense burners to induce intoxication. Zend-Avesta of ancient Persia (600 B.C.) refered to an intoxicating resin, presumably marijuana.

In the ninth century B.C. the Assyrians were using cannabis as incense. In ancient Greece Galen reported the use of marijuana at parties. On the African continent it was used by many native cultures for both social and religious purposes. Known as Kif or Duagga, its vapors were inhaled by devotees from burning hemp. The Kasai tribes of Congo smoked marijuana from calabash pipes. The Tepecano Indians of northwest Mexico are reported to have substituted cannabis for peyote when the latter was not available. Mexican natives still use cannabis under the name "Santa Rosa" in a Christian ceremony that involves the Virgin Mary.

The Scythians, a warlike Middle Eastern nomadic group, cherished the plant and were responsible for spreading its use. The Scythians were closely related to the Semites, and there has been a great deal of controversy as to whether the ancient Jews knew of cannabis. The holy oil God instructed Moses to make from "myrrh, sweet cinnamon, kaneh bosn, and kassia" is believed to have contained cannabis. The previous translation of Kaneh Bosn as "calamus," a marsh plant, was found to be erroneous; the Hebrew Kaneh Bosn and Scythian cannabis were probably the same. The Scythian obsequies, which include cleansing by burning cannabis seeds, are still practiced. Scythians took cannabis into Egypt via Palestine and north into Russia and Europe.

Islam firmly banned all intoxicating agents, including marijuana, with the possible exception of opium. However, Sufis, an unorthodox offshoot of Islam who considered spiritual experiences and communication with the Almighty central to their belief, used hashish on a large scale. Orthodox Muslims do not look upon Sufism favorably, and its followers are often considered to be on the outer fringes of Islam.

Marijuana, also known as Indian hemp, has a close and intimate association with the Indian subcontinent. The earliest Indian text that refers to the drug is the fourth Veda (ancient Hindu scripture), *Atharva Veda* (Kishore, 2001). *Atharva Veda* is believed to have been the forerunner of Ayurveda, the Indian system of medicine (Svoboda, 1992). Despite the Vedic (scriptural) references to the drug, there is no evidence that it was used as part of the orthodox Vedic religion. Although never a component of Hindu orthodoxy, it has been an integral part of the unorthodox antinomian revolutionary movements within the far-flung mosaic of Hinduism (Abel, 1980; McKim, 1991; Schultes & Hofmann, 1992; Mathew, 2001).

The Indian subcontinent was inhabited by two separate ethnic groups: the original Indus Valley dwellers and the Aryan nomads who invaded them from Central Asia around 1500 B.C. (Radhakrishnan, 1989; Kochhar, 2000). Ancient Indians associated at least two plants with their religious ceremonies, soma and cannabis. The Aryans extolled soma in their Vedas over and over again, but cannabis is scarcely mentioned except in the apocryphal last Veda, *Atharva Veda,* which many believe is non-Aryan in origin (Radhakrishnan, 1989). The true identity of soma is controversial, and we shall return to this later in the chapter.

Cannabis grows in abundance throughout India, especially in the northern region. *Atharva Veda,* which probably derived from the people who inhabited the pre-Aryan Indus Valley, mentions cannabis (Abel, 1980). Therefore, it is likely that cannabis was a drug that the Indus Valley inhabitants used. The Aryan tribes seem to have preferred soma.

Cannabis was apparently popular in the Indus Valley. The Hindu god Siva, who some believe to be a later version of Pasupathy, an Indus Valley deity, became associated with cannabis. He is called the Lord of Bhang, a mild liquid extract made from marijuana leaves. Ritual use of cannabis in India is most popular among people who practice Tantrism, an antinomian movement within both Hinduism and Buddhism. In rituals involving the goddess Kali, Bhang is consumed to heighten the senses in order to accomplish union with the goddess. Tantric Buddhism, which is popular in Tibet, also uses cannabis in its meditative rituals. Cannabis is a popular recreational drug in Tibet in general (Schultes & Hofmann, 1992; Mathew, 2001; Abel, 1980).

Cannabis contains a number of chemicals, collectively referred to as cannabinoids, of which Delta-9 tetrahydrocannabinol (THC) is considered principal. THC is a resinous material of high solubility in fats and oils and very low solubility in water. The most common mode of administration is smoking, although the drug may be ingested as a beverage or baked into a cookie. The smoked drug is rapidly absorbed from the lungs, and inebriation occurs within a few minutes. The effects of the drug are usually gone in about three hours (Hollister, 1986; McKim, 1991; Schultes & Hofmann, 1992; Mathew, 2001).

Marijuana smoking results in a wide variety of symptoms—euphoria, anxiety, lethargy, drowsiness, confusion, memory defects, altered time sense, depersonalization, impaired performance, cognitive changes, and psychosis. Dysphoric symptoms, especially panic, are common among inexperienced users or following intoxication with unusually large quantities of the drug (Hollister, 1986; Moran, 1986; Johnson, 1990; McKim, 1991; Schultes & Hofmann, 1992; Mathew, 2001). In recent years significant progress has been made in understanding the effects of cannabis on the brain. The principal ingredient, THC, binds to the cannabinoid receptors in the brain. Two types of receptors, CB1 and CB2, have been identified. Naturally occurring compounds that bind to the cannabinoid receptors have also been isolated. While a great deal of information is available on the cannabinoid receptors and their mechanisms of effect, little is known about how cannabis produces altered feelings of self (Welch & Martin, 2003).

We measured degrees of depersonalization induced by marijuana (Mathew et al., 1999) using a scale devised by Dixon (1963). After marijuana smoking, depersonalization peeked in 30 minutes and returned to the baseline in about 120 minutes. The degree of depersonalization was a function of the THC content of the marijuana leaf. All participants did not report this effect; about 30% definitely had it, while another 30% had some. The others did not have any such effect.

We used positron emission tomography (PET) to identify the brain regions responsible for mediating depersonalization (Mathew et al., 1999). Depersonalization was found to be closely associated with activation of the right anterior cingulate. The anterior cingulate may be the brain region that renders conscious awareness to otherwise unconscious activities of the brain. It has been described as "the seat of dynamic vigilance by which emotional experiences are endowed with conscious awareness" (Papez, 1937). This brain region, transposed between cortical and subcortical structures, may be responsible for integrating the evolutionarily newer and older brain structures that contribute to the composite feeling of self.

Selective functional impairment of this region may result in the decoupling of these mechanisms, and dissociation may be the resultant behavioral manifestation. Electrical stimulation of the human cingulate has been reported to elicit a broad variety of behavioral changes, including altered states of consciousness. Some subjects reported euphoria and a sense of well-being. Seizures with onset in the cingulate region also produce altered consciousness (Mathew et al., 1999).

Marijuana was also found to produce altered time sense. We used a 14-item questionnaire developed by Melges and associates (1970, 1974) to confirm altered time perception after marijuana smoking. We found an association between slowing of the passage of time and decreased activity of the cerebellum (Mathew et al., 1998). The correlation approached statistical significance but did not quite achieve it. However, it is of interest that the association between decreased cerebellar activity and impaired time sense was reported by other investigators. The cerebellum has been found to be involved in the temporal sequencing of motor activity. In human subjects cerebellar lesions were associated with impairment in rhythmic tapping, a time-dependent task. Patients with cerebellar atrophy were found to be deficient at judging the relative durations of time intervals (Ivry, Keele, & Diener, 1988; Ivry & Keele, 1989; Keele & Ivry, 1991; Ivry, 1993). Traditionally, the cerebellum has been associated with maintaining balance and coordination of movements. Our findings indicated that it may also be responsible for the timing function essential to both balance and coordination. Although a number of other investigators reported depersonalization and altered time sense after marijuana and THC use, to the best of my knowledge nobody else has tried to identify the brain regions responsible. Thus, these studies badly need confirmation.

Lysergic Acid Diethylamide

Lysergic acid diethylamide (LSD) is a hallucinogenic drug that has been extensively studied in the laboratory. The drug was developed by Albert Hofmann of Sandoz Pharmaceuticals in Basel, Switzerland. Dr. Hofmann was pursuing the effects of ergot on uterine contractions when he discovered the compound, but he had no idea about its effects on the brain. He accidentally got some of the drug on his skin and experienced some very strange sensory phenomena. This made him suspect that the drug had mental effects. To verify this he took what he considered a small dose, 0.25 mg, before he left for home on a bicycle. Unknowingly, he had

taken a whopping dose, several times higher than what is required to cause a powerful hallucinatory experience. Upon the completion of what must have been one of
the most bizarre bicycle trips in history, he called his family physician (McKim,
1991; Schultes & Hofmann, 1992; Mathew, 2001).

Dr. Hofmann was not actually the first to experiment with lysergic acid amide.
The drug is present in the seeds of *Turbina corymbrosa,* commonly known as morning glory. The Aztecs called it *ololiuqui.* Lysergic acid amide is approximately a
tenth as potent as LSD. The drug causes a dreamlike state without any changes in
the level of awareness. In moderate doses the drug does not produce intense hallucinations like LSD. However, it is used by the natives of Oaxaca in Mexico to
aid in prophecy and the divination of disease (Schultes, 1978; Stafford, 1978;
McKim, 1991; Schultes & Hofmann, 1992; Mathew, 2001).

Like marijuana, LSD produces depersonalization and altered sense of time. In
most instances it also gives a sense of happiness, although "bad trips" are also known
to occur. However, depersonalization and altered time perception are usually lost
in the cacophony of sensory phenomena. Perception is altered in quantity as well
as quality. Illusions and hallucinations are common. Boundaries between sensory
modalities break down, and synesthetic experiences are known to occur (Strassman, 1984; 1994). Total psychotic breakdowns have also been reported (Kenna &
Sedman, 1964).

Mescaline

Although not as rigorously studied in laboratories as marijuana and LSD, a great
deal of clinical information is available on mescaline. Mescaline is present in the
cacti *Lophophora williamsii, Lophophora diffusa, Trichocereus pachanoi* (the San
Pedro cactus), and several others. Natives of South America found ceremonial use
for the drug more than 8000 years ago. Rock carvings of the peyote ceremony and
archaeological discoveries in dry caves and rock shelters in Texas suggest that its
use is more than 3000 years old. It intrigued the Spanish conquistadores. It titil-
lated sufficient interest in Europe for King Phillip II of Spain to send his personal
physician, Dr. Francisco Hernandez, to study the drug and its effects. In his report
Dr. Hernandez claimed that the drug enabled the user to foresee and predict the future (Stafford, 1978; McKim, 1991; Schultes & Hofmann, 1992; Mathew, 2001.)

Its ceremonial use did not sit well with the conservative Spanish missionaries.
They found the drug, its use, the ceremonies during which the drug was ingested,
and the religion of which the ceremonies were part repulsive. They also did not
approve of the singing, dancing, and wine drinking, which were tied to the ceremonial use of the peyote cactus. They equated peyote use with cannibalism and
vampirism, and severe punishment was imposed upon the users.

North American tribes enthusiastically adopted peyote use from their South
American cousins for use in their own religious ceremonies. The Kiowa and Co-
manche were the first North American tribes to emulate their South American
counterparts. Soon peyote use swept across the plains, peyote became an integral
part of Christianity as it was practiced by many Native American churches. Native
Americans found straight-laced Christian ceremonies imported from Europe bland,
bleak, and boring. Bedecked in vibrant paints and festooned with exotic plumage

under the rising Prairie moon, they swayed to the beat of drums and danced around roaring campfires to find union with the Great Spirit. It was a far cry from sitting tight-lipped and neatly clad in Sunday best on finely polished benches arranged in rows with fine geometric precision in spotlessly clean churches singing to the sonorous hum of organ music. As might be anticipated, Ecclesiastes saw the use of peyote, in particular its ceremonial use in Christian ritual, as blasphemous and soon the U.S. lawmakers criminalized its use. The Native American's view of Christianity sharply differed from the European Christians who brought Christianity to them. The natives did not acquiesce; in fact, they took the matter to court. After a series of unfavorable decisions and appeals, in 1960 Judge Yale McFate of Arizona, in a round house ruling, overturned all previous federal and state laws that banned peyote use and granted First and Fourteenth Amendment protection to Native American's on the grounds of religious freedom. In 1970 by a special act of the U.S. congress, the use of peyote as a sacrament by the Native American Church was made legal. The members of the church can grow, purchase, transport, and use the drug (Stafford, 1978; McKim, 1991; Schultes & Hofmann, 1992; Mathew, 2001).

Peyote ceremonies highlight a variety of religious and social events including birthdays, baptisms, funerals, memorial services, Easter, Thanksgiving, Christmas, and New Year. Both men and women participate, but children are not allowed to consume the drug. Drumming, singing, and dancing enter into the celebrations, and peyote consumption is regarded as a sacrament. To many peyote symbolizes the power of Jesus.

Scientific study of peyote started in the latter part of the 1800s, when Parke-Davis and other pharmaceutical houses took an interest in it. The Philadelphia physician Weir Mitchell and Havelock Ellis, a research psychologist, provided the first scientific description of peyote inebriation. In 1897 Arthur Heffter identified mescaline as the active ingredient of the peyote cactus (Stafford, 1978; McKim, 1991; Schultes & Hofmann, 1992; Mathew, 2001). Since then there have been a number of descriptions of mescaline intoxication, of which the most vivid was provided by the famous novelist Aldous Huxley (1963). His picturesque description of mescaline inebriation increased its popularity with a number of well-known people.

Dissociation, especially depersonalization, is extremely common after mescaline ingestion. Time and space are distorted and altered. Time usually slows down and may even come to a screeching halt or may become irregular, moving in fits and starts.

Perception is altered at all levels, from the basics to the most refined. Perceptual distortion is more common, vivid, and varied compared to that caused by LSD. Eidetic and spectral images of protean shades and colors appear, disappear, and melt into one another. Colors take on an intensely pleasing, unearthly hue and glow. Hallucinations of familiar and unfamiliar objects occur: heaps of glittering diamonds, smoke-puffing dragons, and winged angels have all been reported. Synesthetic experiences, in which different sensory modalities commingle, occur. One may see music come out of a trumpet or smell the bright red of a rose.

Body perception is qualitatively and quantitatively altered. This has also been reported with LSD but not with marijuana. The body may seem to shrivel down to the size of a midget or balloon into a giant. It may become luminous or transparent. Out-of-body experiences are frequent accompaniments to peyote intoxication. This is associated with sensations of floating and flying.

There is a sense of detachment, peace, and freedom, and all negative emotions are expunged. A sensation of buoyancy and expansion are often present. For most people spiritual and religious themes become the hub and center of their thought processes. Creativity and aesthetic appreciation are enhanced, and the eidetic images seen during peyote experiences find expression in tribal art forms (Stafford, 1978; Schultes & Hofmann, 1992; Mathew, 2001).

Ecstasy
MDMA, 1-3, 4-methylenedioxymethamphetamine, deserves some discussion. It was developed by Merck as an appetite suppressant, but it was of greater interest to psychiatrists than to internists and gastroenterologists. It produced minimal perceptual distortions, but it induced altered time sense and produced depersonalization and ecstasy. It loosened the boundaries between self and not self and became known as the "hug drug" or "love drug." It has been labeled an "empathogen" with amphetaminelike stimulant side-effects (Glennon, 2003). The drug was put under Schedule I when several serious toxicity problems, especially serotonin neuron degeneration and hyperpyrexia, were identified (Glennon, 2003).

PCP and Ketamine
No account of depersonalizing agents would be complete without at least some mention of the dissociative anesthetics phencyclidine and ketamine (Domino, 2003). Phencyclidine, also known as PCP (short for "peace pill"), was synthesized by Parke Davis as an analgesic and anesthetic in 1963. It induced a trancelike state rather than an unconscious state. The subjects were dissociated from their sensory experiences. While the effects of the drug were of great heuristic significance, clinically its mental effects were too toxic. It induced a delirium with severe agitation and psychosis that made postoperative care difficult. While it disappeared from the operating rooms, it made its appearance in the streets under the name angel dust. The drug is often mixed with other drugs and seldom taken alone.

It has multiple mental and physical effects. It induces relaxation, warmth, tingling, and a sense of numbness. Body image is often distorted, and out-of-body experiences are quite common. In higher doses it may induce "coma with eyes open" or deeper states of coma. It also is known to induce psychotic states that may last several days. It has a reputation for causing unprovoked violence.

Ketamine is a drug with similar effects but is less potent. Dextromethorphan, which is marketed as an antitussive, has similar effects in high doses. Noncompetitive blockade of the NMDA receptor (N-methyl-D-aspartate) is the primary mechanism of action at low concentrations. Glutamte, the major excitatory neurotransmitter in the brain, binds to the NMDA receptor (Domino, 2003).

Other Agents
A number of chemicals, mostly present in various plants, have been found to produce similar depersonalizing effects (De Ropp, 1961; Schultes, 1978; Stafford, 1978; McKim, 1991; Schultes & Hofmann, 1992; Strassman, 1984; 1994; 1995).

However, they have not been as well described as have marijuana, LSD, and mescaline. Psilocybin mushrooms, otherwise known as "magic mushrooms" or "Mexican mushrooms," contain psilocybin and psilocin (De Ropp, 1961). Psilocybin is less potent than LSD or mescaline. As with soma (see below), after oral ingestion some 25% is excreted unchanged in the urine.

Dimethyltryptamine is found in plants. Plants of the species *Virola* contain the chemical in their bark. The bark is boiled and pounded to a powder. It is then sniffed for a variety of purposes, including spell casting and producing miracles. The compound can be synthesized in a laboratory, and it is affectionately known as "the businessman's LSD" because of its short duration of effect and less intense perceptual distortions.

The hallucinogen bufotenin is present in plants as well as animals. Beans of several species of trees of the genus *Anadenanthera* contain it. It has also been identified in the flesh of the "dream fish" from the Norfolk Islands. The skin of the Colorado River toad contains bufotenin. When agitated the toad secretes it. In a piquant practice known as "doing the toad," teenagers toss the toad in the air a few times and lick it to get bufotenin. However, the hallucinogenic effect occurs only when it is injected or inhaled. Usually it is mixed with ashes or lime and inhaled.

Harmine and harmaline, found in several plants of the genus *Bainsteriopsis,* induce a trance associated with colorful images. They are usually consumed as a drink prepared from the bark of the vine and are known by many names, including *coapi, ayahuasca, and yage.*

The National Institute on Drug Abuse (NIDA) became interested in ibogamine, the principle ingredient in the root of *Tabernanthe iboga* found in Central and West Africa. Some individuals with addiction found the *iboga*-induced state of mind so captivating that they lost their desire to ingest their drugs of addiction. Toxicity problems identified in laboratory animals precluded human research and use.

Space restraints limit the discussion of a number of other synthetic and naturally occurring compounds with similar effects. 2,5-dimethoxy-4-methyl-amphetamine (DOM), 2,5-dimethoxyethylamphetamine (DOET), 3,4-methylenedioxyamphetamine (MDA), 3-methoxy-4,5-methylenedioxyamphetamine (MMDA), 2,5-dimethoxyamphetamine (DMA), 3,4,5-introduction of an alpha methyl group to mescaline (TMA), myristicin, and elemicin are just a few (De Ropp, 1961; Schultes, 1978; Stafford, 1978; McKim, 1991; Schultes & Hofmann, 1992; Strassman, 1984; 1994; 1995).

Drugs That Influence the Core Self

Taittriya Upanishad's model of the mind comprises the central core of Atman surrounded by sheaths that represent mind and body. Atman is the only reality, and the rest is phantasmal. Thus, the true self is Atman, and self-realization is identification with Atman and release from the rest. Dissociative drugs that pull apart bonds among the components of the mind are those that are most useful. However, drugs with different modus operandi have also been used in religious ceremonies. In the Taittriya Upanishad model, stimulants amplify Atman, the central core.

Soma

The ancient Aryans who came to India from Central Asia (probably Baluchistan) used a plant called soma in their religious ceremonies. The Aryans deified soma, which purportedly catalyzed communication between humans and gods. All Vedas (Hindu scriptures) make references to it. More than 100 hymns from the anthology *Rig Veda* (1500 B.C.) are about soma and its use (Griffith, 1995). Soma is a vegetal derivative, and *Rig Veda* provides details about pressing the plant between stones in wooden bowls and extracting it via filtration with wisps of wool. The use of Soma was enshrouded in elaborate ceremonies, and rigid rules controlled who consumed it and how. Of the ecstasy induced by the drug it is said: "Where there are joys and pleasures, gladness and delight, where the desires of desire are fulfilled, there make me immortal" (*Rig Veda* 9.113). Another *Rig Veda* verse says: "We have drunk soma; we have become immortal: we have gone to the light; we have found the gods. What can hatred and malice of a mortal do to us now?" (8.48). Soma use was by no means restricted to the Aryans who came to the Indus Valley. References to *hoema* can be found in the *Zend-Avesta* of ancient Persia, which also was inhabited by Aryans (Mills, 1887). The drug was also associated with religious ceremonies among the Koryak tribe in Siberia and among the Native American tribes who lived around the Great Lakes (Wasson, 1968).

After much speculation by various scientists, Gordon Wasson of the Botanical Museum of Harvard University identified the mythical soma as the *Amanita muscaria* mushroom, also known as Fly Agaric: it intoxicates and induces sleep in flies. It is a red mushroom speckled with white (Wasson, 1968; Stafford, 1978; Riedlinger, 1993.)

Unlike other psychedelic drugs, *Amanita muscaria* seems to produce sound sleep followed by visions. After ingesting the mushroom eaters describe a sleep that is beautiful and splendid. The most wonderful images, such as they never see in their lives otherwise, pass before their eyes and lull them into a state of the most intense enjoyment. The effect is largely described as calming, comforting, and tranquilizing. Half an hour after ingestion, twitching, dizziness, and sometimes nausea occur. The twilight state induced by this drug lasts approximately 2 hours. Apparently, ingestors are hard to arouse. The predominant mood during this state is euphoria. Hallucinations occur after waking up, and changes in the size, shape, texture, and color of things have also been reported. The effects of the drug may last a total of 6 to 8 hours. No clear descriptions of depersonalization or altered time sense have been reported (Stafford, 1978).

Amanita muscaria has been found to contain the psychoactive agents ibotenic acid, muscimol, and muscazone. The psychoactive agents of the mushroom are still active when excreted in urine. *Rig Veda* references to people drinking urine from earlier ingestors to get intoxicated have been used to substantiate the identity of soma as *Amanita muscaria* (Stafford, 1978; Schultes & Hofmann, 1992; Mathew, 2001).

The assumption that soma was *Amanita muscaria* seems to be primarily based on the Western model of spiritual experiences such as LSD intoxication. Eastern ideas of spiritual experience are quite different. Most Western scientists accepted Wasson's identification of soma as Amanita muscaria. However, Indian authors have raised a number of what seem to be very valid objections (Mahdihassan, 1977; Kochhar, 2000).

First, none of the Vedas make any mention of the soporific and hallucinogenic effects of the mushroom. On the contrary, it is clearly stated in more than one place that it produces sleeplessness (Kochhar, 2000). The hallucinogenic effects are very prominent, and therefore their omission has to be taken seriously. The Aryans knew and used sedatives such as alcoholic beverages: sura (Kolhatkar, 1999). There was never any confusion between soma and sura. Soma was never mixed with alcohol, marijuana, or opium poppy (Kochhar, 2000). The mushroom can be eaten, as the Koryak tribe does, but there is no mention anywhere in the Vedas or *Zend-Avesta* of eating soma; it is pounded between stones, and the filtered juice is mixed with water, milk, curd (yogurt), barley, clarified butter, and perhaps honey (Kochhar, 2000). There is one *Rig Vedac* reference to chewing it (8.80). It is leafless and is described as a ray, finger, tube, and cane (Kochhar, 2000). *Zend-Avesta* describes it as golden hued with bending sprouts (*yasna* 9.16), and it can also be ruddy or brown (Kochhar, 2000). Both *Rig Veda* (9.97, 9.107) and *Zend-Avesta* (*yasna* 10.4) refer to the sweet scent of the plant and its extract. Pure soma juice is *tivra,* or astringent. None of these characteristics fit *Amanita muscaria.* Soma is more likely to be a stem than a soft mushroom.

Several passages from the Vedas, *Zend-Avesta,* and other ancient treatises suggest that soma was a stimulant. *Rig Veda* says "Have mercy on us for our well being. Know that we are devoted to your laws. Passion and fury are stirred up" (8.79). In *Zend-Avesta:* "I make my claim on thee for strength; I make my claim on thee for victory—and vigor of the entire frame." (yasna 9.17–21) From the passages that follow it is obvious that soma was consumed for strength, energy, vigor, fearlessness, and valor before battles. *Rig Veda* calls Soma "restless," a "strong defense against the enemy," and that which "rushes out and drives out the enemy" (8.79). It is compared to a newborn (9.74), racehorse (9.74), bull (10.94), and eagle ((4.26). It energizes and invigorates, and it produces insomnia (8.2; 8.92; 9.36; 9.44; 9.106). *Rig Veda* claims that soma speeds up thinking and increases creativity and productivity; it is called a poet (9.95; 9.96; 9.107; 3.43). The Veda links soma with Indra, the god of war, who "intoxicated with Soma destroyed nine and ninety fortresses" (4.26) (O'Flaherty, 1981). It would seem highly unlikely that a hallucinogenic mushroom that induces sleep would fit the bill. I also note that some soma ceremonies may last 12 days or more. These events are quite complex and involve rites and rituals that call for a great deal of concentration (Heesterman, 1993). The priests chant long mantras from memory, as Sanskrit did not have a script until around 400 B.C. Even now it is very unusual for a priest to read mantras from a book during circumambulation and oblation. A sedating, hallucinogenic drug imbibed by the priests during the ceremony would definitely get in the way. A stimulant, on the other hand, would come in very handy.

Several sources of evidence support the view that soma belongs to the *Ephedra* genus of plants, native to the mountainous regions of Iran, Afghanistan, and north India. It is probably *Ephedra pachyclada.* In that region the plant is called *hum* and *som* (Kochhar, 2000). They emit a pinelike fragrance and have an astringent taste.

They contain ephedrine, the well-known adrenergic stimulant. These plants do not grow in the Indian subcontinent, which would account for the disappearance of soma and the appearance of soma substitutes as the Aryan nomads moved in an easterly direction across the Gangetic plain.

Indians who regard the waking experience as a bad dream would not be impressed by its additional disfigurement with hallucinogenic drugs, but a stimulant that invigorates the mind and body would substantiates their belief in a central core that energizes the rest. In fact, *Zend-Avesta* considers soma "most nutritious for the soul" (yasna 9.16).

Stimulants such ephedrine produce no dissociation. The self is not detached from mind or body, and one does not feel like an outside observer. The sense of self is not only preserved but also amplified.

Cocaine

In South America stimulants, especially cocaine, have a long history of ceremonial use. Burial middens in Peru dating from 2500 B.C. contain coca leaves. Natives of Colombia believe that from the Milky Way an anaconda pulled to earth a canoe with a man, a woman, and several mind-altering plants, including coca. After they conquered the region the Incas took on the coca-chewing habit. They canonized the plant, and its use was primarily limited to the priestly class and nobility. The sprit of coca was conceptualized as a lovely maiden, "Mama Coca." The Spaniards and the Catholic Church saw coca leaf chewing as idolatrous. However, they permitted its use when they found out that it caused the natives to work long and hard hours. It also suppressed appetite, which was an added benefit. It reduced the cost of feeding the laborers. In 1749 the coca plant was named Erythroxylon coca. Albert Niemann of Gottingen isolated the active principle, cocaine, in 1860 (Hollister, 1988; McKim, 1991).

The drug energizes both the mind and body. The predominant mood is one of euphoria. There is a clear sense of excitement. The individual becomes overtalkative, overactive, and restless. The stream of thought is accelerated, and the content becomes expansive and grandiose. Depersonalization is very rare. Hallucinations may occur, especially with very high doses and in inexperienced users. It energizes, amplifies, and expands the sense of self. The individual totally and fully identifies with the cocaine experience and does not feel like an outside observer. Since we do not have any means of identifying and quantifying the core self, its putative augmentation by cocaine is speculative.

Discussion

This chapter has considered drugs that disrupt the composite self through the mechanism of dissociation and drugs that amplify the core self. Although the dissociative drugs differ in their effects, they do induce some common manifestations. Most of them induce perceptual distortions, with marijuana producing the least and mescaline producing the most. Marijuana and its active ingredient, tetrahydrocannabinol, produce illusions and hallucinations, especially in high doses. Distortion of time perception is yet another common characteristic. The commonest abnormality is slowing of time, although irregularities in the flow of time have also been reported. All of them produce depersonalization.

Depersonalization is a form of dissociation. The term *dissociation* implies separation. According to DSM IV, the disruption is in the usually integrated functions of consciousness, memory, identity, and perception of the environment. The neurophysiologic basis for the separation is unclear. Our research on marijuana-induced depersonalization pointed to the anterior cingulate as the site of the abnormality. The anterior cingulate has been identified as the part of the cortex that gives conscious awareness to such subcortical functions as emotions.

Such common expressions as "my body" and "my mind" would seem to separate "me" from the body and the mind. Depersonalization is a loosening of the bonds between one's self and the mind and body. It would seem safe to assume that in order to experience the self, thus defined, in full, one would have to turn off the mind and the body image completely. This happens, at least to some extent, in two states of mind, dreamless sleep and meditation.

Dreamless sleep, also known as slow-wave sleep, is characterized by relative inactivity of the brain. The slow waves on the electroencephalogram indicate relative electrical silence of the brain (Hobson, 1989). More recent investigations involving functional neuroimaging also support this idea of decreased brain activity (Madsen & Vorstrup, 1991). Since everyone cycles through deep sleep every night, it should be possible to make some statements about the associated state of mind. There is most definitely a decreased sense of time and decreased sense of space. In fact, there are no boundaries and no subdivisions and therefore no clear self and not-self separations. Dreamless sleep is associated with a sense of peace and tranquility. Most people find this sensation pleasurable and look forward to it.

Studies of meditation (with the possible exception of zen) have also shown decreased levels of electrical activity of the brain and brain metabolism (Mathew, 2001). The subjective experience of the meditative trance is ineffable. There is general consensus that the experience transcends time and space and is associated with bliss (Kasamatsu & Hirai, 1969; Anand, Chinna, & Singh, 1969; Mathew 2001).

If dissociation results in the separation of the core self from the rest, it should be associated with bliss as are slow-wave sleep and meditation. Yet depersonalization is usually regarded as an unpleasant state of mind. However, drug-induced depersonalization is often, but not always, a pleasant sensation. In the clinic depersonalization is associated with such unpleasant states of mind as fatigue, sleep deprivation, sensory deprivation, anxiety, depression, temporal lobe migraine, temporal lobe epilepsy, and so on. When depersonalization occurs on its own it is called depersonalization disorder, which, according to DSM IV, causes "clinically significant distress or impairment."

Depersonalization has been explained as a defense against such dysphoric mood states as anxiety and depression. However, drug-induced depersonalization appears to be at variance with this hypothesis (Good, 1989; Castillo, 1990). We administered a number of addictive drugs to human subjects to study their behavioral and neurophysiologic manifestations. Few of the subjects who reported depersonalization after administration of marijuana, THC, and mescaline found the experience unpleasant. Depersonalization is a common accompaniment of meditation. Most meditation practitioners look forward to the depersonalization experience and find it highly pleasurable. Similarly, individuals who undergo sensory deprivation also look forward to depersonalization and the associated sense of peace. Depersonalization is a common experience among normal people (Dixon, 1963; Sedman, 1966).

If the experience of the core self is associated with a sense of well-being, then amplification of the core self should also lead to euphoria. Indeed, such is the case with cocaine (and possibly soma) intoxication. We hypothesized that cocaine intoxication is associated with augmentation of the core self.

If we accept the DSM IV description of depersonalization as detachment of one's self from one's mental processes and body, we would also have to accept the argument that feelings of self are independent of mental operations and the body. We would also have to ascribe the feeling of the self to a brain region or regions independent of those that mediate mental processes and body image. Such a region would have to be phylogenetically older than areas dedicated to higher order mental processes.

This must be so since feelings of the self are not exclusively human. Few people would disagree with the notion that animals, even primitive amoeba, have a sense of self. If the amoeba did not have a sense of self it would not volitionally move away from noxious stimuli and move toward food particles. Although its experience of self may be extremely limited, it still has to have one.

The term *self* is meaningful only when and if it can be differentiated from "not-self." In other words, the perceiving self has to be differentiated from the perceived not-self. How the brain perceives itself is a complex issue. There has to be a master region that serves as the subject that perceives the parts that mediate the body and mind. Mind and body have to be wired to this master region. That preeminent part has to be indivisible, as the quintessential self cannot be divided further into subject and object. That brain region has to be primary and everything else, secondary. It also should be the oldest. Is it a critical collection of neurons in the brain stem or something even more primitive?

As we have seen, the experience of the core self is associated with bliss. The brain stem contains norepinephrine and serotonin, and both are believed to mediate normal happiness; most antidepressants act on these chemicals (McKim, 1991; Stahl, 2000). Serotonin has been implicated in intoxication with hallucinogenic drugs and spiritual states (Borg et al., 2003).

The self, bereft of the mind and body, is intensely subjective and outside the realm of objectivity and science. Language, which is largely a tool to describe the phenomenal world, is ill-equipped to deal with such intense subjectivity. Individuals who claim to have known such states of mind also claim experiences and abilities that are difficult to prove or disprove. Paranormal and supernatural abilities and experiences have been claimed (Mathew, 2001).

However, one such phenomenon is often enough associated with dissociative drugs that it merits some discussion. Several investigators have reported "out-of-body" experiences after the ingestion of dissociative agents (Stafford, 1978). One of our research subjects, a staff member, reported such an experience after the ingestion of ketamine in our laboratory. He clearly felt separated from his physical body and was able to "see" his body from outside. He could identify from "outside" his facial features and the attire that he was in. Such experiences are difficult to explain in neurophysiological terms. Obviously, it cannot be simple, straightforward perception. It cannot be reactivation of memory, since it is related to the present, in real time. It may be simple imagination. However, what such subjects "imagine" often corresponds to what others who are present observe. It also seems strange that so many people would have the same type of imagination—out-of-body experiences—over and over again.

It is equally strange that such experiences are also reported by people who are declared dead (Kubler-Ross, 1970; Moody, 1975). One of my patients, a Vietnam veteran, vividly described his out-of-body experience after he was accidentally electrocuted by a 440 volt, 5 amp DC charge while on a military excursion in Vietnam. When he was out of his body, looking down on his jerking, burned, smoking body, he did not feel any pain. When he "returned" to his body, the intense burning pain came back with a vengeance. While it is conceivable that these people did not experience total brain death and that some region of the brain that was still alive created the experience, it is also conceivable that the same brain region may be responsible for the out-of-body experiences associated with drug induced depersonalization.

Since the out-of-body experience involves detailed and vivid sensory impressions, it cannot be subcortical. However, as we have seen, other evidence suggests that the self is probably mediated by a phylogenetically old brain region. At the moment we have to concede that we do not have s satisfactory neurological explanation for this.

Out-of-body experiences are also associated with a unique sense of happiness similar to the peace and tranquility that accompany intoxication with dissociative drugs, slow-wave sleep, and meditation. *Taittriya Upanishad* attributes ontological significance to this bliss: "Bliss is the essence of the Absolute. Infusion of the Absolute infuses one with bliss" (II.7.I).

One thing appears to be clear. The core self is independent of the mind and body. It also is beyond time and space constraints. It does not have boundaries, so there is no clear demarcation between the self and not-self. Thus, the true self would seem to be selfless. According to the *Brihad-Aranyaka Upanishad,* composed sometime around 500 B.C., "He who knows the self, he knows everything" (1, 7, 1) (Radhakrishnan, 1994).

References

Abel, E.L. (1980). *Marijuana: The First Twelve Thousand Years.* New York: Plenum Press.
Anand, B.K., Chinna, G.S., & Singh, B. (1969). Some aspects of electroencephalographic studies in yogis. In: C.T. Tart (Ed.) *Altered States of Consciousness.* New York: John Wiley.

American Psychiatric Association (1994). *Diagnostic and Statistical Manual of Mental Disorders,* 4th ed. Washington, DC: American Psychiatric Association.

Borg, J., Andree, B., Soderstrom, H., & Farde, L. (2003). The serotonin system and spiritual experiences. *American Journal of Psychaitry, 160,* 1965–1969.

Castillo, R.J. (1990). Depersonalization and meditation. *Psychiatry, 53,* 158–168.

Crick, F. & Koch, C. (1992). The problem of consciousness. *Scientific American, September,* 153–159.

De Ropp, R.S. (1961). *Drugs and the Mind.* New York: Grove Press.

Dixon, J.C. (1963). Depersonalization phenomena in a sample population of college students. *British Journal of Psychiatry, 109,* 371–375.

Domino, E.F. (2003). The pharmacology of NMDA antagonists: Psychotomimetics and dissociative anesthetics. In: A.W. Graham, T.K. Schultz, M.S. Mayo-Smith, R.K. Ries & B.B. Wilford (Eds.) *Principles of Addiction Medicine,* (3rd ed.) (pp. 287–294). Chevy Chase, MD: American Society of Addiction Medicine.

Gazzaniga, M.S. (1998). *The Mind's Past.* Los Angeles: University of California Press.

Glennon, R.A. (2003). The pharmacology of serotonergic hallucinogens and "designer" drugs. In: A.W. Graham, T.K. Schultz, M.S. Mayo-Smith, R.K. Ries, & B.B. Wilford (Eds.) *Principles of Addiction Medicine,* (3rd ed.) (pp. 271–285). Chevy Chase, MD: American Society of Addiction Medicine.

Good, M.I. (1989). Substance induced dissociative disorders and psychiatric nosology. *Journal of Clinical Psychopharmacology, 9,* 88–93.

Griffith, R. (1995). *The Hymns of the Rig Veda.* New Delhi: Motilal Banarsidass Publishers.

Gupta, B. (1995). *Perceiving in Advaita Vedanta. Epistemological Analysis and Interpretation.* New Delhi: Motilal Banasidass Publishers.

Heesterman, J.C. (1993). *The Broken World of Sacrifice. An Essay in Ancient Indian Ritual.* Chicago: University of Chicago Press.

Hobson, J.A. (1989). *Sleep.* New York: Scientific American Library.

Hogan, R.E. & Kaiboriboon, K. (2003). The "dreamy state": John Hughlings-Jackson's ideas of epilepsy and consciousness. *American Journal of Psychiatry, 160,* 1740–1747.

Hollister, L.E. (1986). Health aspects of cannabis. *Pharmacological Reviews, 38,* 1–20.

Hollister, L.E. Cocaine–1988. (1988). *Human Psychopharmacology, 3,* 1–2.

Huxley, A. (1963). *The Doors of Perception.* New York: Harper & Row.

Ivry, R.B. (1993). Cerebellar involvement in the explicit representation of temporal function. *Annals of the New York Academy of Sciences, 682,* 214–230.

Ivry, R.B., Keele, S.W. & Diener, H.C. (1988). Dissociation of the lateral and medial cerebellum in movement timing and movement execution. *Experimental Brain Research, 73,* 167–180.

Ivry, R.B. & Keele, S.W. (1989). Timing functions of the cerebellum. *Journal of Cognitive Neuroscience, 1,* 136–152.

Johnson, B.A. (1990). Psychopharmacological effects of cannabis. *British Journal of Hospital Medicine, 43,* 114–122.

Kasamatsu, A. & Hirai, T. (1969). An electroencephalographic study of zen meditation (zazen). In: C.T. Tart (Ed.) *Altered States of Consciousness.* New York: John Wiley.

Keele, S.W. & Ivry, R.B. (1991). Does the cerebellum provide a common computation for diverse tasks? A timing hypothesis. *Annals of the New York Academy of Sciences, 608,* 179–211.

Kenna, J.C. & Sedman, G. (1964). The subjective experience of time during lysergic acid diethylamide (LSD-25) intoxication. *Psychopharmacologia, 5,* 280–288.

Kishore, B.R. (2001). *Atharvveda.* New Delhi: Diamond Pocket Books.

Kochhar R.(2000). *The Vedic People. Their History and Geography.* Hyderabad, India: Orient Longman.

Kolhatkar, M.B.(1999). *Sura. The Liquor and the Vedic Sacrifice.* New Delhi: D.K. Printworld.

Kubler-Ross. E. (1970) *On Death and Dying.* London: Tavistock Publications.

Madhihassan, S. (1977). *Indian Alchemy or Rasayana. In the Light of Asceticism and Geriatrics.* Delhi: Motilal Bararsidass Publishers.

Madsen, P.L. & Vorstrup, S. (1991) Cerebral blood flow and metabolism during sleep. *Cerebrovascular and Brain Metabolism Reviews, 3,* 281–296.

Mathew, R.J. (2001) *The True Path. Western Science and the Quest for Yoga.* Cambridge, MA: Perseus Publishing.

Mathew, R.J., Wilson, W.H., Turkington, T.G., & Coleman, E.R. (1998). Cerebellar activity and disturbed time sense after marijuana. *Brain Research, 797,* 183–189.

Mathew, R.J., Wilson, W.H., Chiu, N.Y., Turkington, T.G., Degrado, T.R. & Coleman, R.E. (1999). Regional cerebral blood flow and depersonalization after tetrahydrocannabinol administration. *Acta Psychiatria Scandinavica, 100,* 67–75.

McKim, W.A. (1991). *Drugs and Behavior: An Introduction to Behavioral Pharmacology,* 5th ed. Upper Saddle River, NJ: Prentice-Hall.

Melges, F.T., Tinklenberg, J.R., Hollister, L.E., & Gillespie, H.K. (1970). Marijuana and temporal disintegration. *Science, 168,* 118–120.

Melges, F.T., Tinklenberg, J.R., Deardorff, M., Davis, M.H., Anderson, R.E., & Owen, C.A. (1974). Temporal disorganization and delusion-like ideation. *Archives of General Psychiatry, 30,* 855–861.

Mellor, C.S. (1988). Depersonalization and self perception. *British Journal of Psychiatry, 153 (Suppl. 2),* 15–19.

Mills, L.H. (1887). The Zend-Avesta. In: M.F. Muller (Ed.) *The Sacred Books of the East,* vol. 31. New Delhi: Motilal Benarsidass Publishers.

Moody, R.A., Jr. (1975). *Life after Life.* New York: Bantam Books.

Moran, C. (1986). Depersonalization and agoraphobia associated with marijuana use. *British Journal of Medical Psychology, 59,* 187–196.

O'Flaherty, W.D. (1981). *The Rig Veda.* London: Penguin Books.

Papez, J.W. (1937). A proposed mechanism of emotion. *Archives of Neurology and Psychiatry, 38,* 725–743.

Radhakrishnan, S. (1989). *Indian Philosophy,* vol. 1. New Delhi: Oxford University Press.

Radhakrishnan, S. (1994). *The Principal Upanishads.* New Delhi: Indus, Harper Collins.

Ramachandran, V.S. & Blakeslee, S. (1998). *Phantoms in the Brain.* New York: William Morrow.

Riedlinger, T.J. (1993). Wasson's alternate candidates for soma. *Journal of Psychoactive Drugs, 25,* 149–156.

Sedman, G. (1966). Depersonalization in a group of normal subjects. *British Journal of Psychiatry, 112,* 907–912.

Schultes, R.E. (1978). Plants and plant constituents as mind-altering agents throughout history. In: L.L. Iverson, S.D. Iverson, & S.H. Snyder (Eds.) *Handbook of Psychopharmacology,* vol. 11 (pp. 219–242). New York: Plenum.

Schultes, R.E. & Hofmann, A. (1992). *Plants of the Gods: Their Sacred, Healing, and Hallucinogenic Powers.* Rochester, NY: Healing Arts Press.

Stafford, P. (1978). *Psychedelics Encyclopedia,* 3rd ed. Berkeley: Ronin Publishing.

Stahl, S.M. (2000). *Essential Psychopharmacology.* Cambridge: Cambridge University Press.

Strassman, R.J. (1984). Adverse reactions to psychedelic drugs: A review of the literature. *Journal of Nervous and Mental Disorders, 172,* 577–595.

Strassman, R.J. (1994). Human psychopharmacology of LSD, dimethyltryptamine and related compounds. In: A. Pletscher & D. Ladewig (Eds.) *Fifty Years of LSD: Current Status and Perspectives of Hallucinogens. A Symposium of the Swiss Academy of Medical Sciences.* New York: Parthenon Publishing.

Strassman, R.J. (1995). Hallucinogenic drugs in psychiatric research and treatment. *Journal of Nervous and Mental Disease, 183,* 127–138.

Svoboda, R.E. (1992). *Ayurveda, Life, Health, and Longevity.* London: Arkana, Penguin.

Wasson, R.G. (1968). *Soma: Divine Mushroom of Immortality.* Orlando: Harcourt Brace Jovanovich.

Wasson, R.G. (1972). The divine mushroom of immortality. In: P.T. Furst (Ed.) *Flesh of the Gods* (pp. 185–200) New York: Praeger.

Welch, S.P. & Martin, B.R. (2003). The pharmacology of marijuana. In: A.W. Graham, T.K. Schultz, M.S. Mayo-Smith, R.K. Ries, & B.B. Wilford (Eds.) *Principles of Addiction Medicine* (3rd ed.) (pp. 271–285). Chevy Chase, MD: American Society of Addiction Medicine.

16

Meditation and the Self

HANS C. LOU AND TROELS W. KJAER

The study of meditation is an obvious choice in attempting to gain insight into the neurobiological correlate of consciousness and the self. A wide variety of meditation techniques exist, and all involve voluntary changes in states and contents of consciousness. In this chapter we first present the results of a positron emission tomography (PET) investigation of yoga nidra relaxation meditation compared with the normal resting conscious state. Yoga nidra is a condition in which the subject experiences almost complete relaxation, with minimal demands of attention or preparedness to act, but with vivid sensory imagination. Our aim was to study the neural basis of consciousness by separating its two main aspects: intention and sensory experience. We found that meditation was accompanied by relatively increased perfusion in the hippocampus and sensory and higher-order association regions. Decreased perfusion was seen in bilateral inferior parietal regions, the dorsolateral prefrontal cortex, and other executive regions. Increased striatal dopamine binding to D2 receptors during meditation suggested the decreased dorsolateral prefrontal perfusion to be caused by dopaminergic activity.

A principal component analysis of the results separated the blood flow data into two groups, explaining 25% and 18% of their variance. One group corresponded to the executive system and the other to the systems that support sensory imagery. A small group of regions contributed considerably to both networks: the medial parietal and medial prefrontal cortices together with the striatum. We interpreted these cortical regions to be a medial core of consciousness, possibly essential for unity of consciousness and self-representation.

To test this hypothesis, we then investigated the neural networks that support retrieval of earlier judgments about individuals with different degrees of self-relevance: self, best friend, and the Danish queen. We found all conditions activated the medial core, together with an increasing activation in the right inferior parietal cortex and a decreasing activation in the right lateral temporal cortex according to the degree of self-relevance. Transcranial magnetic stimulation was applied to the medial parietal region to transiently disrupt its normal neural function. This resulted in specific decreased efficiency of retrieval of self-judgment when applied with a latency of 80–160 ms after presenting visual adjectives. We concluded that the medial parietal cortex is essential for self-representation in interaction with the medial prefrontal and right lateral parietal cortices.

Meditation and the Medial Core of Consciousness

Meditation is a term covering a large variety of mental practices that involve voluntary changes in states and contents of consciousness (Ballantyne & Deva, 1990). It is a constituent of major religions such as Hinduism and Buddism, particularly in its Zen form, and variants are encountered in Christianity as well. An early expression of increased globalization after World War II has been the expansion of these practices in Western societies, with or without religious contexts.

Early physiological studies on its effects on physiological homeostasis appeared in the 1960s and 1970s. Particularly influential were a series of studies by Wallace on oxygen consumption and EEG (Wallace, 1970), which led him to conclude that "the physiological changes during meditation differ from those during sleep, hypnosis, auto-suggestion, and characterize a wakeful, hypometabolic physiologic state" with characteristic effects (increase in theta activity combined with essential preservation of alpha activity). This claim has since been corroborated by some researchers (Benson, Beary, & Carol, 1974) and disclaimed by others (Pagano & Warrenburg, 1983). The reason for this variability of physiological data may be the phenomenological variability of the condition.

In spite of the surging interest in recent years in the study of the neural correlates of consciousness, neuroimaging methods have been used in the study of meditation in only a handful of studies. Again, the results have been heterogeneous, possibly reflecting the differences in phenomenological contents involved in the meditation practices used. The first study was reported in 1990 by Herzog and colleagues using [F18]-fluorodeoxyglucose as a tracer to measure glucose metabolism during self-induced yoga relaxation meditation. This investigation failed to reveal detailed regional differences but found a significant frontal-occipital ratio of cerebral metabolism, mainly due to a marked decrease in metabolism in the occipital and superior parietal lobes. Using another attention-demanding meditation technique, Newberg and colleagues (2001) also found increases in frontal lobe activity. This finding was in accordance with the increased activity in the prefrontal cortex during attention-focusing tasks (Frith, Friston, & Frackowiak, 1991; Pardo, Fox, & Raichle, 1991).

In 1999 we reported a study with a different meditation technique, voice-induced yoga nidra relaxation meditation (Lou et al., 1999). In this study the participants listened to a tape that guided them through the meditation sequence, thus requiring less attention and willful concentration. Structured interviews confirmed that the participants experienced a reduced drive to act and an increase in imagery during the meditation procedure (Kjaer et al., 2001). We originally attempted to use this technique to study separately the neurological correlates of "passive" and "active" consciousness (Taylor, 1999). The activation pattern changed with the focus of meditation: meditation on the sensation of the weight of limbs and other body parts, presumably related to "motor attention," was supported mainly by the supplementary motor area in the superior medial prefrontal cortex (Martin et al., 1996). Parietal and occipital activation was also noted. An abstract sensation of "joy" was almost exclusively accompanied by left-hemisphere activation of parietal and superior temporal cortices when compared to the normal resting conscious state, and visual imagery by strong activation of the lateral parietal and occipital lobe, with sparing of the primary visual region (V1). The activated regions in these tasks are similar to those previously shown to be active during voluntary visual imagery (Kosslyn et al. 1993). These findings also demonstrate important similarities to the activation pattern seen during REM sleep and dreaming without the anterior cingulate activity seen in this condition (Braun et al., 1998). The lack of anterior cingulate activation during our meditation technique probably reflects the subjective loss of the motivation to act. The meditation on the symbolic representation of the self was supported by bilateral parietal activity in accordance with the role attributed to these regions in representation of the physical (Adair et al., 1995) and mental (Lou et al., 2004) self. This was not found during meditation on other items during the sequence. Common to most meditative situations in our study was a strong bilateral hippocampal activation. This was also apparent in the combined meditation measurements, which in addition were characterized by activity in parietal and occipital association and sensory regions.

Relaxation meditation was accompanied by a relative *decrease* of activation in bilateral orbital and dorsolateral prefrontal, anterior cingulate, temporal, inferior parietal cortices, and caudate nucleus, thalamus, pons, and cerebellar vermis and hemispheres, structures subserving executive functions and, particularly in the case of the dorsolateral prefrontal cortices, working memory (Mehta et al., 2000). Reduction of perfusion in prefrontal cortical regions, together with increased proficiency of working memory, is seen in dopaminergic activation during methylphenidate administration (Mehta et al., 2000). We therefore hypothesized that dopaminergic release could be responsible for the reduced prefrontal perfusion during meditation. We found increased D2 receptor occupancy in the ventral striatum during yoga nidra relaxation meditation, an indication of dopamine release, at least in the striatum (Kjaer et al., 2002). The striatum is active in selection and inhibition of cortical activity in the control of actions (Posner & Rothbart, 1994), an effect that is dopamine-mediated by increasing the signal-to-noise ratio (see Horvitz, 2002, for review). In slow-wave sleep decreased activity has been noted in a similar set of regions, including the anterior cingulate gyri, prefrontal cortex, basal ganglia, and brain stem (Maquet et al., 1997). Maquet and coworkers proposed that one characteristic of all sleep stages is the lack of dorsolateral frontal activity, similar to our findings during meditation, an activity similarly characterized by decreased executive activity. Thus, our findings demonstrated an experimentally induced separation of the neural substrates of the complementary "active" and "passive" aspects of consciousness (Taylor, 1999).

We found that meditation, in general, shifted cortical activity from prefrontal to posterior regions (Figs. 16–1 and 16–2). However, the most important finding

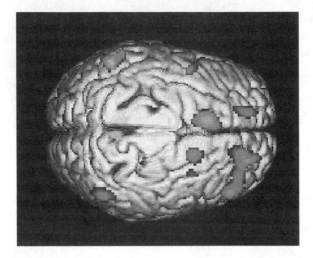

Figure 16–1. Cortical regions with relatively decreased perfusion during meditation: bilateral prefrontal dorsolateral and bilateral inferior parietal. The right parietal is included after revision in light of its participation in self-representation evident after our recent study (Lou et al., 2004). It was originally omitted due to cluster size below an arbitrarily defined threshold (Lou et al., 1999). A marked striatal and cerebellar contribution is not shown here.

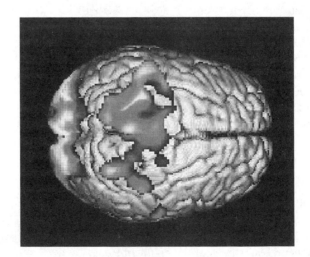

Figure 16–2. Cortical regions with increased perfusion during meditation: superior parietal and occipital sensory and association cortices. A marked hippocampal contribution is not shown here.

of our study occurred to us only after its original publication. It concerned how these constituents of the neural correlate of consciousness interact to achieve mental unity: We reanalyzed the blood flow data from 29 regions in the above study with the principal component method. The first principal component explained 25% of the regional cerebral blood flow (rCBF) variability and consisted primarily of regions differentially active during the normal resting conscious state. The second component explained 18% of the variability and consisted primarily of posterior sensory and association regions differentially active during meditation. Three structures contributed markedly to both networks: right precuneus, middle prefrontal frontal gyri (Brodmann area 10), and the right striatum (Table 16–1, Fig. 16–3). We first presented this data at the Association for Scientific Study of Consciousness (ASSC4) conference in Brussels in 2000 (Kjaer & Lou, 2000), and we interpreted this set of regions as a robust medial core of the resting conscious states, hypothetically assuring coherence and unity across their variations. With its central anatomical location, this network would be optimally suited to connect not

Table 16–1. Comparison of PC Analysis to SPM Analysis of Regions According to Increase (m) or Decrease (c) During Meditation.

| Region | PC Analysis | | | SPM Analysis |
Brodman area in ( )	PC1 + PC2	PC1 (PC1 + PC2)	Group	Condition
Pons	2	100	1	c
R thalamus	5	98	1	c
L thalamus	6	98	1	c
L cerebellum	5	97	1	c
L temp pole (38)	2	92	1	—
R cerebellum	7	91	1	c
L striatum	4	90	1	c
L orbito-frontal g (11)	2	88	1	c
R cingulate g (24)	2	85	1	—
R mid frontal g (10)	3	59	3	c
L mid frontal g (10)	3	47	3	c
R striatum	2	39	3	—
R precuneus (7)	3	36	3	—
L hippocampus	2	11	2	m
L occipital lobe (17, 18)	5	7	2	m
L postcentral gyrus (1, 2, 3, 5)	4	6	2	m
R hippocampus	8	4	2	—
R occipital lobe (17, 18)	6	3	2	m
R sup temp g (22)	6	1	2	m
R. postcentral gyrus (1, 2, 3, 5)	3	0	2	—
L sup temp g (22)	6	0	2	m

PCA analysis of regional cerebral blood flow during relaxation meditation and normal resting consciousness: allocation of regions with respect to participation in each of two groups explaining 25% and 18% of variability (Groups 1 and 2). A small medial set of regions contribute about equally to both groups, indicating participation in both meditation and normal resting consciousness (Group 3).

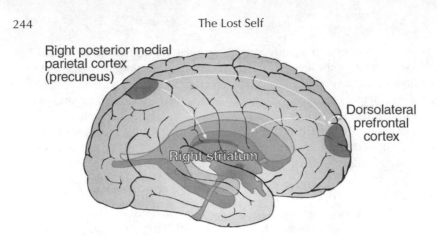

Figure 16–3. Artist´s drawing of medial core regions that participate in both anterior (executive) and posterior aspects of consciousness: anterior prefrontal and medial parietal regions, together with the striatum.

only the posterior and anterior brain, but also right and left hemispheres and limbic and neocortical regions. If this assumption were correct, we further reasoned that the medial core would be active in self-reference, considered to be pivotal in the phenomenological unity of consciousness (Taylor, 1999).

The Medial Core and Self-Representation

All subjective experience may be seen as self-conscious in the *weak* sense that there is something it feels like for the subject to have that experience. We may at times be self-conscious in a *deep* way, for example, when we are engaged in figuring out who we are and what we are going to do with our lives, a distinctly human experience giving organization, meaning, and structure to life. In its absence, our representation of ourselves and our world becomes kaleidoscopic and our life chaotic (Flanagan, 1995). Such explicit "autonoetic consciousness" is thought to emerge by retrieval of memories of personally experienced events (episodic memory) (Tulving, 1972; Gardiner, 2001). The cerebral activation pattern during episodic memory retrieval differs from that of semantic retrieval of common knowledge: for example, activation of the medial parietal cortex is characteristic of the former, and of the left lateral temporal lobe of the latter (Cabeza & Nyberg, 2000).

To test the hypothesis that self-representation is based on interaction of the medial parietal and medial prefrontal cortices, we compared rCBF changes in three subjects making judgments with different degrees of self-relevance (self, best friend, and the Danish queen) using a simple nonmemory loaded condition with identical input and output as a control. Prior studies have used related retrieval methodology but have not attempted to distinguish mental self from other (Johnson et al., 2002; Kircher et al., 2000). In addition, we used transcranial magnetic stimulation (TMS) (Keenan, 2001) to transiently disrupt normal neural activity in the medial parietal region to see if such disruption would affect the task.

The major finding was the demonstration of a distinct neural correlate of the mental self, or explicit "autonoetic consciousness (Gardiner, 2001; Posner & Rothbart, 1998; Stuss & Levine, 2002), related to activity in the parietal cortex and interacting with the medial prefrontal cortex. The results were surprisingly clear: the massive activation of the medial prefrontal and medial parietal/posterior cingulate regions in all three tasks compared to the control condition was in agreement with their episodic nature (Lou et al., 2004). The medial prefrontal cortex is the classical region involved in self-reference (Posner & Rothbart, 1998). Earlier studies of lesions have shown deficient self-awareness and self-control in lesions of this structure (Stuss & Levine, 2002), and increased activity has been seen in first-person reports of mental states such as emotions, self-generated thoughts, and intentions to speak (Cabeza & Nyberg, 2000). In addition, "theory of mind," or attributing mental states to others, are functions that have been associated with activity in this region (Vogeley et al., 2001). The medial prefrontal cortex is also highly active during the resting state. It was early suggested by David Ingvar that this activity expressed a "rehearsal," or "simulation of behavior" (1979), while the Frith's concluded that dorsal medial prefrontal regions are concerned with explicit representations of states of the self (Frith & Frith, 1999). In our study we extend the responsibility for self-reference to a medial paralimbic network of parietal–prefrontal regions in interaction with the (right) inferior lateral parietal cortex.

The medial parietal/posterior cingulate region has repeatedly been associated with episodic memory retrieval (for review, see Cabeza & Nyberg, 2000). It has been suggested that perfusion in the medial parietal region (precuneus) is correlated with linking new information with prior knowledge in a memory processing and retrieval system (Maguire, Frith, & Morris, 1999), with an important role for precuneus in *retrieval* of episodic memory compared to episodic *encoding* (Kelley et al., 2002) and *semantic* retrieval (Henson et al., 1999; Wiggs, Weisberg, & Martin, 1999).

Our findings suggest that the medial parietal cortex is particularly important for self-representation, in spite of our finding of similar hemodynamic activation during all three tasks. Thus, TMS impaired the retrieval of highly self-referential information selectively at this site with a latency of 160 ms. In other regions neural activity with a latency of 160 ms includes non–phase-locked visually elicited gamma oscillations that have been suggested to be important for the emergence of visual awareness of *physical* objects (Tallon-Baudry et al., 1996). The differential importance of the medial parietal cortex for self-representation is in agreement with our coherence analysis of synchrony, which showed functional correlation between the precuneus and the right inferior parietal cortex, selectively active in explicit self-reference, and not with the left temporal region, selectively active in other-reference. Extended TMS studies will be needed to ascertain whether the effect of TMS at the medial parietal site is truly specific for self-representation.

The finding that the right inferior parietal cortex was particularly active during retrieval of self-referential information was unexpected. However, several studies provide circumstantial evidence for a role of the right inferior parietal region in self-representation. First, there is a right hemisphere preference for self-recognition (Keenan et al., 2001). Second, a number of recent studies on physical first-person perspective such as position in space, imagination of agency, and body representation have shown activation in the right inferior parietal region (Maguire et al., 1998; Maguire, Burgess, & O'Keefe, 1999; Vogeley & Fink, 2003). Last, illusory own-body perceptions have even been produced by direct electrical stimulation of the right inferior parietal cortex during surgical treatment for epilepsy (Blanke et al., 2002). These studies point to a role for the right lateral parietal region in representation of the *physical* self. With our present results showing that this is also the case for the *mental* self, we conclude that the right inferior parietal cortex is selectively activated in self-representation in general. It should be noted, however, that the degree of activity was not significantly different from our simple control task and was solely apparent when compared to memory-loaded retrieval of representations of the other. Although the present study was not specifically designed to test the hypothesis of a medial prefrontal and lateral and medial parietal "default mode" system with high activity during rest and self-related activity (Gusnard et al., 2001), our results support that hypothesis. It may also be noted that we found decreased activity in the right inferior parietal region during combined meditation tasks only when revising our meditation study in the light of the new data on self-representation (Fig. 16–1). This is in accordance with a view of meditation as a means of decreasing self-awareness (Ballantyne & Deva, 1990).

An important contribution of a semantic retrieval network not related to self-reference was apparent in the activity of the left lateral temporal region. Activity in this region is a hallmark of semantic retrieval. The region is activated not only for words but also for pictures (Martin et al., 1995; Martin et al., 1996; Vandenberghe et al., 1996) and faces (Sergent, Ohta, & MacDonald, 1992; Gomo-Tempini et al., 1998), in accordance with involvement in higher-level semantic processes that are independent of input modality.

The hypothesis that not only medial anterior but also medial posterior regions are essential for subjectivity is a new development. The concept was proposed recently by Raichle and coworkers with a metaanalysis of spontaneous rCBF and oxygen consumption in the resting brain (Raichle et al., 2001; Gusnard & Raichle, 2001). They stated that high activity in medial frontal and medial parietal regions is "consistent with the continuity of a stable, unified perspective of the organism relative to the environment (a "Self")" (Gusnard & Raichle, 2001). The tonic activity decreases during engagement in non–self-referential goal-directed actions (i.e., "default mode") (Gusnard et al., 2001). Regional CBF depends on afferent function (i.e., all aspects of presynaptic and postsynaptic processing) but is independent of the efferent function (i.e., the spike rate of the same region) (Lauritzen, 2001). Even if that were not the case, increased cognitive expediency of a given region cannot be inferred from increased regional CBF or oxidative metabolism. There are, in fact, several examples of the opposite (Mehta et al., 2000). Therefore, these important suggestions from regional CBF studies have lacked decisive experimental support.

The present evidence for an essential role of the medial parietal region in self-reference connects the right (and left) lateral inferior parietal cortex with the medial prefrontal cortex, already known to be essential for self-representation (Stuss & Levine, 2002). There are abundant anatomical connections between the medial parietal/posterior cingulate region and the medial prefrontal/anterior cingulate region (Cavada & Goldman-Rakic, 1989), and these regions are functionally integrated in reflective self-awareness (Kjaer et al., 2001) and the resting conscious state (Greicius et al., 2003). Together these findings point to a new principle of regulation of subjectivity and conscious self-monitoring.

The self may act as a core in the unity of conscious experience (Gusnard & Raichle, 2001). This is in agreement with the proposed role of these medial regions in such unity (Kjaer & Lou, 2000). The medial structures not only integrate the anterior and posterior brain but also the left and right hemispheres (Goldman-Rakic & Schwartz, 1982) and limbic and neocortical structures (Posner & Rothbart, 1998). They have also been shown to provide gateways for the spread of information in the brain from lateral cortical regions (Lou et al., 2004). We speculate that such local brain activity may gain access in this way to a "global workspace" of consciousness proposed by Baars (2002).

References

Adair, K.C., Gilmore, R.L., Fennell, E.B., Gold, M., & Heilman, K.M. (1995). Anosognosia during intracarotid barbiturate anestesia: Unawareness or amnesia for weakness. *Neurology, 45,* 241–243.

Baars, B.J. (2002). The conscious access hypothesis: Origins and recent evidence. *Trends in Cognitive Science, 6,* 47–51.

Ballantyne, J.R. & Deva, G.S. (1990). Yoga sutras of Panjali Delhi. *Parimal,* 48–87.

Benson, H., Beary, J.R., & Carol, M.K. (1974). The relaxation response. *Psychiatry, 37,* 37–46.

Blanke, O., Ortigue, S., Landis, T., & Seeck, M. (2002). Stimulating illusory own-body perceptions. *Nature, 149,* 269–270.

Braun, A.R., Balkin, T.J., Wesensten, N.J., Gwadry, F., Carson, R.E., Varga, M., Baldwin, P., Belenky, G., & Herscovitch, P. (1998). Dissociated patterns of activity in visual cortices and their projections during human rapid eye movement sleep. *Science, 279,* 91–95.

Cabeza, R. & Nyberg, L. (2000). Imaging cognition II:An empirical review of 275 PET and fMRI studies *Journal of Cognitive Neuroscience, 12,* 1–47.

Cavada, C. & Goldman-Rakic, P.S. (1989). Posterior parietal cortex in rhesus monkey: II. Evidence for segregated corticocortical networks linking sensory and limbic areas with the frontal lobe. *Journal of Comparative Neurology, 287,* 422–445.

Flanagan, O. (1995). *Consciousness Reconsidered.* Cambridge MA: MIT Press.

Frith, C.D., Friston, K., & Frackowiak, R.S.J. (1991). Willed action and the prefrontal cortex in man. A study with PET. *Proceedings of the Royal Society of London, 244,* 241–246.

Frith, C.D. & Frith, U. (1999). Interacting minds — a biological basis. *Science, 286,* 1692–1695.

Gardiner, J.M. (2001).Episodic memory and autonoetic consciousness: A first person approach. *Philosophical Transactions of the Royal Society of London, B, 356,* 1351–1361.

Goldman-Rakic, P.S. & Schwartz, P.S. (1982) Interdigitation of contralateral and ipsilateral columnar projections to frontal association cortex in primates. *Science, 216,* 755–757.

Gomo-Tempini, M.L., Price C.J., Josephs, O., Vandenberghe, R., Cappa, S.F., Kapur, N., & Frackowiak, R.S. (1998). The neural systems sustaining face and proper-name processing. *Brain, 121,* 2103–2118.

Greicius, M.D., Krasnow, B., Reiss, A.L., & Menon, V. (2003). Functional connectivity of the resting brain: A network analysis of the default mode hypothesis. *Proceedings of the National Academy of Sciences (USA), 100,* 253–258.

Gusnard, D.A. & Raichle, M.E. (2001). Searching for a baseline: Functional imaging and the resting human brain. *Nature Reviews Neuroscience, 2,* 685–694.

Gusnard, D.A., Akbudak, E., Shulman, G., & Raichle M.E. (2001). Medial prefrontal cortex and self-referential mental activity: Relation to a default mode of brain function. *Proceedings of the National Academy of Sciences, (USA), 98,* 4259–4264.

Henson R.N., Rugg M.D., Shallice, T., Josephs, O., & Dolan R.J. (1999). Recollection and familiarity in recognition memory: An event-related functional magnetic resonance study. *Journal of Neuroscience, 19,* 3962–3972.

Horvitz, J.C. (2002). Dopamine gating of glutamatergic sensorimotor and incentive motivational input signals to the striatum. *Behavioural Brain Research, 137,* 65–74.

Ingvar, D.H. (1979). "Hyperfrontal" distribution of the cerebral grey matter flow in resting wakefulness, on the functional anatomy of the conscious state. *Acta Neurologica Scandinavica, 60,* 12–25.

Johnson, S.C., Baxter, L.C., Wilder, L.S., Pine, J.G., Hiesemann, J.E., & Prigatano, G.P. (2002). Neural correlate of self-reflection. *Brain, 125,* 1808–1814.

Herzog, H., Lele, V.R., Kuwert, T., Langen, K.J., Kops, E.R., & Feinendegen, L.E. (1990). Changed pattern of regional glucose metabolism during yoga meditative relaxation. *Neuropsychobiology, 23(4),* 182–187.

Keenan J.P., Nelson A., O'Connor M., & Pasqual-Leone A. (2001). Self-recognition and the right hemisphere. *Nature,* 409, 305.

Keenan, J.P. (2001). A thing well done. *Journal of Consciousness Studies, 3,* 31–34.

Kelley, W.M, Macrae, C.N., Wyland, C.L., Caglar, S., Inati, S., & Heatherton, T.F. (2002). Finding the self? An event-related fMRI study. *Journal of Cognitive Neuroscience, 14,* 785–794.

Kircher, T.T., Senior, C., Phillips, M.L., Benson, P.J., Bullmore, E.T., Barummer, M., Simmonds, A., Williams, S.C.R., Bertels, M., & David, A.S. (2000). Towards a functional neuroanatomy of self-processing: Effects of faces and words. *Cognitive Brain Research, 10,* 133–144.

Kjaer, T.W. & Lou, H.C. (2000). Interaction between precuneus and dorsolateral prefrontal cortex may play a unitary role in consciousness—a principal component analysis of rCBF. *Consciousness and Cognition, 9,* S59.

Kjaer, T.W. Nowak, M., Kjaer, K.W., Lou, A.R., & Lou, H.C. (2001). Precuneus-prefrontal activity during awareness of visual verbal stimuli. *Consciousness and Cognition, 10,* 356–365.

Kjaer, T.W., Nowak, M., & Lou, H.C. (2002). Reflective self-awareness and conscious states: PET evidence for a common midline parietofrontal core. *Neuroimage, 17,* 1080–1086.

Kjaer, T.W., Bertelsen, C., Piccini, P., Brooks, D., Alving, J., & Lou, H.C. (2002). Increased dopamine tone during meditation-induced change of consciousness. *Brain Research Cognitive Brain Research, 13,* 255–259.

Kosslyn, S.M., Albert, N.M., Thompson, W.L., Maljkovic, V., Weise, S.B., Chabris, C.F., Hamilton, S.E., Rauch, S.L., & Buanno, F.S. (1993). Visual mental imagery activates topographically organized visual cortex. *Journal of Cognitive Neuroscience, 5,* 263–287.

Lauritzen, M. (2001). Relationship of spikes, synaptic activity, and local changes of cerebral blood flow. *Journal of Cerebral Blood Flow Metabolism, 21,* 1367–1383.

Lou, H.C., Kjaer, T.W., Friberg, L., Wildschiodtz, G., Holm, S., & Nowak, M. (1999). A ^{15}O-H$_2$O PET study of meditation and the resting state of normal consciousness. *Human Brain Mapping, 7,* 98–105.

Lou, H.C., Luber, B., Crupain, M., Keenan, J.P., Nowak, M., Kjaer, T.W., Sackeim, H.A., & Lisanby, S.H. (2004). Parietal cortex and representation of the mental self. *Proceedings of the National Academy of Sciences (USA), 101,* 6827–6832.

Maguire, E.A., Burgess, N., & O'Keefe, J. (1999). Human spatial navigation: Cognitive maps, sexual dimorphism, and neural substrates. *Current Opinion in Neurobiology, 9,* 171–177.

Maguire, E.A., Burgess, N., Donnett, J.G., Frackowiak, R.S., Frith, C.D., & O'Keefe, J. (1998). Knowing where and getting there. A human navigation network. *Science, 280,* 921–924.

Maguire, E.A., Frith, C.D., & Morris, R.G. (1999). The functional neuroanatomy of comprehension and memory: The importance of prior knowledge. *Brain, 122,* 1839–1850.

Maquet, P., Degueldre, C., Delfiore, G., Aerts, I., Peters, J.M., Luxen, A., & Franck, G. (1997). Functional neuroanatomy of human slow wave sleep. *Journal of Neuroscience, 17,* 2807–2812.

Martin, A., Haxby, J.V., Lalonde, F.M., Wiggs, C., & Ungerleider L.G. (1995). Discrete cortical regions associated with knowledge of color and knowledge of action. *Science, 5233,* 102–105.

Martin, A., Wiggs, C.L. Ungerleider, L.G., & Haxby, J.V. (1996). Neural correlates of category-specific knowledge. *Nature, 379,* 649–652.

Mehta, M.A., Owen A.M., Sahakian, B.J., Mavaddat, N., Pickard, J.D., & Robbins, T.W. (2000). Methylphenidate enhances working memory by modulating discrete frontal and parietal lobe regions in the human brain. *Journal of Neuroscience, 20,* 1–6.

Newberg, A., Alavi, A., Baime, M., Pourdehnad, M., Santanna, J., & d'Aquili, E. (2001). The measurement of regional cerebral blood flow during the complex cognitive task of meditation: A preliminary SPECT study. *Psychiatry Research, 106,* 113–122.

Pagano, R.R. & Warrenburg, S. (1983). Meditation In search of a unique effect. In: R.J. Davidson, N.D. Schwartz, & D. Shapiro (Eds). *Consciousness and Self-Regulation. Advances in Research and Theory,* vol. 3. New York: Plenum Press.

Pardo, J.V., Fox, P.T., & Raichle, M.E. (1991). Localization of a human system for sustained attention by positron emission tomography. *Nature, 349,* 61–64.

Posner, M.I. & Rothbart, M.K. (1994). Large-scale neuronal theories of the brain. In: C. Koch, & J.L. David (Eds). *Constructing Neuronal Theories of the Mind.* Cambridge, MA: MIT, pp. 183–201.

Posner, M.I. & Rothbart M.K. (1998) Attention, self-regulation and consciousness. *Philosophical Transactions of the Royal Society of London. B, 353,* 1915–1927.

Raichle, M.E, MacLeod, A.M., Snyder, A.Z., Powers, W.J., Gusnard, D.A, & Shulman, G.L. (2001). A default mode of brain function. *Proceedings of the National Academy of Sciences (USA), 98,* 676–682.

Sergent J., Ohta, S., & MacDonald, B. (1992). Functional neuroanatomy of face and object processing: A positron emission tomography study. *Brain, 115,* 15–36.

Stuss, D.T. & Levine, B. (2002). Adult clinical neuropsychology: Lessons from studies of the frontal lobes. *Annual Review Psychology, 53,* 401–433.

Tallon-Baudry, C., Bertrand, O., Delpuech, C., & Pernier, J. (1996). Stimulus specificity of phase-locked and non–phase-locked 40 Hz visual responses in human. *Journal of Neuroscience, 16,* 4240–4249.

Taylor, J. (1999). *The Race for Consciousness,* Cambridge, MA: MIT press.

Tulving, E. (1972). Episodic and semantic memory. In: E. Tulving & W. Donaldson (Eds). *Organization of Memory* (pp. 781–403). New York: Academic Press.

Vandenberghe, R., Price, C., Wise, R., Josephs, O., & Frackowiak, R.S. (1996). Functional anatomy of a common semantic system for words and pictures. *Nature, 383,* 254–256.

Vogeley, K., Bussfeld, P., Newen, A., Herrman, S., Happe, F., Falkei, P., Maier, W., Shah, N.J., Fink, G.R., & Zilles, K. (2001). Mind reading: Neural mechanisms of theory of mind and self-perspective. *NeuroImage, 14,* 170–181.

Vogeley, K. & Fink, G.R. (2003). Neural correlates of the first person perspective. *Trends in Cognitive Science, 7,* 38–42.

Wallace, R.K. (1970). Physiological effects of trascendental meditation. *Science, 167,* 1751–1754.

Wiggs, C.L., Weisberg, J., & Martin A. (1999). Neural correlates of semantic and episodic memory retrieval. *Neuropsychologia, 37,* 103–118.

17

The Enduring Self: A First-Person Account of Brain Insult Survival

J. ALLAN HOBSON

The purposes of this communication are to describe how I survived two unexpected and life-threatening cocomplications of lateral medullary infarct and to explain why I believe that all of these events are related to one another. Throughout the chapter, I emphasize the durability of the self in the face of these major insults. An important subtext of this chapter is that self-observation is an important adjunct to third-person accounts in medical research.

My first point is to suggest that following a medullary infarct there is compensation but not true recovery either of swallowing or of normal cardiorespiratory functioning. Both of these weakenings of the nutritional and oxygen supply systems of my body are due to the original stroke insult to the brainstem and its coordinating modulatory systems, which mediate autonomic control in the heart, lungs, and other viscera.

When the acute illness that is the focus of this account was triggered, the previously injured brain stem was once again compromised. It then reverted back to its strokelike condition, and many of the sensorimotor symptoms that were present following the initial insult reemerged. For example, the sleep disturbance returned again, and dreaming was once again suppressed. Diplopia was again present, and the ataxia, the facial pain, and all my other paresthesias intensified. In response to the many drugs that were used to deal with the severe medical situation, numerous new, bizarre psychological experiences were triggered. However, except when I lost consciousness, my self remained intact. I am therefore happy to be alive and to be able to tell this tale.

My Brain Recovers

I have published an account of the changes in sleep and dreaming that immediately followed my lateral medullary infarct incurred on February 1, 2001 (Hobson, 2002b). During the five months that transpired between my discharge from Spaulding

251

Rehab Hospital on April 15, 2001, and October 5, 2001, when I was readmitted to Brigham and Women's Hospital, I had enjoyed a pleasant summer. Quite satisfyingly, I was able to resume a relatively full range of activities. I first traveled to Sicily with my wife on June 16 and spent the summer there in our apartment in Messina until about August 15. In late June and early July we had a wonderful vacation in Stromboli with our 5-year-old twin boys.

In retrospect, I probably made a great mistake in trying so hard to recover my swallowing so completely and so quickly. I was pleased to be able to have the peg tube taken out in mid-May. By that time I relied entirely on oral ingestion of food as a dietary source. I was back, I thought, to my old gourmand self. Flush with success in this domain, I ate everything that I pleased over the summer and into the fall. This inevitably led to increasing aspiration and contributed to the pneumonia that brought me down in early October.

Before going to Sicily, home-based rehab and nursing had helped me, but once the peg tube was out I did not use them anymore and was more or less able to do whatever I wanted to do. I was on coumadin to prevent embolic phenomena. Wanting to avoid a fall and a bleeding accident, I did not ride bicycles, nor did I garden with my usual freedom, but I was nonetheless able to drive, to cut the grass, to go to work every day, to review my grant resubmission, and to enjoy the press reception of two books: *Out of Its Mind: Psychiatry in Crisis* (Hobson, & Leonard, 2001) (that I wrote together with Jonathan Leonard) and *The Dream Drugstore* (Hobson, 2001) (that I wrote for MIT Press). This, together with the publication of our massive *Behavioral and Brain Sciences* (Hobson, Pace-Schott, & Stickgold, 2000) review of dreaming, were deeply satisfying signs of continued creativity and productivity. The most important part of my self, my critical and creative mind, was intact.

In Messina that summer I was even able to complete writing a first draft of a short book on dreaming (Hobson, 2002a) for Shelley Cox at Oxford University Press. Shelley had been wanting me to write a book for the last couple of years, but I had declined her invitation until the other two books had been published. It was fun to write the Oxford book, especially to show that I could function as I had before, writing in the morning either in my office in Messina or on the dining porch at the Hotel Miramare in Stromboli. I even made a good start on *Experimental Animal,* a book about my life, my dreams, and my scientific career. We had a very full range of social activities, having dinner with friends and spending long weekends with several of them. Taormina was a particularly exciting venue that year with Bob Dylan in concert. In general, I was feeling really very good about the future and completely unprepared for what was going to happen to me in October.

There were, however, some important premonitory signs. One was that my attempt in Messina to stop the 20-mg daily dose of Ritalin that I had been taking since early April was unsuccessful. I simply could not make it from 10 mg to 5 mg without finding that my motor system had begun to behave in a very Parkinsonian manner. For instance, it was practically impossible for me to initiate movement without the help of the stimulant until I went back to 20 mg. The telephone in our hallway would ring four times before I could get out of my chair in an adjoining office! After four rings the fax and/or the phone message mode was triggered and my lame trip was useless!

When I got to Boston in September and saw my doctor, Jamie Winshall, it was clear that I had gone back into atrial fibrillation (AF). The initial defibrillation, which had occurred prior to my transfer from Brigham and Women's Hospital to Spaulding on March 15, had not held, and my heart reverted to AF at some point during the summer. We obviously do not know when, but there was already evidence that two processes were involved whose causal connection must be considered. One is that I had become Ritalin-dependent and/or that my system so badly needed the aminergic boost that it could not get along without it. In order to try to reduce the propensity to arrhythmia, Winshall had strongly backed my Ritalin withdrawal. This seemed to set the stage for the second process, the acute illness I describe below. By the time I finally did withdraw from Ritalin, my motor and cardiorespiratory systems had acquired a major vulnerability.

In retrospect, I may have been wise to resist taking Ritalin in the first place. To overcome my lassitude and inability to stay awake at Spaulding during late March and early April, Dr. Wu had persuaded me to try it in small doses. They helped, so we increased to 20 mg, and I got out of Spaulding by April 15 (which was about the time my insurance coverage ran out). Now I wonder if my cardiovascular and cardiopulmonary motor system had become dependent on the externally supplied dopaminelike agent. It is also possible that my withdrawal campaign was too vigorous. In both attempts, I would typically spend four days at each drug level: 20, 15, 10, 5, and then 0. That means complete withdrawal was occurring in four steps, from 20 mg to 15 mg, from 15 mg to 10 mg, from 10 mg to 5 mg, and from 5 mg to 0 mg over the course of two weeks. But I did not have any particular difficulty the second time around, so it is not at all clear what the contribution of Ritalin and/or its withdrawal was to the clinical picture that I will now describe.

My Heart Fails

On October 2, a Friday (exactly 8 months to the day after my initial stroke symptoms in Monte Carlo), I drove with my twin sons, Andy and Matty, to Vermont. We left in the early morning, a time when I would normally feel extremely refreshed. Instead I felt drowsy. I had to stop at least three times to avoid going off the road. I presumed that this was a hangover from Ritalin withdrawal. When I got to Vermont, I met Nick Tranquillo, and we had a lovely Friday afternoon and evening together. We enjoyed all of Saturday as well, as our friends came to join us from Boston. This was the famous Columbus Day weekend retreat for the Laboratory of Neurophysiology staff, which had been neglected for the past 2 years owing to the death of my wife, Lia's, parents, and this year was particularly exciting because I felt that I had been granted a second life. Work was going well at the lab, and it was an absolutely glorious foliage year.

One of my hopes was to be able to recruit the visitors to do some work picking up small branches from my wood lots that had been cleared recently by Roger

Laramee and his brother, Roland, but when I walked out through the fields to examine them, I was very aware of feeling not only too tired to do so but tired in a specifically cardiac sense. There is something distinctive about fatigue when the heart is the culprit. You know that you do not have enough energy and that your muscular system is being oxygen starved when it is asked to deliver more. Primed by my father's experience with cardiovascular arrhythmia and fatigue, I remember sitting down two or three times in the field. I really felt better only when I was seated on the ground, asking nothing of my motor system. I quickly abandoned the idea of cleaning the woods because I knew I could not even supervise the job, much less participate as I would have liked. I went back to the house determined at least to be a jovial host.

This was easy for me because the guests were so delightful, and people piled in one after the other up to a total of 17 for our magnificent sit-down dinner on Saturday night. I was feeling quite giddy and wonderful, not a bit tired. It is true that I had a cough, but no fever, no malaise, no chills, nothing to suggest that I was developing pneumonia. Once the dinner was over, I retired to my bed but slept extremely poorly. The next day, for the first time in my life, I really felt that I did not want to get out of bed. Indeed, I could not get out of bed. When I went downstairs to look around and noticed that no one else was up, I went back upstairs and stayed in bed for most of the day. I ate no breakfast, fixed my guests a lobster bisque for lunch, ate a token amount of that, but skipped dinner altogether.

By then I knew I was very sick but still did not correctly assess what was going on. Although my self felt the same, my critical judgment was certainly impaired. On Monday I was so weak that I knew I could not successfully drive my car back to Boston, and I asked Ed Pace-Schott to do so for me. When we got back to Brookline, Ed called Jamie Winshall, who suggested that I go to Brigham and Women's the next morning in an ambulance. We got in touch with Lia, and she began a hurried return to Boston from Sicily.

Via ambulance and the emergency ward, I was admitted to Brigham and Women's Hospital on Tuesday morning, October 6. I was then begun on massive doses of IV antibiotics because a chest film revealed that no less than three of the lobes of my lungs were infiltrated with pneumonia. This kind of pneumonia is called "atypical" in that it is not isolated to a single lobe, nor does it arise quickly. It is not associated with chills, fever, and the intense sense of illness that typical pneumonias evince. It was nonetheless malicious, probably caused by multiple episodes of aspiration of food as my dietary indiscretions increased over the summer and fall. I did not like it much in the hospital but after 2 days of antibiotic treatment was beginning to feel better. I thought that I would be discharged in a week or so, go home, and resume my life. How wrong I was.

The Bottom Falls Out

On the night of Thursday, October 9, while asleep or unconscious for some other reason, I suffered an acute cardiovascular collapse characterized by a failure to respond and by blood pressure readings of 60/0. In this emergency situation, I was transferred to the ICU and spent 5 days there in a critical, near death, condition. I have no memory of those 5 days, although informants tell me that I appeared to be conscious much of the time. The reason for my amnesia is probably pharmacologic. I was on high doses of Versed and Fentomil. According to Dr. Winshall, I may have had an acute aspiration event (although I was taking no food by mouth and being fed only through IV tubes). Or perhaps the acute toxic state of the pneumonia precipitated this major setback. We will never know for sure.

Dr. Winshall described my first 2 days in the ICU as a "touch and go" adventure, implying that he was not sure whether I was going to live or die. When I finally regained consciousness in the morning hours of Tuesday October 13, I found myself with my hands tied and an intubation tube in my trachea. By then I was breathing on my own, and the nurses were waiting until dawn to remove the incredibly uncomfortable breathing tube. My sleep and dreams were totally disrupted, and many of my stroke symptoms were exacerbated.

The Heart and the Brain

The unanswerable question is: which comes first, the chicken (my brain) or the egg (my heart)? As in the case of the development of the stroke and atrial fibrillation in Monaco, which came first, my heart trouble or my brain trouble? Obviously, we cannot know, but since most people favor the primacy of cardiac pathology, I will emphasize the possible primacy of central nervous system dysfunction in giving my own account. On this view, the cardiovascular symptoms are secondary to the dyscontrol that results when large areas of the brainstem subserving autonomic functions are lost due to a stroke.

This pathophysiology must at least play a role, if not a uniquely causative one. Even the pulmonary difficulties are in part conditioned or primed by a stroke, as the lungs no longer function normally. As my oropharynx hypersecreted and hypersalivated, it was more difficult to cough effectively and to remove the increased number of foreign bodies taken into my lungs. This vicious cycle leads to pneumonia. In parallel, there is a collapse of cardiovascular function.

One of the greatest unexplained mysteries is: why did I go into congestive heart failure? When I sat down in my Vermont field, I did not just feel that I was having cardiac limitation of motion but was, in fact, on the point of severe congestive cardiac decompensation. According to my model, this weakening of cardiac function is also due to changes in the autonomic nervous system. The alternative hypothesis, which is favored by my doctors, is that I had an acute myocarditis associated with the pneumonia.

The most significant evidence that one of these two theories may be correct is the completely negative cardiac catheterization, which was performed on October 2. Although my cardiac output was poor, my coronary arteries were described by the physician who did the study as "superhighways large and wide open enough to drive trucks through." So there is no explanation for my defective cardiovascular function in terms of the most common culprit, arteriosclerotic heart disease. What did happen? That is an open question, but there can be no doubt that these events led to the first major threats to the waking state mental functions that constitute my "self."

Chemical and Behavioral Alterations of My Self

My psychological experiences during my hospitalization reveal the potent effects of benzodiazepines and my idiosyncratic reaction to them. First, there were the 5 days of total amnesia that were associated with the heavy doses of Versed (midazolam) and Fentomil. Then there were my stereotyped reactions to Ambien and Serax when these were given as sedatives. Finally, there was the extraordinary response to antihistamines that occurred when I was on the ICU.

Fentomil and Versed Effects on Consciousness

I have absolutely no recollection whatsoever of 5 successive days in the ICU, during which time I was intermittently conscious, unconscious, and most probably delirious. Because of the amnesia, I would say that my self was totally lost during that ICU episode, but the fact that others related to "me" as if I were intact qualifies this judgment. Who is correct, "I" or "they"? The answer must be both, meaning that a self is a dynamic construct of an individual and those in his or her immediate social surround.

After I began to recover and the automatic physiological control of breathing resumed, I had the same sort of insomnia that I had experienced during the original poststroke period: total, wall-to-wall, upright waking all through the night. It is for that reason that I was seeking relief through various sedatives and finding very little indeed. Instead, I experienced the many interesting side effects that I now recount.

These experiments of nature were cooked up for me by circumstances that I knew how to exploit and enjoy. The writing of *The Dream Drug Store* (Hobson, 2001) over the previous 2 years had made me wonder why had I never taken drugs. "Fear" was my honest answer. Now I had good clinical reasons to take them, but I was surprised by the intensity and variety of the experimental effects. My "self" was radically altered by these psychoactive drugs.

Serax (oxazepam)
This is a short-acting benzodiazepine with sedative hypnotic properties that I have prescribed over the years without recognizing that it might have the effects on patients that it had on me. Serax induced in me a kind of somnolent confusional state during which I experienced a very specific symptom that troubled me greatly. Thinking myself to be awake, I would reach for the bedside table only to find the glass that I was reaching for did not exist. My hand would pass right through it. The same disturbing insubstantiality characterized numerous other objects that I perceived. In retrospect, this must have been due to hallucinatory construction of an unreal glass that would vanish as I tried to grasp it. I have no insight whatso-

ever about what causes this disturbing effect except to say that it is neither normal sleep nor normal waking, but rather a hybrid state with elements of both waking and dreaming. In a word, I was in a microscopic but robust delirium.

Ambien (zolpidemtartrate) has been associated with confusional states in the elderly, and it certainly confused me. I took it twice, and on both occasions I had similar reactions. I was convinced that instead of being in my hospital bed, I was sleeping in a very attractively designed summer camp. I was convinced that there were other families present that I might or might not know, but it seemed that I should. And there were women talking in what I took to be a kitchen about making provisions for me and the other campers. In retrospect, these voices were the nurses outside my hospital room door. The room that I thought was a summer camp room was my hospital bedroom, and the rooms that I thought were occupied by fellow campers were in reality the rooms of my patient colleagues on pod 10A of Brigham and Women's Hospital at the time. The fantasy that this was a very special camp was totally convincing.

During these long episodes I experienced an almost euphoric sleeplike transformation of my consciousness. Instead of being in a hospital bed, I felt that I was on the top of a huge pile of mattresses, perhaps rolled and stacked on end, but very soft. I could sink down into whatever level I chose and then have my consciousness follow me down these lovely deep folds in the pillowlike surface of the bed. In reality, of course, I was on the plain old hospital bed all the time, it just did not feel that way. So I accepted the reality of the camp scenario as if it were fully explanatory. It was extremely pleasant and reassuring to hear the women talking outside my door, in part because so many of them spoke with accents that sounded "Latin" (just like my wife, Lia). In fact, many of them were Latin, but they were Hispanic, not Italian, and some were very lovely nurses who knew how to deliver care in the hands-on fashion that I had so much appreciated during my original stay at the Princess Grace Hospital in Monaco.

Thalamo-Saurus: My Idiosyncratic Reaction to Benadryl

"In the intensive care unit sooner or later everyone becomes psychotic," according to its director, Dr. Lowenfeld, who spoke with me after my own dramatic episode of delirium. I had begun to experience hypnagogic hallucinations, but it is the more distinctive and stereotyped effects of Benadryl (diphenhydramine) that I want to emphasize here.

On Wednesday, the night after my recovery from shock and respiratory failure, I had been unable to sleep despite taking both trazodone (Desyrel) and Ambien. Bob, my nurse, reminded me on Thursday night that I really should not be taking any pills by mouth. In order to achieve sedation, he suggested giving me morphine via the intravenous line that was in my arm. Thinking this might provide an interesting opportunity for a description of the subjective effects of narcotics, I assented, but there was absolutely no effect of morphine either on my perceptions or on my sleep. Even after a second 25-mg dose of morphine, I was still wide awake and lucid. I felt neither euphoric nor high, just wide awake.

It was then that Bob suggested that we try the antihistamine Benadryl. Benadryl has been a popular over-the-counter drug that has been used as a clinical sedative for years. I thought this was an interesting idea, especially since the specific arrest of histaminergic neurons in REM sleep had been described by my colleague Cliff Saper and his group (Sherin et al., 1998). Histaminergic neurons belong in the same category as the serotonin and norepinephrine-containing REM-off cells that we discovered 25 years ago (Hobson, McCarley, & Wyzinski, 1975). From this experiment I thought I might learn what the sudden and acute effects upon sleep and/or perception of the blockade of histaminergic neuronal system would be. Of course, it must be admitted that my inferences about this drug are tainted by the massively dirty chemical conditions of this experiment (especially the pretreatment with morphine), but the effects were so spectacular and so specific as to warrant detailed notation.

One of the advantages of using Benadryl intravenously is that the recipient is immediately aware of the drug entering the circulatory system because it causes a strong sense of warming of the vein into which it is being injected. No sooner had my right anticubital vein begun to heat up than there appeared the first of a succession of images that recurred for almost an hour on the ceiling over my bed. The images appeared to be computer animated sketches of imaginary reptiles. They were visually complete, with the title "Thalamo-Saurus" rendered in very artistic computer graphics. There was a sequence of four characteristic reptiles. The one that I remember best is the blue and red crocodile, but there were several others. There was a green and yellow lizard that typically followed the red and blue fellow, and there were a couple of other smaller ones. There were also some butterflies, some birds, and some fish, but mostly exotic reptiles. With my eyes open (and only with my eyes open), these images would form typically on the right side of the ceiling over the foot of my bed and then proceed diagonally left to behind my head as I watched and wondered.

By and large, they were friendly little beasties. I quite enjoyed them, especially when I realized that I could alter their speed and location to some degree by making voluntary eye and head movements. Their trajectory was otherwise consistent, their appearance stereotyped and clear, and their artistic characteristics quite internally harmonious and even beautiful. Amazingly, there also appeared the name of the studio in Tokyo that had made this little tape. The very apt and imaginative title, Thalamo-Saurus, obviously suggests imaginary reptiles conjured up by my own drug soaked thalamus! As far as I know I had never heard this very creative and apt neologism before. It came, unbidden, from my unconscious self.

My Thalamo-Saurus experience is similar to that reported by well-known writers such as Robert Louis Stevenson, who claimed that "dream brownies" gave him some of his best literary ideas. Unfortunately, I am not a great writer and I do not have creative hallucinosis in waking unless I am sick and taking drugs. Are my visions a product of my "self"? Am I a closet novelist needing only a boost from an antihistamine to realize my full creative potential? I leave this question for the reader to answer.

I noted that the hallucinated creatures were mostly friendly, meaning I experienced pleasure in looking at them. However, they did occasionally become distinctly unfriendly, when the ceiling would assume a kind of a parachutelike filamentous character and appear to float down toward the bed. The images then would become distorted on the falling ceiling and sometimes even separate away from it. This was the case of one particularly menacing goldfish and butterfly combination that threatened to fly off the projection surface and enter my room space. This lack of boundaries made me anxious and fearful.

Only artistic drawings could convey the exotic abstract patterning of these forms, but you will have a good idea if you simply imagine that every animal image was composed of geometrically organized units with two color outlines. In the case of the red and blue reptile, these looked like little plastic building blocks, the red outlined around the blue. This pattern was repeated over and over again. In forming the various components of the animals, the color blocks were very fascinating and beautiful to look at; they were also very stereotyped and did not change from the start of the show to its end. Whether "I" am creative is difficult to say, but my brain certainly is. Am "I" my brain?

MRI Hallucinosis

Once I had again developed diplopia and told the neurologists about it, the question of anatomical extension of my lateral medullary infarct was raised, and so I was sent to the brain imaging unit for a repeat MRI. The results were reassuring: there was no evidence of spread of the infarct in my medulla. I am nonetheless convinced that my stroke was already functionally worse, and my disability has since progressed markedly. This is likely due to cerebral anoxia associated with heart failure.

The experience of having the MRI was unnerving. This was the third MRI exam, and the previous two, in Monaco, were equally stressful but free of the psychotic effects I experienced at Brigham and Women's Hospital. There I was convinced that a young child and his mother were in the magnet with me.

Lying quiet and still in the dark as MRI images are being collected is a special case of sensory isolation. After about 30 minutes of magnet whines and cranks one is ready to get out, but the technician's voice admonished me, "Please don't move, the session is almost over." She said this several times before admitting that we still had 10 minutes to go! By then I was sure that the young boy (who was whimpering) and his mother (who was reassuring him) were suffering more than I, so I began to reach out to them and to reassure them that our torture would soon end and we would all escape unharmed.

At one point my hallucinatory perception of voices convinced me that there were numerous other people, all standing up, under the magnet at the same time! As a physician, I know perfectly well that MRIs must be highly focused on one and only one subject's brain at a time. That subject was me — and I was lying down, not standing up — but my brain was still easily tipped over into the delirious mode probably because I was still anoxic, still under the influence of drugs, and now sensorially isolated in the magnet.

A Sequential Model

It should be made clear that the episode of pulmonary and cardiovascular dysfunction that occurred in October was discrete and quite different from anything that had occurred before. Since it was part of a sequence that was continuous with the previous events, I will attempt to develop the argument that there was a cause-and-effect relationship between the links in this temporal chain.

What is unequivocally clear is that in the two weeks between September 15 and October 5, 1 simultaneously and in parallel developed both a severe pulmonary infection and heart failure. The pneumonia may have had a long incubation period, as microaspiration after microaspiration set the stage for the development of widespread pneumonia. This is understandable, as I had been eating freely and with almost perverse pleasure since early July. In fact, I had regained *all* of my poststroke weight of 200 lbs! That is 35 lbs in 6 months.

At the same time my cardiovascular function was going downhill. This is extremely interesting and puzzling. Could the fact that my pulmonary function was deteriorating progressively due to coughing and regurgitating food at least over the past two months have had something to do with it? Was I developing an infection of both heart and lungs, or were both systems dysfunctional because of the brain stem lesion? About 2 weeks before I was hospitalized, I noticed that I could not finish mowing my lawn, a task I performed easily before I got sick. Because my fatigue was associated with abstention from the stimulant Ritalin, I interpreted it that way. And it is true that my development of cardiovascular symptoms was most immediately tied to my abrupt weaning from Ritalin in early September. It is ironic to imagine that this move, which was strongly urged as being in the interest of my heart, could have contributed to my heart failure.

In any case, it is clear that I was rapidly becoming a cardiovascular invalid. On October 4, I went to Vermont and could not walk across the fields. I found that I had to sit down to regain any sense of equilibrium and strength.

Brain, Heart, and Lung Dysfunction: A Dysautonomia Hypothesis

The most conservative scientific position to take account of all of these problems is that they had no relationship with one another but were simply coincidental. In other words, I had one tendency to develop the stroke or embolic or thrombotic occlusion of my cerebrovascular system, another tendency to develop pneumonia, and still a third tendency to develop heart muscle disease.

An alternative model, and one that I favor, is that the problems of all three systems were not only sequential but also causally interconnected. Here is one way such a causal sequence might work.

As a first and initiating episode, there was a thrombus in the vertebral artery secondary to atherosclerotic disease of the great vessels of my neck. This caused a partial occlusion of the posterior inferior cerebellar artery (pica) and produced my stroke onset syndrome. There was anoxic destruction 24 hours later of many structures in the lateral medullary and pontine tegmentum region on the right side of my brain stem. The structures include parts of the oculomotor system, the trigeminal sensory system, and the seventh nerve motor enervation of the face. More specifically and more severely, there was damage to vestibular, cerebellar, glossopharyngeal, and vagal neurons, all of which are associated with autonomic control of the brain itself, the lungs, the heart, and other viscera. The vagus is a major source of cholinergic input to the heart, which it slows dramatically.

Today I still have a problem with cardiac rhythm and rate. My heart beats too irregularly and too rapidly to be efficient. Why? The doctors say it is idiopathic, meaning, "We don't know." To the extent that cell loss occurred in the pons, norepinephrine-containing neurons might also have been killed, as well as sensorimotor neurons. This would set the stage for failure of the sympathetic autonomic systems that innervate the brain itself as well as the heart and lungs.

The glossopharyngeal and vagal impairments could plausibly have led to a secondary impairment in pulmonary regulation. The ability to clear my lungs of fluid was compromised, and the propensity toward pneumonia was increased not only because of the swallowing defects due to glossopharyngeal cell loss but also to a weakening of the defensive reactions to aspiration. This could explain the pooling of fluid and the excessive secretions of mucus, and this process could, in turn, provide a causal link between the stroke and the pneumonia. Most of my doctors accept this hypothesis.

What could be the more precise cause of the cardiovascular effects? It has been clear right from the start that autonomic functions previously controlled by the right vagus may have been impaired given that my voice is still hoarse. The vagus contributes to the control of secretions from the salivary glands and stomach, and it contributes to the way in which these secretions are moved up and out of the lungs and then down to the gastrointestinal tract. Could it be that because this transoropharyngeal traffic was so badly upset I developed pneumonia? However, the vagus does not innervate only the pulmonary system, it also has powerful slowing effects on the heart. It is this propensity that allowed Otto Loewi to demonstrate neurotransmission by a chemical substance, the "vagustuff" which turned out to be acetylcholine. By the way, Loewi claimed that the idea of his definitive crossed-heart perfusion experiment occurred to him in a dream.

We can thus hypothesize that the cardiac arrhythmia first experienced in Monaco was the acute effect of the thrombus in the brainstem via the dampening of vagal output. The vagus is one of the major contributions to heart slowing, and that is what I cannot do anymore. I cannot slow my heart and I cannot keep it regular. I need medications for that.

More than that, I cannot maintain effective cardiovascular output. My cardiac output is badly compromised. This is due in part to the arrhythmia, no question about it, but could it also be due to some other trophic functions normally medi-ated by the neuromodulatory systems on the heart muscle itself? In other words, does heart muscle tone depend on trophic effects mediated by autonomic inputs? These trophic effects could well be second or third messenger phenomena medi-ated by the cholinergic neurons of the medulla and the sympathetic neurons of the pons. On this view, heart muscle is trophically dependent on sympathetic and para-sympathetic maintenance. When the central sympathetic systems are shut down in REM sleep, the neurons regain sensitivity to aminergic regulation on waking, but when they are not there at all, the heart not only loses its rhythmic control but fails altogether. This is what my doctors called "idiopathic" heart failure.

However fanciful it may be, I prefer this integrated model to no model at all. This speculative, theoretical bent has always characterized my science, and I feel both impelled and pleased to apply it to myself now that I am a patient. In fact, having a model that is related to my life's work and that integrates such a wild concatenation of symptoms is, in itself, not only intellectually gratifying but also therapeutic. In other words, my illness has provoked a dramatic challenge to my "self" as physician and scientist.

The Fragility and Durability of the Self

My experience and my ability to describe and analyze it constitute strong testi-mony to the durability of my "self." Despite life-threatening insults to my brain-stem, my lungs, and my heart, the essence of my self as an observing, reasoning scientist is intact. Even when I am hallucinating, I can self-observe and analyze the perceptual aspects of my consciousness. Only when memory is impaired and/or sleeplike states are induced is my observing self temporarily put out of commis-sion. This means that the stroke itself did not touch my brain-mediated self and that even drugs that markedly altered parts of my consciousness did not disrupt my self in functional terms. What does all this imply?

With respect to localization, it implies that my sense of self is engendered by my forebrain and most probably by anterior structures in my forebrain (because these continue to function and watch the perceptual disturbances mediated by the more posterior structures that are damaged). Putting my self-observational data to-gether with recent data concerning the effects of sleep on the self, I hypothesize that the self that writes this paper is localized (at least in part) to my frontal cortex and more specifically to my dorsolateral prefrontal cortex.

With respect to functional mediation, my frontocortical "self" needs to be in a certain state to operate properly. That state is waking, implying specific levels of regional brain activation, input–output gating, and modulation, none of which have been crippled by my horrendous illnesses. In other words, I am still able to acti-vate my frontal brain, to control the flow of information in and out of it, and to chemically modulate its constituent circuits in such a way as to be fully conscious, that is to say, sentient and analytical.

On this view, my "self" can be defined as a specific functional state of specific brain structures. While it cannot be reduced to brain tissue per se, it is reducible to dynamic aspects of brain activity. The fact that my "self" differs from your "self" in specific historical ways is a function of the role of brain-based memories of our particular autobiographical experiences. To boil it down to an easily remembered aphorism: the brain is a subjective object, and a state-dependent change in the self is an objective subject.

Acknowledgment

Although I disagree with many of them, I am grateful to all the many physicians who participated in my treatment. I am also grateful to my nurses, some of whom were very supportive and nurturing of my wounded body. My wife, Lia, and my children, especially my twin sons, Andrew and Matthew, have been unswervingly tolerant and encouraging.

Some of the material presented here has been previously published in *Cerebrum:* Hobson, J.A. (2002). Shock waves: A scientist studies his stroke. *Cerebrum, 4(2),* 39–57.

References

Hobson, J.A., McCarley, R.W., & Wyzinski, P.W. (1975). Sleep cycle oscillation: Reciprocal discharge by two brain stem neuronal groups. *Science, 189,* 55–58.

Hobson, J.A.. (1988). *The Dreaming Brain.* New York: Basic Books.

Hobson, J.A., Pace-Schott, E.F., & Stickgold, R. (2000). Dreaming and the brain: Toward a cognitive neuroscience of conscious states. *Behavioral and Brain Sciences, 23,* 793–842.

Hobson, J.A. (2001). *The Dream Drugstore.* Cambridge, MA: MIT Press.

Hobson, J.A. & Leonard, J. (2001). *Out of Its Mind: Psychiatry in Crisis.* Cambridge, MA: Perseus Publishing.

Hobson, J.A. (2002a). *Dreaming: An Introduction to the Science of Sleep.* Oxford: Oxford University Press.

Hobson J.A. (2002b). Sleep and dream suppression following a lateral medullary infarct: A first-person account. *Consciousness and Cognition, 11(3),* 377–390.

Sherin, J.E., Elmquist, J.K., Torrcalba, F., & Saper, C.B. (1998). Innervation of histaminergic tuberomammillary neurons by GABAergic and galaninergic neurons in the ventrolateral preoptic nucleus of the rat. *Journal of Neuroscience, 18(12),* 470–521.

Index